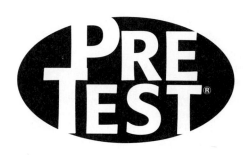

Anatomy, Histology, & Cell Biology

PreTest® Self-Assessment and Review

Notice

Medicine is an ever-changing science. As new research and clinical experience broaden our knowledge, changes in treatment and drug therapy are required. The authors and the publisher of this work have checked with sources believed to be reliable in their efforts to provide information that is complete and generally in accord with the standards accepted at the time of publication. However, in view of the possibility of human error or changes in medical sciences, neither the authors nor the publisher nor any other party who has been involved in the preparation or publication of this work warrants that the information contained herein is in every respect accurate or complete, and they disclaim all responsibility for any errors or omissions or for the results obtained from use of the information contained in this work. Readers are encouraged to confirm the information contained herein with other sources. For example and in particular, readers are advised to check the product information sheet included in the package of each drug they plan to administer to be certain that the information contained in this work is accurate and that changes have not been made in the recommended dose or in the contraindications for administration. This recommendation is of particular importance in connection with new or infrequently used drugs.

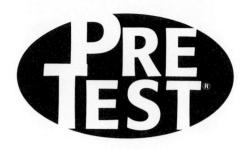

Anatomy, Histology, & Cell Biology
PreTest® Self-Assessment and Review

Robert M. Klein, Ph.D.
Professor of Anatomy and Cell Biology
University of Kansas Medical Center
Kansas City, Kansas

James C. McKenzie, Ph.D.
Associate Professor of Anatomy
Howard University College of Medicine
Washington, District of Columbia

Student Reviewers
Christopher A. Heck
University of South Alabama College of Medicine
Mobile, Alabama
Class of 2001

Christopher T. Lang
State University of New York at Buffalo School of Medicine
and Biomedical Sciences
Buffalo, New York
Class of 2002

McGraw-Hill
Medical Publishing Division

New York   Chicago   San Francisco   Lisbon   London   Madrid   Mexico City
Milan   New Delhi   San Juan   Seoul   Singapore   Sydney   Toronto

McGraw-Hill

A Division of The **McGraw·Hill** Companies

Anatomy, Histology, & Cell Biology: PreTest® Self-Assessment and Review

1 2 3 4 5 6 7 8 9 0   DOC/DOC   0 9 8 7 6 5 4 3 2 1

ISBN 0-07-137087-0 (alk. paper)

This book was set in Berkeley by North Market Street Graphics.
The editor was Catherine A. Johnson.
The production supervisor was Phil Galea.
Project management was provided by North Market Street Graphics.
The cover designer was Li Chen Chang / Pinpoint.
R.R. Donnelley & Sons was printer and binder.

This book is printed on acid-free paper.

Library of Congress Cataloging-in-Publication Data

Anatomy, histology, and cell biology: PreTest self-assessment and review /
Robert M. Klein, James C. McKenzie; student reviewers, Christopher A. Heck,
Christopher T. Lang; contributors, Mohammed M. Aziz, Vincent H. Gattone II, Dwayne
A. Ollerich.
    p.; cm.
  Includes bibliographical references and index.
  ISBN 0-07-137087-0 (alk. paper)
    1. Histology—Examinations, questions, etc. 2. Human anatomy—Examinations,
questions, etc. 3. Cytology—Examinations, questions, etc. I. Klein, Robert M. (Robert
Melvin), 1949– II. McKenzie, James C., 1947–
    [DNLM: 1. Anatomy—Examination Questions. 2. Cytology—Examination Questions. 3.
Histology—Examination Questions. QS 18.2 A53603 2001]
  QM554 .A52 2001
  611'.0076—dc21   2001034278

To my wife, Beth, and our children Melanie, Jeffrey, and David, for their support and patience during the writing of this text, and to my parents, Nettie and David, for their emphasis on education and the pursuit of knowledge—RMK

To my mother, Inge McKenzie, for her unfailing love and support, and to the authors of all those books about medical research and researchers that I read as a child, for putting my feet irrevocably on this path. Also, deepest thanks to Alyce Smith and my friend, Bob Klein, for literally saving my life. Deepest gratitude to Bev, Denise, and the rest of the family and thanks to Willard and Glendora Conway for their love and support—JCM

In memoriam, for Howard and Anna Dunn.

Contents

Reproductive Systems

Urinary System

Eye and Ear

Head and Neck

Thorax

Abdomen

Pelvis

Extremities

Contributors

Mohammed M. Aziz, Ph.D.

Associate Professor of Anatomy
Howard University College of Medicine
Washington, District of Columbia

Vincent H. Gattone II, Ph.D.

Professor of Anatomy and Cell Biology
Indiana University School of Medicine
Indianapolis, Indiana

Dwayne A. Ollerich, Ph.D.

Professor of Anatomy and Cell Biology
University of Kansas Medical Center
Kansas City, Kansas

Preface

In this first edition of *Anatomy, Histology, & Cell Biology: PreTest® Self-Assessment and Review,* a significant number of changes and improvements have been made from previous Anatomy and Histology and Cell Biology PreTest® reviews. First, this PreTest® reviews all of the anatomic disciplines encompassing early embryology, cell biology, histology of the tissues and organs, as well as regional human anatomy of the head and neck, thorax, abdomen, pelvis, and extremities. This PreTest® is not just a compilation of two separate texts, but a comprehensive effort to integrate the anatomic disciplines with clinical scenarios and cases. The sections on cell biology and microscopic anatomy have been updated to include important new knowledge in cell and tissue biology. There is also a greater focus on clinically related questions, problems, and scenarios. New and improved light micrographs have been added, and the number of matching questions has been dramatically reduced in keeping with recent changes in USMLE format.

New for this PreTest® is the addition of many radiographs and MRIs. These radiologic methods have become an important part of medical practice. It is imperative that students be able to recognize structures and relationships as part of their radiological anatomy knowledge base.

A High-Yield Facts section is provided to facilitate rapid review of specific areas of anatomy that are critical to mastering the difficult concepts of each subdiscipline: embryology, cell biology, histology of tissues and organs, and regional human (gross) anatomy.

The authors express their gratitude to their colleagues who have greatly assisted them by providing light and electron micrographs as well as constructive criticism of the text, line drawings, and micrographs. They also acknowledge Karen Chinn and Eileen Roach for their painstaking care in the preparation of line drawings and photomicrographs. Thanks to Drs. H. Clarke Anderson, Nancy E.J. Berman, George C. Enders, Kuen-Shan Hung, George Varghese, Anne W. Walling, and John K. Young for their contribution of micrographs and ideas for question development. The authors remain indebted to their students and colleagues at the University of Kansas Medical Center and Howard University College of Medicine, past and present, who have challenged them to continuously improve their skills as educators.

Introduction

Each *PreTest® Self-Assessment and Review* allows medical students to comprehensively and conveniently assess and review their knowledge of a particular medical school discipline, in this instance anatomy and cell biology. The 500 questions parallel the format and degree of difficulty of the questions found on the United States Medical Licensing Examination (USMLE) step 1. Although the <u>main emphasis of this PreTest® is preparation for step 1</u>, the book will be very beneficial for medical students during their preclinical courses whether they are enrolled in a medical school with a problem-based, traditional, or hybrid curriculum. This PreTest® focuses on an interdisciplinary approach incorporating numerous clinical scenarios so it will also be extremely valuable for students preparing for USMLE step 2 who need to review their anatomic knowledge. Practicing physicians who want to hone their basic science skills and supplement their knowledge base before USMLE step 3 or recertification will also find this book to be a good beginning in their review process.

This book is a comprehensive review of early embryology, cell biology, histology (tissue and organ biology), and human (gross) anatomy with some neuroanatomic topics covered through cases that integrate neuroanatomic tract information with regional anatomy of the head and neck. In keeping with the latest curricular changes in medical schools, as much as possible questions integrate macroscopic and microscopic anatomy with cell biology, embryology, and neuroscience as well as physiology, biochemistry, and pathology. This PreTest® begins with early embryology including gametogenesis, fertilization, implantation, the formation of the bilaminar and trilaminar embryo, and overviews of the embryonic and fetal periods. This first section is followed by a review of basic cell biology with separate chapters on membranes, cytoplasm, intracellular trafficking, and the nucleus. There are questions included to review the basics of mitosis and meiosis as well as regulation of cell cycle events. Tissue biology is the third section of the book, and it encompasses the tissues of the body: epithelium, connective tissue, specialized connective tissues (cartilage and bone), muscle, and nerve. Organ biology includes separate chapters on respiratory, integumentary (skin), digestive (tract and associated glands), endocrine, urinary, male and female reproductive systems, as well as eye and ear. The topics in tissue and organ histology and cell biology include light and electron microscopic micrographs of appropriate structures that students should be able to identify. The last section of the book contains questions reviewing the basic concepts of regional anatomy of the head and neck, thorax, abdomen, pelvis, and extremities. For each section, appropriate x-rays including MRIs are included to assist the student in reviewing pertinent radiologic aspects of the anatomy. Where possible, information is integrated with development and histology of the organ system.

Each question is accompanied by an answer, a detailed explanation, and a specific page reference to an appropriate textbook. A bibliography listing sources can be found following the last chapter of this PreTest®.

High-Yield Facts

Embryology

Embryological development is divided into three periods:

The **Prenatal Period** consists of **gamete formation** and maturation, ending in fertilization.

The **Embryonic Period** begins with fertilization and extends through the **first eight weeks** of development. It includes implantation, germ layer formation, and organogenesis. This is the critical period for susceptibility to **teratogens.**

The **Fetal Period** extends from the **third month** through birth.

THE PRENATAL PERIOD

The **development of gametes** begins with the duplication of chromosomal DNA followed by two cycles of nuclear and cell division (**meiosis**).

Genetic variability is assured by **crossing over** of DNA and by **random assortment** of chromosomes during the first meiotic division. Errors can result in duplication or deletion of all or part of a specific chromosome.

Spermatogenesis

During puberty, primordial stem cells in the walls of the seminiferous tubules of the testes undergo mitotic divisions to replenish their population and form a group of **spermatogonia** that will undergo meiosis.

Primary spermatocytes are spermatogonia that have duplicated their DNA (4N).

Secondary spermatocytes result from the first meiotic division (2N).

Spermatids are formed by the second meiotic division (1N).

Spermiogenesis

During this phase, spermatids mature into sperm by losing extraneous cytoplasm and developing a head region consisting of an **acrosome** (giant lysosome) surrounding the nuclear material.

The processes of spermatogenesis and spermiogenesis are **continuous** and last about two months.

Oogenesis

Oogenesis begins in the fetal period in females and is a **discontinuous** process involving both meiosis and maturation.

Oogonia form **primary oocytes** but stop in the metaphase of the first meiotic division until puberty.

The second meiotic division is not concluded until fertilization occurs.

Maturational events include retention of protein synthetic machinery in the surviving oocyte, formation of **cortical granules** that participate in events at fertilization, and development of a protective glycoprotein coat, the **zona pellucida.**

Fertilization
Fertilization occurs when sperm and oocyte cell membranes fuse and the male pronucleus is injected into the oocyte. Following coitus, exposure of sperm to the environment of the female reproductive tract causes **capacitation,** removal of surface glycoproteins from the sperm membrane enabling fertilization to occur.

Binding of the first sperm initiates the **zona reaction.** Release of **cortical granules** causes biochemical changes in the zona pellucida and oocyte membrane that prevent **polyspermy.**

EMBRYONIC DEVELOPMENT
The embryo forms one **germ layer** during each of the first three weeks.

During the second week, the **embryoblast** differentiates into two germ layers, the **epiblast** and the **hypoblast.** This establishes the dorsal (epiblast)–ventral (hypoblast) body axis.

During the third week, the process of **gastrulation** occurs by which epiblast cells migrate toward the **primitive streak** and ingress to form the **endoderm** and **mesoderm** germ layers below the remaining epiblast cells (**ectoderm**).

Lateral body folding at the end of the third week causes the germ layers to form three concentric tubes with the innermost layer being the endoderm, the mesoderm in the middle, and the ectoderm on the surface.

GERM LAYER DERIVATIVES
Mesoderm Derivatives
The mesoderm is divided into four regions (from medial to lateral): axial, paraxial, intermediate, and lateral plate.

Axial mesoderm is midline and forms the notochord.

Paraxial mesoderm forms somites. Somites are divided into **sclerotomes** (bone formation), **myotomes** (muscle precursors), and **dermatomes** (dermis).

Intermediate mesoderm gives rise to components of the genitourinary system.

Lateral plate mesoderm forms bones and connective tissues of the limbs and limb girdles (**somatic layer**) and the smooth muscle lining viscera and the serosae of body cavities (**splanchnic layer**).

Intermediate mesoderm is *not found* in the head region, and the lateral plate mesoderm is *not divided* into layers there.

Germ Layer Derivatives		
Ectoderm Derivatives	Epithelium of skin (superficial epidermis layer)	
	All nervous tissue: formed by neuroectoderm: Brain and spinal cord (neural tube) Peripheral nerves and other neural crest derivatives	
Endoderm Derivatives	Epithelial linings of:	The gastrointestinal tract
		Organs that form as buds from the endodermal tube: Pharyngeal gland derivatives* Respiratory system Digestive organs (liver, pancreas) Terminal part of urogenital systems
	Hypoblast Endoderm: Gametes migrate to gonads	
Mesoderm Derivatives	All connective tissues**	General connective tissues
		Cartilage and bone
		Blood cells (red and white)
	All muscle types:	Cardiac, skeletal, smooth
	Epithelial linings of:	Body cavities
		Some organs: Cardiovascular system Reproductive and urinary systems (most parts)

*Pharyngeal derivatives: palatine tonsils, thymus, thyroid, parathyroids
**Some connective tissues in the head are derived from neural crest

Ectoderm Derivatives

Formation of the primitive central nervous system is induced in the ectoderm layer by cells forming the **notochord** in the underlying mesoderm.

The neural plate ectoderm (**neuroectoderm**) forms two lateral folds that meet and fuse in the midline to form the neural tube (**neurulation**).

Cells from the tips of the folds (**neural crest**) migrate throughout the body to form many derivatives including the peripheral nervous system.

FORMATION OF THE HEAD REGION

Neural crest contributes significantly to formation of connective tissue elements in the head.

The bony skeleton of the head is comprised of the **viscerocranium** and the **neurocranium**.

The neurocranium (cranial vault) is composed of a base formed by **endochondral ossification** (chondrocranium) and sides and roof bones formed by **intramembranous ossification.**

The chondrocranium is derived from both **somitic mesoderm** (occipital) and neural crest.

The viscerocranium (face) is derived from the first two **pharyngeal (branchial) arches** (neural crest).

LIMB FORMATION

The limbs form as ventrolateral buds under the mutual induction of ectoderm [apical ectodermal ridge (AER)] and underlying mesoderm beginning in the fifth week. *The AER influences proximal-distal development.*

Somatic lateral plate mesoderm forms the bony and connective tissue elements of the limbs and limb girdles while skeletal muscle of the appendages is derived from somites.

Cranio-caudal polarity is determined by specialized mesoderm cells [**zone of polarizing activity** (ZPA)] that release inducing signals such as **retinoic acid.**

Homeobox genes are the targets of induction signals.

Rotation of the limb buds establishes the position of the joints, the location of muscle groups, and the pattern of sensory innervation.

MATURATION OF THE CENTRAL NERVOUS SYSTEM

Both neurons and glia develop from the original neurectoderm forming the neural tube.

Microglia are the exception: they develop from the monocyte-macrophage lineage of mesodermal (bone marrow) origin and migrate into the CNS.

Induction of regional differences in the developing CNS is regulated by **retinoic acid** (vitamin A). Overexposure of the cranial region to retinoic acid can result in "caudalization," i.e., development more similar to the spinal cord.

During development, the spinal cord and presumptive brainstem develop three layers: (1) a germinal layer or **ventricular zone,** (2) an **intermediate layer** containing neuroblasts and comprising gray matter, and (3) a **marginal zone** containing myelinated fibers (white matter).

Other layers are added in the cerebrum and cerebellum by cell migration along glial scaffolds.

The notochord induces the establishment of **dorsal-ventral polarity** in the neural tube. Ventral portions of the tube will become the **basal plate** and give rise to motor neurons, whereas the dorsal portions become the **alar plates** and subserve sensory functions.

Meninges are formed by mesoderm surrounding the neural tube with contributions to the arachnoid and pia from neural crest.

Defects in the CNS may result from several causes including high maternal blood glucose levels and vitamin A overexposure and often involve bony defects (e.g., **spina bifida** and **anencephaly**). Defects are most common in the regions of **neuropore** closure.

PERIPHERAL NERVOUS SYSTEM

Sensory neurons of the spinal ganglia, as well as autonomic postganglionic neurons and their supporting cells, are derived from neural crest.

Focal deficiencies in neural crest cell migration may result in lack of innervation to specific organs or parts of organs. In **Hirschsprung disease,** failure of neural crest cells to migrate to a portion of the colon results in a localized deficiency in parasympathetic intramural ganglia that may cause a loss of peristalsis and fatal bowel obstruction.

DEVELOPMENT OF THE HEAD AND NECK

The cartilages, bones, and blood vessels of the face (viscerocranium) develop from the **pharyngeal (branchial) arches.** Each arch receives its blood supply from a specific aortic arch and its innervation from a specific cranial nerve. The **skeletal muscles** of the head and neck primarily arise from the pharyngeal arches and have a unique innervation (special visceral efferent).

The face develops from a midline **frontonasal prominence** and bilateral **maxillary and mandibular prominences.** Failure of the prominences to fuse results in various facial malformations.

Teeth originate from both ectodermal (enamel) and neurectodermal (neural crest: dentin, pulp, cementum, and periodontal ligament) derivatives.

Pouch and cleft 1:	Epithelial lining of middle and outer ear canals and tympanic membrane
Pouch 2:	Epithelial lining of palatine tonsils
Pouch and cleft 3:	
Ventral Portion:	Epithelial components of thymus gland
Pouch 3: Dorsal Portion:	Epithelial cells of inferior parathyroid glands
Pouch 4: Ventral Portion:	Epithelial parafollicular cells (incorporate into thyroid gland)
Dorsal Portion:	Epithelial cells of superior parathyroid glands
Clefts 2 and 4:	No derivatives

DERIVATIVES OF PHARYNGEAL POUCHES AND CLEFTS

The anterior portion of the pituitary is derived from oral ectoderm arising from the roof of the oral cavity (Rathke's pouch) anterior to the buccopharyngeal membrane and migrating through the sphenoid anlagen to unite with a downgrowth (posterior pituitary) from the hypothalamus.

The eye is derived from three different germ layers:

Neurectoderm: Vesicular outgrowths of the forebrain differentiate into **retina and optic nerve.**

Surface ectoderm: Contributes to the **lens, cornea,** and epthelial coverings of the lacrimal glands, eyelids, and **conjunctiva.**

Mesoderm: The **sclera** and **choroid** are derived from lateral plate mesoderm.

The **extraocular muscles** are formed by myotomes of **cranial somitomeres.**

Structures of the **outer and middle ear** are derived from the first and second **pharyngeal arches** and the **first pharyngeal cleft.**

Structures of the **inner ear** are derived from the **ectodermal otic placode.**

Maternal rubella can cause defects in both eye (fourth to sixth weeks of gestation) and ear (seventh to 8th weeks).

FORMATION OF THE CARDIOVASCULAR SYSTEM

All components of the cardiovascular system, including the epithelia, are derived from **splanchnic lateral plate mesoderm.**

The heart tubes forming on either side of the endodermal tube are brought together by **lateral body folding.**

Looping of the heart tube occurs while the tube is being divided into left and right portions by interatrial and interventricular septa.

In the interatrial septum, the **septum primum** and **septum secundum** do not close off the **foramen ovale** until birth.

Failure of the **atrioventricular endocardial cushions** to fuse can result in septal and valve defects.

Neural crest cells contribute to septation of the truncus arteriosus and the formation of the aortic and pulmonary outflows, as well as the aortic arches.

The "**Tetralogy of Fallot**" is the most common defect of the conus arteriosus/truncus arteriosus and involves stenosis of the pulmonary trunk, ventricular septal defect, right ventricular hypertrophy, and overriding aorta.

Vasculature

The endothelial lining of most blood vessels forms by coalescence of **mesodermal cells** and subsequent **vacuolization** to form a lumen. Subsequently, smooth muscle cells and connective tissue elements are supplied by local mesoderm.

The paired doral aortae and the five aortic arches form an early symmetric arterial system. Regression of portions of these vessels later results in the asymmetrical adult arterial system.

The **vitelline arteries** connect the yolk sac to the abdominal dorsal aorta. They will form the arteries of the GI tract: **celiac, superior mesenteric, and inferior mesenteric.**

Blood islands formed during etiology of the vitelline arteries are the first sites of **hematopoiesis** and seed other hematopoietic tissues.

The paired **umbilical arteries** develop from the caudal end of the dorsal aorta and invade the mesoderm of the placenta. They carry deoxygenated blood from the fetus to the placenta.

The **caval venous system** is derived mostly from the right anterior and posterior **cardinal veins.**

The **vitelline veins** form the veins of the digestive system, including the **portal vein,** and the terminal part of the inferior vena cava.

No components of the **umbilical veins** remain patent after closure of the ductus venosus.

DEVELOPMENT OF THE HEMATOPOIETIC SYSTEM

Onset of **hematopoiesis** begins with formation of **blood islands** in the wall of the yolk sac (derived from the hypoblast) during week 3.

Pluripotent stem cells from the blood islands seed the other hematopoietic sites. These are, in succession, the **liver** (week 5), **spleen** (week 5), and **bone marrow** (month 6).

All components of hematopoietic organs are derived from **mesoderm** except for the **epithelium of the thymus,** which is derived from endoderm of the **third pharyngeal pouch.**

DEVELOPMENT OF THE DIGESTIVE SYSTEM

The epithelium of the digestive tract and associated organs is formed by the **endoderm tube,** whereas connective tissue and smooth muscle are derived from **splanchnic lateral plate mesoderm.** The mesoderm induces regional specialization in the endoderm.

The midgut endoderm is the last to fold into a tube and remains connected to the yolk sac via the yolk stalk.

Formation of the mesodermal **urorectal septum** divides the cloaca into the **urogenital sinus** and **primitive rectum.**

Cell proliferation results in closure of the endodermal tube lumen during week 6. The lumen is reopened by **recanalization** in week 8.

Failure to recanalize can result in **stenosis,** preventing the passage of amniotic fluid swallowed by the fetus (**polyhydramnios**).

Peristalsis begins in week 10 when cells of neural crest origin invade the muscular layer to form the enteric nervous (autonomic) system. Failure of neural crest cell migration to the distal hindgut results in **aganglionic mega-colon (Hirschsprung disease**), which may cause fatal intestinal obstruction.

The adult pattern of GI organ distribution is achieved by **physiologic herniation** and then retraction of the midgut during the second month.

Failure of the midgut loop to return to the abdominal cavity may result in an **omphalocele or umbilical hernia.**

Associated digestive organs (liver, gallbladder, and pancreas) originate as outgrowths of the endodermal tube. Connective tissue components of the liver are derived from both splanchnic and somatic (septum transversum) lateral plate mesoderm. Lateral plate mesoderm also forms the peritoneum and mesenteries of the abdominal cavity.

FORMATION OF THE RESPIRATORY SYSTEM

The first part of the respiratory system is lined by ectoderm derived from the nasal **ectodermal placodes.**

In the fourth week, a **respiratory diverticulum** arises as an outgrowth of the ventral **endodermal tube.**

Endoderm will form the respiratory epithelium, whereas **splanchnic lateral plate mesoderm** will form connective tissue elements including cartilage, smooth muscle, and blood vessels.

Mesoderm directs the branching pattern of the developing airways.

Although most alveoli do not form until after birth, the lungs are capable of sufficient gas exchange after 6.5 months' gestation. **Respiratory distress syndrome** develops in premature births if **surfactant** levels are inadequate.

Abnormal septation of the trachea and esophagus can result in stenosis, atresia, or tracheoesophageal fistulas.

DEVELOPMENT OF THE URINARY SYSTEM

Epithelial structures of the urinary system are derived from two sources: **intermediate mesoderm and urogenital sinus endoderm.**

Three pairs of kidneys develop in cranio-caudal sequence in the urogenital ridge of intermediate mesoderm: **pronephros, mesonephros, and metanephros.**

The caudal end of the mesonephric duct gives rise to the **ureteric bud.** The ureteric bud induces surrounding intermediate mesoderm to form the metanephric cap, which forms the excretory units of the kidney. The ureteric bud will form the collecting ducts.

The epithelial lining (transitional epithelium) of the **ureters**, as well as their muscular and connective tissue components, are derived from **intermediate mesoderm.**

The transitional epithelium of the **bladder** and most of the **urethra** (transitional) is derived from hingut **endoderm of the urogenital sinus.** Connective tissue and muscle are derived from splanchnic lateral plate mesoderm.

DEVELOPMENT OF THE REPRODUCTIVE SYSTEMS

Intermediate mesoderm forms the epithelia, connective tissues, and smooth muscle of the indifferent **sex cords** and their ducts.

The **endoderm of the urogenital sinus** gives rise to the epithelia of distal organs of the reproductive system and the external genitalia. As in the urinary system, connective tissue and smooth muscle of these terminal elements is provided by splanchnic lateral plate mesoderm.

Germ cells migrate from their origins in yolk sac endoderm into the indifferent sex cords of the **urogenital ridge** by week 6. Further differentiation of both the immature sex cords and the germ cells depends on **mutual induction.**

The *Sry* **gene** on the **Y chromosome** directs the differentiation of the medullary sex cords into **testes.** If this gene (or a Y chromosome) is not present, the cortical sex cords will develop as ovaries.

Production of **Müllerian inhibiting substance** by Sertoli cells induces presumptive Leydig cells to produce **testosterone** and other sex hormones that regulate further **male differentiation.**

In the absence of testosterone, developing **follicular cells** of the ovaries direct the **differentiation** of germ cells into **oogonia.**

Two pairs of genital ducts develop in both sexes. **Wolffian (mesonephric)** ducts develop first as part of the urinary system.

Paramesonephric (Müllerian) ducts develop next and are open to the pelvic cavity at their cranial ends. The mesonephric system will persist in the male and the paramesonephric system in the female.

In **males,** the **urogenital sinus endoderm** gives rise to the epithelia of the **urethra** and associated **prostate and bulbourethral glands.**

In the **female,** the endoderm of the **urogenital sinus** is the origin of the epithelium of the **lower vagina,** the upper portion being formed by the **paramesonephric ducts.**

Male differentiation of external genitalia requires testosterone. Female differentiation requires **placental estrogen.**

DEVELOPMENT OF THE PLACENTA AND FETAL MEMBRANES

The fetal portion of the placenta forms from the **trophoblast**.

Syncytiotrophoblast cells are in direct contact with maternal tissue, whereas the embryo proper is separated from the **cytotrophoblast** by **extraembryonic mesoderm** (together, **the chorion**).

Primary villus: syncytiotrophoblast with a cytotrophoblast core.

Secondary villus: Cytotrophoblast core invaded by extraembryonic mesoderm.

Tertiary villus: Fetal blood vessels invade the mesoderm (week 3).

The presumptive **umbilical blood vessels** form in the wall of the **allantois**, an endodermal outpocket of the urogenital sinus.

The **amnionic membrane** develops from **epiblast** and is continuous with embryonic ectoderm. The lining of the **yolk sac** develops from **hypoblast** and is continuous with embryonic endoderm.

The yolk sac gives rise to the first **blood islands** that will form the **vitelline vessels**.

Passive immunity is transfered to the fetus by diffusion of **immunoglobulin G** from the maternal to the fetal circulation.

Excess amniotic fluid is swallowed by the fetus, absorbed by the fetal GI tract, transferred to the fetal circulation, and finally crosses the placental membranes to the maternal circulation.

Hormones secreted by the placenta include **chorionic gonadotropin,** estrogen, progesterone, and **chorionic somatostatin** (placental lactogen).

High-Yield Facts

Histology and Cell Biology

CELL MEMBRANES

Cell membranes consist of a **lipid bilayer** and associated proteins and carbohydrates. In the bilayer, the hydrophilic portions of the lipids are arranged on the external and cytosolic surfaces, and the **hydrophobic tails** are located in the interior. **Transmembrane proteins** are anchored to the core of the bilayer by their hydrophobic regions and can be removed only by detergents that disrupt the bilayer. **Peripheral membrane proteins** are attached to the surface of the membrane by weak electrostatic forces and are easy to remove by altering the pH or ionic strength of their environment.

CYTOPLASM AND ORGANELLES

Cytoplasm is a dynamic fluid environment bounded by the cell membrane. It contains various membrane-bound organelles, nonmembranous structures (such as lipid droplets, glycogen, and pigment granules), and structural or cytoskeletal proteins in either a soluble or insoluble form. The **endoplasmic reticulum** (ER) is a continuous tubular meshwork that may be either smooth (SER) or rough (RER) where studded with ribosomes. The discoid stacks of the **Golgi apparatus** are involved in packaging and routing proteins for export or delivery to other organelles, including lysosomes and peroxisomes. **Lysosomes** degrade intracellular and imported debris, and **peroxisomes** oxidize a variety of substrates, including alcohol. Only the **nucleus**, which is the repository of genetic information stored in deoxyribonucleic acid (DNA), and the **mitochondria**, which are the storage sites of energy for cellular function in the form of adenosine triphosphate (**ATP**), are enclosed in a double membrane. Also included in the cytoplasm are three proteins that form the **cytoskeletal infrastructure: actin bundles** that determine the shape of the cell; **intermediate filaments** that stabilize the cell membrane and cytoplasmic contents; and **microtubules** (**tubulin**), which use molecular motors to move organelles within the cell.

NUCLEUS

The nucleus consists of a nuclear envelope that is continuous with the ER, chromatin, matrix, and a nucleolus rich in ribosomal ribonucleic acid (rRNA). The **nuclear envelope** contains pores for bidirectional transport and is supported by intermediate filament proteins, the **lamins**. **Chromatin** consists of euchromatin, which is an open form of DNA that is actively transcribed, and heterochromatin that is quiescent. During cell division, DNA is accurately replicated and divided equally between two daughter nuclei. Equal distribution of chromosomes is accomplished by the microtubules of the mitotic spindle. The separation of cytoplasm (cytokinesis) occurs through the action of an actin contractile ring. The cell cycle consists of interphase (G_1, S, G_2, and M), prophase, prometaphase, metaphase, anaphase, and telophase. The cell cycle is regulated at the G_1/S and G_2/M boundaries by phosphorylation of complexes of a protein kinase [cyclin-dependent kinase (Cdk) protein] and a cyclin (cytoplasmic oscillator).

INTRACELLULAR TRAFFICKING

The key event in exocytosis is translocation of newly synthesized protein into the cisternal space of the rough ER (signal hypothesis). Proteins and lipids reach the Golgi apparatus by vesicular transport. Using carbohydrate-sorting signals, proteins are sorted from the *trans*-face of the Golgi apparatus to secretory vesicles, the cell membrane, and lysosomes. Lysosomal enzymes are sorted by using a mannose-6-phosphate signal recognized by a receptor on the lysosomal membrane. Nuclear and mitochondrial-sorting signals (positively charged amino acid sequences) are recognized by those organelles.

Endocytosis involves transport from the cell membrane to lysosomes using endosome intermediates. The process originates with a clathrin-coated pit that invaginates to form a coated vesicle that fuses with an endosome. This internalization can be receptor-mediated (e.g., uptake of cholesterol). Endosomes subsequently fuse with lysosomes. Internalized receptor/ligand complexes may be conserved, degraded, or recycled.

EPITHELIUM

Epithelial cells line the free external and internal surfaces of the body. Epithelia have a paucity of intercellular substance and are interconnected by junctional complexes. Components of the junctional complex include the *zonula occludens* (tight junction), which prevents leakage between the adjoining cells and maintains apical/basolateral polarity; *zonula adherens,* which links the actin networks within adjacent cells; and *macula adherens* (desmosome), which links the intermediate filament networks of adjacent cells. Epithelial cells also form a firm attachment to the basal lamina, which they secrete. Gap junctions or nexi permit passage of small molecules directly between cells. Apical specializations are prominent in epithelia and include microvilli that increase surface area; stereocilia, which are nonmotile modified microvilli; and cilia and flagella, which are motile structures. **Cilia** and **flagella** have the classic "9 + 2" microtubular arrangement emanating from basal bodies.

CONNECTIVE TISSUE

Connective tissue consists of cells and a matrix (fibers and ground substance). The cells include **fibroblasts** (the source of collagen and other fibers), plasma cells (the source of antibodies), **macrophages** (the cells responsible for phagocytosis), **mast cells** (the source of heparin and histamine), and a variety of transient blood cells. **Type I collagen** and elastin make up the predominant fibers found in connective tissue. Ground substance includes proteoglycans and glycoproteins that organize and stabilize the fibrillar network. **Type II collagen** is associated with hyaline cartilage, **type III collagen** forms the collagenous component of reticular connective tissue found in lymphoid organs, and **type IV collagen** forms a sheetlike meshwork of the basal lamina. Other types of collagen exist and include the fibril-associated collagens with interrupted triple helices (**FACIT**). Collagen fibrils are connected to other extracellular matrix molecules by the FACIT collagens.

SPECIALIZED CONNECTIVE TISSUES: BONE AND CARTILAGE

Bone contains three major cell types: **osteoblasts** that secrete type I collagen and noncollagenous proteins; **osteocytes**, which maintain mature bone; and **osteoclasts**, which resorb bone by acidification. Bone deposition is regulated primarily by **parathyroid hormone** (**PTH**), which is secreted in response to low serum calcium levels. **Calcitonin** opposes the actions of PTH, but plays a lesser role overall. Bone is highly vascular and mineralized with **hydroxyapatite**.

In contrast, the three types of cartilage are avascular and contain chondrocytes that synthesize fibers and ground substance. **Hyaline cartilage** covers articular surfaces and forms the cartilage model in long bone development. **Elastic cartilage** is found in the pinna of the ear and in the larynx, while **fibrocartilage** is an intermediate form found in the intervertebral disc, pubic symphysis, and connecting tendon and bone.

MUSCLE AND CELL MOTILITY

Skeletal and cardiac (striated) muscle contract by sliding **myosin** and **actin** filaments past each other in a process facilitated by ATP. Myosin contains a motor that interacts with the actin filament and allows myosin to ratchet along the actin. The filaments are arranged in a banded pattern in individual **sarcomeres**, which act in series. Specialized invaginations of the plasma membrane (**T tubules**) spread the surface depolarization to the interior of the cell to release calcium from the **sarcoplasmic reticulum**, initiating contraction. **Troponin** and **tropomyosin** are specialized proteins that permit contraction of skeletal and cardiac muscle to be regulated by calcium. Skeletal muscle is a syncytium, while cardiac muscle consists of individual cells connected by intercalated disks. The organization of striated muscle is shown below:

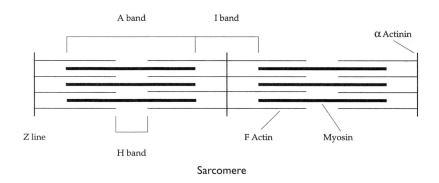

Sarcomere

Smooth muscle contraction closely resembles the cell motility exhibited in other cell types. It also occurs through the action of actin and myosin, which are arranged in a lattice-like pattern.

NERVOUS SYSTEM

Myelin, which insulates neuronal projections and permits rapid (saltatory) conduction, is produced by **oligodendroglia** in the central nervous system (**CNS**) and by **Schwann cells** in the peripheral nervous system (**PNS**). **Microglia** are the macrophages of the brain. **Astrocytes** have a complicated role in physical and metabolic support of neurons. **Neurons** conduct electrochemical impulses and move neurotransmitters to their synaptic termini by **axoplasmic transport**. Transneuronal transmission is accomplished by calcium-regulated release of **synaptic vesicles**. Neurons also synapse with muscle cells. A typical contact between a myelinated neuron and skeletal muscle (**neuromuscular** junction) is shown below.

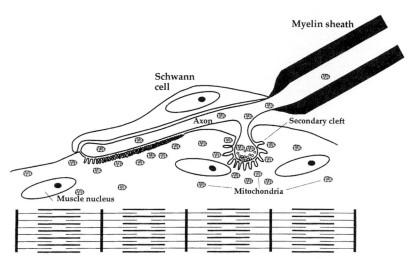

Neuromuscular junction. Axonal terminals (telodendria) rest in shallow depressions (primary clefts) on the surface of the striated muscle fiber. Secondary clefts increase the surface area for interaction with a neurotransmitter (acetylcholine). Muscle cell nuclei and mitochondria are abundant near the junction.

In the **cerebral** and **cerebellar cortices**, **gray matter** (cell bodies and immediately adjacent processes) is located peripherally and **white matter** centrally; this pattern is reversed in the **spinal cord**. Cerebellar cortex consists of **molecular, Purkinje,** and **granular layers** with extensive arborization of the neuronal processes. The cerebral cortex consists of a homogenous **layer I** with multiple deeper layers of large **pyramidal** and other types of **neurons**. The number of layers varies, depending on the cortical region. Neuronal cell bodies (**perikarya**) are also localized in ganglia in the peripheral nervous system and autonomic nervous system (**ANS**).

CARDIOVASCULAR SYSTEM, BLOOD, AND BONE MARROW

In large arteries close to the heart, the *tunica media* contains high amounts of elastin to buffer the heart's pulsatile output. Smaller muscular arteries distribute blood to organs and capillary beds; their contractions are mediated by both the **sympathetic nervous system** (**SNS**) and by humoral factors. **Endothelial cells** lining the vascular lumen secrete vasoactive substances (e.g., endothelin) and factors important in **blood clotting** (e.g., von Willebrand factor). Smooth muscle cells undergo **hyperplasia** and **hypertrophy** in hypertension. The heart contains specialized cardiomyocytes that function as impulse-generating and conducting cells regulated by the ANS. The heart also functions as an endocrine organ, releasing **atrial natriuretic peptides** (ANPs) in response to increased plasma volume. ANPs reduce plasma volume by (1) increasing urinary sodium and water excretion, (2) inhibiting aldosterone synthesis and angiotensin II production, and (3) inhibiting vasopressin release from the neurohypophysis.

Blood cells include **erythrocytes**, which are specialized for oxygen transport; **lymphocytes** that function in cellular and humoral immune responses; **neutrophils**, which are early responders to acute inflammation; **monocytes** that are the precursors of tissue **macrophages**; **eosinophils**, which respond to parasitic infection; and **basophils**, which contain **histamine** and **heparin** and assist mast cell function.

Bone marrow is the site of blood cell development in adults. The erythrocyte lineage includes the following stages: proerythroblasts → basophilic erythroblasts → polychromatophilic erythroblasts → orthochromatophilic erythrocytes. The white cell series includes myeloblasts → promyelocytes → myelocytes → metamyelocytes → mature granular leukocytes.

LYMPHOID SYSTEM AND CELLULAR IMMUNOLOGY

Functional cells include **B lymphocytes** (humoral immunity), **T lymphocytes** (cellular immunity), **macrophages** (phagocytic and **antigen-presenting cells**), and **mast cells**. Lymphoid organs may be either primary (**bone marrow** and **thymus**) or secondary (**lymph nodes** and dispersed **lymphatic nodules**, **spleen**, and **tonsils**). The B lymphocytes are educated in the bone marrow and are seeded to specific **B cell regions** of the secondary lymphoid organs, and T lymphocytes are educated in the thymus and seeded to **T cell-dependent regions** of the secondary lymphoid organs. The thymus is recognized by lobulation, separate cortex and medulla in each lobule, the absence of germinal centers, and the presence of Hassall's corpuscles. The lymph nodes, which **filter lymph not blood**, are characterized by a central medulla and a cortex containing primary and secondary follicles. The spleen, which **filters blood**, is characterized by red and white pulp. The **tonsils** are characterized by an **epithelial lining** on one side.

RESPIRATORY SYSTEM

The respiratory epithelium consists of **conducting pathways** (nasal cavities, naso- and oropharynx, larynx, trachea, bronchi, and bronchioles) and **respiratory portions** (respiratory bronchioles and alveoli). The nasal epithelium includes a region of specialized olfactory receptors. Ciliated cells appear in all portions of the respiratory system except the respiratory epithelium and move mucus and particulates toward the oropharynx. Gas exchange in the lungs takes place across a minimal barrier consisting of the capillary endothelium, a joint basal lamina, and an exceedingly thin alveolar epithelium consisting primarily of type I pneumocytes. Type II pneumocytes are responsible for the secretion of surfactant, a primarily lipid substance that facilitates respiration by reducing alveolar surface tension.

INTEGUMENTARY SYSTEM

The epidermis of thick skin consists of five layers of cells (**keratinocytes**): *stratum basale* (proliferative layer), *stratum spinosum* (characterized by tonofibrils and associated desmosomes), *stratum granulosum* (characterized by keratohyalin granules), *stratum lucidum* (a translucent layer not present in thin skin), and *stratum corneum* (characterized by dead and dying cells with compacted keratin). Specialized structures of the skin include hair follicles (found only in thin skin), nails, and sweat glands and ducts. Nonkeratinocyte epidermal cells include **melanocytes** (derived from the neural crest), **Langerhans cells** (antigen-presenting cells derived from monocytes), and **Merkel cells** (sensory mechanoreceptors). Various sensory receptors and extensive capillary networks are found in the underlying dermis.

GASTROINTESTINAL TRACT AND GLANDS

The epithelium of the gastrointestinal (GI) tract is simple and columnar throughout, except for the stratified squamous epithelia in regions of maximal friction (**esophagus** and **anus**). The **stomach** is a grinding organ with glands in the **fundus and body** that produce **mucus** (**surface and neck cells**), **pepsinogen** (**chief cells**), and **acid** (**parietal cells**). The small intestine is an absorptive organ with folds at several levels (**plicae, villi,** and **microvilli**) that increase surface area for more efficient absorption. Cell types in the small intestine include **enterocytes** (**absorption**), **Paneth cells** (**production of lysozyme**), **goblet cells** (**mucus**), and **enteroendocrine cells** (**secretion of peptide hormones**). All of these cells originate from a single stem cell in the crypt. New cells are born in the crypt, move up the villus, and are sloughed off at the tip. The primary function of the colon, which appears histologically as crypts with prominent goblet cells and no villi, is water resorption.

The major salivary glands (**parotid, submandibular,** and **sublingual**) are exocrine glands that secrete amylase and mucus, primarily regulated by the parasympathetic nervous system. In contrast, the **pancreas** has both **exocrine** (**acinar cells**) and **endocrine** (**islet cells**) components that synthesize pancreatic juice and blood sugar–regulating hormones, respectively. The exocrine pancreas is primarily regulated by the hormones **cholecystokinin (CCK)** and **secretin**, which regulate acinar and ductal secretion, respectively.

The **liver** is also a dual-function gland whose exocrine product is **bile**, which is transported by a duct system to the **gallbladder** for storage and concentration; **bile emulsifies lipids** for more efficient enzymatic access. The endocrine products include **glucose** and major blood proteins.

ENDOCRINE GLANDS

The pituitary is formed from two embryonic sources. The **adenohypophysis** is derived from the **oral ectoderm** of Rathke's pouch and is regulated through a **hypophyseal portal system** carrying factors that stimulate or inhibit secretion. It contains **acidophils**, which produce prolactin and growth hormone (GH), and **basophils** that produce luteinizing hormone (LH), follicle-stimulating hormone (FSH), thyroid-stimulating hormone (TSH), adrenocorticotropic hormone (ACTH), and melanocyte-stimulating hormone (MSH). The **neurohypophysis** is derived from the floor of the **diencephalon** and consists of **glial cells** (**pituicytes**) and expanded terminals of nerve fibers originating in the **paraventricular** and **supraoptic nuclei** of the hypothalamus. It contains **vasopressin** and **oxytocin**.

The adrenal gland consists of two parts. The **adrenal cortex**, derived from intermediate mesoderm, and covered by a connective tissue capsule, consists of three zones: the *zona glomerulosa* produces aldosterone (a mineralocorticoid) and is regulated primarily by angiotensin II; the *zona fasciculata* and *zona reticularis* produce glucocorticoids (e.g., cortisol and weak androgens) and are regulated primarily by ACTH. The **adrenal medulla**, derived from the neural crest, synthesizes epinephrine and norepinephrine (see figure below).

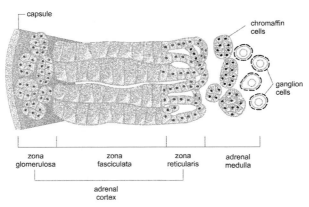

Adrenal (suprarenal) gland. The gland is covered by a connective tissue capsule and divided into a cortex containing steroid-producing cells with prominent lipid droplets (only two are drawn) and a medulla containing chromaffin cells that secrete catecholamines and neuropeptides.

The **thyroid gland** is characterized by an extracellular hormone precursor (**iodinated thyroglobulin**) in the follicles. Scattered between the follicular cells are **parafollicular cells**, which secrete **calcitonin**, a hormone that reduces blood calcium levels. The **parathyroid gland** consists primarily of **chief cells** that secrete PTH that increases blood calcium levels by stimulating osteoclastic activity and affecting kidney excretion and intestinal absorption.

Endocrine cells of the **pancreatic islets** secrete primarily **insulin** and **glucagon**, hormones that regulate blood glucose. Scattered through several organ systems are enteroendocrine cells, which synthesize peptide hormones for local regulation.

URINARY SYSTEM

The filtration apparatus of the renal glomeruli consists of an expanded **basement membrane** and **slit pore** associated with podocytes. Epithelial cells of the **proximal tubule** are specialized for absorption and ion transport. They remove most of the sodium and water from urine, as well as virtually all of the amino acids, proteins, and glucose. The **brush border** of the proximal tubule cells contains proteases. The cells of the **distal tubule**, under the influence of **aldosterone**, resorb sodium and acidify the urine. Specialized cells of the distal tubule (the **macula densa**) monitor ion levels in the urine and stimulate the **juxtaglomerular cells** of the afferent arteriole to secrete **renin**, an enzyme that cleaves angiotensinogen to a precursor of angiotensin II. Collecting ducts contain light and dark (intercalated) cells; they are sensitive to **antidiuretic hormone (ADH)** and are the final mechanism for concentrating urine. Transitional epithelium (allowing for stretch) is found lining the calyces, renal pelvis, ureters, and urinary bladder.

MALE REPRODUCTIVE SYSTEM

The **testes** produce sperm and testosterone under the influence of **LH** and **FSH**, secreted by gonadotrophs of the anterior pituitary. The testicular epithelium contains **Sertoli cells** and precursors of sperm. **Spermatogenesis** involves the following lineage: spermatogonia (germ cells) → (**spermatocytogenesis**) → primary spermatocytes → secondary spermatocytes → (**completion of meiosis**) → **spermatids** (**spermiogenesis**) → mature sperm. Sertoli cells perform several functions: (1) maintenance of the **blood-testis barrier**, (2) phagocytosis, and (3) secretion of androgen-binding protein and inhibin, as well as Müllerian inhibiting hormone in the fetus.

The **epididymis**, like most of the male duct system, is lined by a pseudostratified epithelium characterized by modified microvilli (**stereocilia**). The **seminal vesicles** produce fructose and other molecules that activate spermatozoa.

The **prostate** is a fibromuscular organ that produces the largest fluid component of the ejaculate. Virtually all males over 70 show some form of **prostatic hypertrophy**. Prostatic malignancies are the second most common form of cancer in males.

FEMALE REPRODUCTIVE SYSTEM

The **ovaries** produce **ova**, **estrogen**, and **progesterone** under the influence of LH and FSH. Oocyte (germ cell) maturation involves several stages of follicular development (granulosa cells plus the oocyte): primordial follicle → primary follicle → secondary follicle → mature, or Graafian, follicle. In the secondary follicle, the stroma differentiates into a theca. The *theca interna* synthesizes androgens, which are converted into estradiol by granulosa cells. After ovulation, these thecal cells form the *theca lutein;* the granulosa cells become the *granulosa lutein,* which produces **progesterone** (see figure below). Human chorionic gonadotropin (hCG) in the placenta maintains the **corpus luteum** of pregnancy.

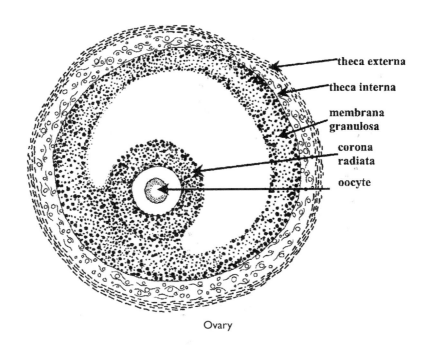

theca externa
theca interna
membrana granulosa
corona radiata
oocyte

Ovary

The **uterine endometrium** goes through a monthly cycle during which the **functionalis** is lost and replaced from the **basalis**. The **menstrual phase** occupies the first four days of the cycle (in the absence of hCG), followed by the **proliferative phase** under the influence of FSH (days 5 to 14) and then the **secretory phase** under the influence of LH (days 15 to 28). During this phase, endometrial cells accumulate glycogen preliminary to the synthesis and secretion of glycoproteins.

Vaginal epithelium is made up of stratified squamous cells and varies with maturity, phase of the menstrual cycle, pregnancy, and cancer (detected by vaginal Pap smear).

When fertilization and implantation occur, the placenta, consisting of the **chorion (fetal part)** and **decidua basalis (maternal part)**, is established for O_2/CO_2 exchange, as well as its endocrine role (e.g., conversion of androgens to estradiol, placental lactogen secretion). During parturition, oxytocin secreted by the neurohypophysis stimulates the contraction of uterine smooth muscle.

The **breast** is a resting alveolar gland except during pregnancy, when the lactiferous ducts proliferate and milk production is initiated. Milk synthesis and ejection are under the influence of prolactin and oxytocin.

EYE

The photosensitive layer of the **retina** is derived from the inner layer of the **optic cup** and contains the **rod** and **cone cells** involved in visual signal transduction. **Rhodopsin** is a visual pigment found within lamellar disks of the outer segment of the rod cell. Rhodopsin consists of **retinal** and **opsin**; photons induce an isomeric change in retinal, leading to dissociation of the retinal/opsin complex. The resulting decrease in the intracellular second messenger, guanosine 3'5'-cyclic monophosphate (**cGMP**), directs closure of membrane sodium channels and leads to **hyperpolarization** of the photoreceptor cell. This signal is transmitted to interneurons within the retina and finally to ganglion cells.

The **lens** arises from **surface ectoderm** during development. Production of lens fibers (elongated, protein-filled cells) continues throughout life without replacement. Increased opacity of the lens (**cataract**) may be caused by congenital factors, excess ultraviolet (UV) radiation, or high glucose levels.

The **choroid** and **sclera** are the supportive, protective coats of the eye. The **aqueous humor**, produced by processes of the ciliary body, flows between the lens and iris to the anterior chamber of the eye toward the iridocorneal angle, where it is drained into the **canal of Schlemm**. Blockage of the canal of Schlemm or associated structures leads to increased intraocular pressure and **glaucoma**.

EAR

The ear functions in two separate but related signal transduction systems, **audition** and **equilibrium**. The **external ear**, largely formed from the first two branchial arches, funnels sound to the tympanic membrane. The **middle ear** is made up of the **malleus, incus**, and **stapes** formed from the first two arch cartilages. The internal ear consists of a membranous and a bony labyrinth filled with **endolymph** and **perilymph**, respectively. The saccule (ventral) and utricle (dorsal), parts of the membranous labyrinth, form from the **otic vesicle** (an ectodermal invagination). The cochlea contains three spaces, the *scala vestibuli, scala media* (cochlear duct, which extends from the saccule), and *scala tympani*. The **semicircular canals** (which extend from the utricle) contain the *cristae ampulares*, made up of cupulae with hair cells embedded in a gelatinous matrix that respond to changes in direction and rate of angular acceleration. The hair cells are located within the **organ of Corti** and respond to different frequencies. In the saccule and utricle, the maculae, along with **stereocilia, kinocilia**, and **otoconia** (crystals of protein and calcium carbonate), detect changes in position with reference to gravity.

High-Yield Facts

Neural Pathways

ASCENDING PATHWAYS

Afferents terminating in the spinal cord and cerebellum are generally ipsilateral. Those ascending to the thalamus and cerebral cortex terminate on the contralateral side.

The funiculi of the spinal cord are dorsal, lateral, and ventral.

Fibers within a funiculus have common origins, termination, and function.

Pain, Temperature, Tactile

Simple receptors, unmyelinated, or poorly myelinated fibers.

Enter via dorsal root and may ascend or descend a few segments.

Secondary fibers cross the midline in the ventral commissure and ascend in ventral and lateral funiculi (**ventral and lateral spinothalamic tracts**).

Terminate in **ventral posterior lateral nucleus of thalamus**.

Tertiary fibers project via the internal capsule to terminate in the postcentral gyrus.

Injury to the spinothalamic tracts results in loss of pain and temperature sensation on the opposite side of the body.

Syringomyelia interrupts pain and temperature fibers crossing in the ventral white commissure and thus results in bilateral sensory deficit.

Proprioception, Tactile Discrimination, and Stereognosis

Primary fibers arising from more complicated receptors are generally well myelinated.

Afferents enter the spinal cord via the dorsal root and ascend in the dorsal funiculus. The dorsal funiculus becomes divided into a medial **fasciculus gracilis** (sacral, lumbar, and lower thoracic inputs) and a lateral **fasciculus cuneatus** (upper thoracic and cervical inputs). Both fasciculi terminate in corresponding midbrain nuclei.

Secondary fibers cross the midline and ascend in the medial lemniscus to terminate in the **ventral posterior lateral nucleus of the thalamus**.

Tertiary fibers terminate in the postcentral gyrus.

Some primary fibers terminate in the dorsal horn. Ascending secondary fibers in the lateral funiculus form the dorsal and ventral spinocerebellar tracts that enter the cerebellum via the inferior and superior cerebellar peduncles, respectively, to terminate in the vermis.

Interruption of primary fibers in the dorsal funiculus will cause loss of proprioception, and so forth, on the same side of the body as the lesion.

Interruption of secondary fibers in the medial lemniscus will give rise to contralateral deficits.

Tabes dorsalis and pernicious anemia attack the dorsal funiculi.

Trigeminal Pathways

On reaching the brachium pontis, afferent primary trigeminal fibers divide into ascending (proprioception, two-point discrimination, light touch) and descending (pain, temperature, light touch) roots.

Primary afferents of the descending root terminate in the **sensory nucleus of CN V.**

Secondary fibers ascend through the medulla and pons as the trigeminal lemniscus to terminate in the **ventral posterior medial (VPM) nucleus** of the thalamus.

The ascending root primary tactile afferents terminate in the main sensory nucleus of CN V.

Secondary fibers ascend in the **trigeminal lemniscus** to the VPM.

Primary proprioceptive afferents from the muscles of mastication enter the pons with the motor division of the nerve and terminate in the **mesencephalic nucleus** of V.

Collaterals are given off to the motor nucleus for reflexes.

Lesion of the descending root of V and the adjacent lateral spinothalamic tract on one side of the medulla will result in pain and temperature deficits on the contralateral side of the body and the ipsilateral side of the head.

Vestibular Pathways

Primary afferents terminate in the vestibular nuclei and in the cerebellum on the same side.

Secondary fibers ascend or descend in the **medial longitudinal fasciculus** or the ventral funiculus of the spinal cord.

In the upper midbrain, fibers terminate in the motor nuclei for extraocular muscles.

In the spinal cord, secondary fibers terminate on internuncial neurons in the intermediate gray.

Unilateral lesions of the vestibular system result in movement of the head, body, and eyes (nystagmus) to the affected (ipsilateral) side. Symptoms include vertigo, nausea, and a tendency to fall to the affected side.

Visceral Afferents

Primary general visceral afferents have cell bodies in the dorsal root ganglia and terminate in the dorsal horn. Ascending secondary neurons make abundant reflex connections with autonomic and somatic pathways and terminate in the **centromedian**, **intralaminar**, and **parafascicular nuclei** of the thalamus.

Central processes of primary general visceral afferents associated with cranial nerves VII, IX, and X enter the solitary fasciculus and terminate in the **nucleus of the solitary tract.** Secondary fibers make reflex connections with visceral motor nuclei or ascend in the medial lemniscus to terminate in the VPM nucleus of the thalamus.

Secondary visceral tracts ascend bilaterally

DESCENDING (MOTOR) PATHWAYS

In the brain, the cell bodies of general somatic efferent neurons are located in columns ventral to the cerebral aqueduct and fourth ventricle and ventrolateral to the central canal. Special visceral efferents are located lateral and ventral to the general somatic efferents. In the spinal cord, they originate in the ventral horn.

These are lower motor neurons, or the "final common pathway." Total, or flaccid, paralysis results from destruction of peripheral nerves or motor nuclei. Destruction of upper motor neurons (from higher centers) results in spastic paralysis and hypo- or hyperreflexia.

Cerebellar Pathways

The dentate nucleus receives fibers from the Purkinje neurons of the cerebellum and projects via the superior peduncle to the reticular formation (descending limb) and to the basal ganglia/thalamus-motor cortex (ascending limb).

The cerebellum is involved with coordination of fine movements.

Lesions to the cerebellum or superior peduncle result in ataxia, hypotonia, hyporeflexia, and/or intention tremor on the same side as the lesion.

Corticospinal (Pyramidal) Pathways

Fibers arise from pyramidal neurons in layer 5 of the precentral gyrus and premotor areas and descend through the internal capsule and basis pedunculi, cross in the lower medulla, and form the **lateral corticospinal tract** in the lateral funiculus of the spinal cord. They terminate on lower motor neurons in the ventral horn or on interneurons of the central grey.

Most muscles are represented in the contralateral motor cortex. However, some (such as the muscles of the upper face and the muscles of mastication and muscles of the larynx) are represented bilaterally.

With the noted bilateral exceptions, lesion of the pyramidal tract above the decussation results in spastic paralysis, loss of fine movements, and hyperreflexia on the contralateral side.

Lesion of the corticospinal tract in the cord results in ipsilateral deficits.

The Extrapyramidal (Basal Ganglia) System

The basal ganglia (caudate, putamen, globus pallidus) and associated nuclei (e.g., substantia nigra) do not project directly to medullary or spinal lower motor neurons but to the motor cortex.

The system controls coarse, stereotyped movements. Lesions result in altered muscle tone (usually rigidity), paucity of movement, and the appearance of rhythmic tremors and writhing or jerky movements.

Reticular Pathways

Nuclei of the reticular system send ascending projections to the hypothalamus and thalamus as well as descending projections to the motor nuclei of cranial, nerves, and the intermediate gray of the spinal cord.

The reticular formation has reciprocal connections with most other areas of the CNS and produces both faciliatory and inhibitory effects on motor systems, receptors, and sensory conduction pathways.

High-Yield Facts

Anatomy

UPPER EXTREMITY

- **Axillary nerve injury** results in deltoid paralysis with total inability to abduct the arm and severe impairment of flexion and extension at the glenohumeral joint.
- **Midhumeral** fracture may involve the deep brachial artery and the radial nerve as they wind about the posterior aspect of the humerus. Arterial injury produces ischemic contracture; nerve injury paralyzes the wrist extensors and extrinsic extensors of the hand.
- Except on the ulnar side, the **forearm flexor compartment** is innervated by the median nerve.
- **Scaphoid fracture** is most common because it transmits forces from the abducted hand directly to the radius. Because the blood supply enters distally, the scaphoid is especially prone to avascular necrosis.
- **Lunate dislocation** is most common in falls on the out-stretched hand, compressing the median nerve within the carpal tunnel and producing carpal tunnel syndrome.
- **Extension of the proximal phalanges** is accomplished by the extensor digitorum in the forearm, innervated by the radial nerve. **Digital extension** at the interphalangeal joints is primarily by dorsal and ventral interossei, both innervated by the ulnar nerve.
- **Proximal phalangeal flexion** is by the interossei and lumbricales (median and ulnar nerves); **middle phalangeal flexion** is by the extensor digitorum superficialis (median nerve); **distal phalangeal flexion** is by the flexor digitorum profundus (median and ulnar nerves).
- **Digital abduction** is a function of the dorsal interossei; **digital adduction** is a function of palmar interossei.
- The **ulnar artery** is the principal supply to the superficial palmar arch in the hand.
- **Lymphatic drainage** from the palmar hand and digits is toward the dorsal subcutaneous space of the hand, explaining the extreme swelling of this region that accompanies infections of the digits or volar surface.
- **Radial sensory function** is tested in the web space of the thumb; **ulnar sensory function** is tested along the fifth digit. The **digital branches** of the median and ulnar nerves lie along the sides of the fingers where they may be anesthetized (see figure below).

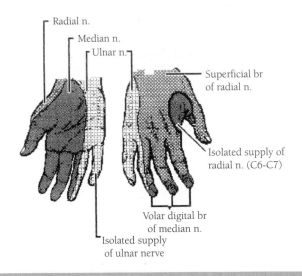

Radial n.

Median n.

Ulnar n.

Superficial br
of radial n.

Isolated supply of
radial n. (C6-C7)

Volar digital br
of median n.

Isolated supply
of ulnar nerve

Nerve Function, Tests, and Dysfunction

Nerve	Muscle Group	Reflex Test	Sign or Functional Deficit
Long thoracic	Serratus anterior		Wing scapula
Suprascapular	Supraspinatus, infraspinatus		Difficulty initiating arm abduction
Axillary	Deltoid		Inability to fully abduct arm
Radial	Extensors of forearm, wrist, proximal phalanges, and thumb	Triceps and wrist extension reflexes	Loss of arm extension; loss of forearm extension, supination, abduction; loss of wrist extension (**wrist-drop**); loss of proximal phalangeal extension and thumb extension
Musculocutaneous	Flexors of arm, forearm	Biceps reflex	Weak arm flexion, weak forearm flexion, weak forearm supination
Median	Wrist and hand flexors	Wrist flexion reflex	Paralysis of flexor, pronator, and thenar muscles; inability to fully flex the index and middle fingers (**sign of benediction**)
Ulnar	Wrist and hand flexors, phalangeal extensors		Inability to extend the distal and middle pha-langes (**clawhand**); loss of thumb adduction

BACK

- **Fracture of the dens** of the axis with posterior dislocation may crush the spinal cord at the level of the first cervical vertebra with terminal paralysis of respiratory musculature.
- The **cruciform ligament** is the principal structure preventing subluxation at the atlantoaxial joint because the articular surfaces between the axis and atlas are nearly horizontal and there is no intervertebral disk.
- **Herniation** usually occurs in the fourth or fifth intervertebral disks because of the pronounced lumbar curvature and the considerable body mass superior to this region.
- The **anterior** and **posterior longitudinal ligaments** reinforce the underlying annulus fibrosus but do not meet posterolaterally, resulting in a weak area predisposed to herniation.
- **Lumbar puncture** and intrathecal anesthesia should be introduced below the third lumbar vertebra as the spinal cord usually terminates between the first and second lumbar vertebrae.
- **Posterolateral disk prolapse** impinges on the spinal nerve of the next lower vertebral level, causing symptoms associated with the dermatomic and myotomal distributions of that nerve.

Hernia Involvement, Signs, and Reflex Test			
Hernia	**Involvement**	**Signs**	**Reflex Test**
C3-C4	C4 (Phrenic, C3-C5)	Weak diaphramatic respiration	
C4-C5	C5 (Suprascapular, C4-C6)	Weak arm abduction	
C5-C6	C6 (Musculocutaneous, C5-C6)	Weak forearm flexion	Biceps
C6-C7	C7 (Radial, C6-C8)	Weak forearm extension	Triceps
C7-C8	C8 (Ulnar, C7-T1)	Weak thumb adduction	
L1-L2	L2 (Genitofemoral, L1-L2)	Weak hip flexion	Cremaster
L2-L3	L3 (Obturator, L2-L4)	Weak hip adduction	
L3-L4	L4 (Femoral, L1-L4)	Weak leg extension	Knee jerk
L4-L5	L5 (Fibular, L4-S1)	Weak dorsiflexion	
L5-S1	S1 (Tibial, L5-S2)	Weak plantar flexion	Ankle jerk

LOWER EXTREMITY

Neurovascular Contents of the Buttock		
Quadrant	Contents	Symptoms
Upper lateral	No major vessels or nerves; A preferred location for intramuscular injection	
Upper medial	Superior gluteal neurovascular bundle	Abductor lurch
Lower lateral	Inferior gluteal neurovascular bundle	Difficulty climbing stairs or rising from a chair
Lower medial	Sciatic nerve	Foot-drop

- **Intracapsular fractures** of the femoral neck or hip dislocations tear the retinacular arteries that supply the proximal fragment; avascular necrosis may result.
- The **femoral triangle** is bounded by the inguinal ligament, the sartorius muscle, and the adductor longus muscle. A **femoral pulse** is palpable high within the femoral triangle just inferior to the inguinal ligament. The femoral vein, lying just medial to the femoral pulse, is a preferred site for insertion of venous lines.
- The **anterior cruciate ligament** is a key stabilizer of the knee joint, preventing posterior movement of the femur on the tibial plateau.
- The **medial meniscus,** being more mobile and attached to the medial collateral ligament, is most likely to be injured. Twisting movements that combine lateral displacement with lateral rotation pull the medial meniscus toward the center of the joint where it may be trapped and crushed by the medial femoral condyle.
- The **adductor canal,** the location of popliteal aneurysms, contains the femoral artery, femoral vein, and saphenous nerve.
- The **deep fibular nerve** innervates the muscles of the anterior compartment (dorsiflexors of the foot and pedal digits). The **superficial fibular nerve** innervates the lateral crural compartment (plantar flexors and everters of the foot). The **tibial nerve** innervates the posterior crural muscles which plantarflex and invert the foot.
- The **posterior tibial artery** descends posteriorly to the medial malleolus where the **posterior tibial pulse** is normally palpable.
- **Inversion sprains,** the most common ankle injury, involve the lateral collateral ligaments.
- The **plantar calcaneonavicular (spring) ligament** supports the head of the talus and thereby maintains the longitudinal plantar arch. Laxity of this ligament results in fallen arches or "flat feet."
- **Sensory distribution of the anterior leg:** the web space between the first and second toes is specific for the fibular nerve (L5) (see following figure).

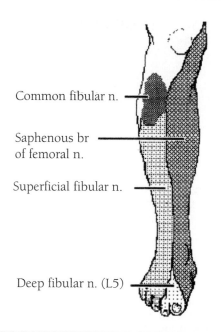

Common fibular n.

Saphenous br
of femoral n.

Superficial fibular n.

Deep fibular n. (L5)

Nerve Function, Tests, and Dysfunction			
Nerve	**Muscle Group**	**Reflex**	**Sign or Functional Deficit**
Genito-femoral	Cremaster	Cremasteric (L2-L3)	Cremaster paralysis
Femoral	Anterior thigh	Patellar (L4)	Weakness of hip flexion and loss of knee extension
Obturator	Medial thigh		Loss of thigh adduction
Superior gluteal	Gluteus medius and minimus		Abductor lurch (inability to keep pelvis level when contralateral foot is raised)
Inferior gluteal	Gluteus maximus		Difficulty rising from seated position and difficulty climbing stairs
Sciatic	Hamstrings	Hamstring (L5)	Weakness of hip extension and knee flexion
Fibular	Anterior and lateral crural compartments		Foot slap, inability to stand back on heels.
Tibial	Posterior crural compartment	Achilles (S1)	Inability to stand on tip-toes

THORAX

Thoracic Cage and Lungs

Respiratory Musculature	
Function	**Muscles**
Inspiration	External intercostals, interchondral portion of internal intercostals, and the diaphragm
Expiration	Internal intercostals proper, transverse thoracic, and abdominal muscles

- The **anterior border of the left pleural cavity** deviates laterally between the fourth and sixth ribs to form the cardiac notch—a preferred route for needle insertion into the pericardial cavity.
- When upright, excess fluid tends to collect in the **costodiaphragmatic recess.**
- Introduction of air into the pleural space results in **pneumothorax** with loss of lung ventilation. Fluid or blood produce hydrothorax and hemothorax, both of which limit expansion of the lung with reduced ventilation/perfusion ratio.
- The **right mainstem bronchus** is wider, shorter, and more vertical than the left mainstem bronchus, and therefore, is where large aspirated objects commonly lodge.
- The **right lower lobar bronchus** is most vertical, most nearly continues the direction of the trachea, and is larger in diameter than the left, and therefore, is where small aspirated objects commonly lodge, causing segmental atelectasis.
- A **bronchopulmonary segment** is defined by a segmental bronchus and accompanying segmental artery that lie centrally, as well as by intersegmental veins that form a peripheral venous plexus.
- Because the **superior segmental bronchi** of the lower lobes are the most posterior, and therefore dependent, when the patient is supine, they are most frequently involved in aspiration pneumonia (Mendelson's syndrome).

Heart

- The **transverse cardiac diameter** varies with inspiration and expiration but normally should not exceed one-half the diameter of the chest.
- An **apical pulse** is palpable at the point of maximal impulse (PMI) in the fifth intercostal space just beneath the nipple.
- **Ventricular coronary flow** occurs during ventricular diastole when a pressure differential occurs between the left ventricle and the aorta.

Cardiac Features		
Landmark	**Location**	**Contents**
Coronary sulcus	Between atria and ventricles; nearly vertical behind sternum; marks the annulus fibrosus that supports the valves	Right side contains the right coronary artery, and small cardiac vein; crossed by anterior cardiac veins
		Left side contains circumflex branch of the left coronary artery and coronary sinus
Anterior interventricular sulcus	Between left and right ventricles; marks the interventricular septum	Contains the anterior interventricular branch of the left coronary artery and the great cardiac vein
Posterior interventricular sulcus	Delineates the interventricular septum, posteriorly	Contains the posterior interventricular branch of the right coronary artery and the middle cardiac vein

- The **papillary muscles** take up the slack in the chordae tendineae to maintain the competence of the valvular closure as ventricular volume is reduced during blood ejection. The valves close passively.
- A **ventricular septal defect** produces a serious right-to-left shunt with cyanosis—"blue-baby" syndrome—because left ventricular pressure exceeds that in the right ventricle. A large VSD is the principal factor in **tetralogy of Fallot.**

Heart Valves		
Valve	**Auscultation**	**Comment**
Tricuspid	Right of sternum in sixth intercostal space	
Pulmonary	Left of sternum over second intercostal space	
Mitral	Apex of heart in fifth intercostal space in left midclavicular line	**Insufficiency** produces a low-pitched, late systolic blowing murmur
Aortic	Right of sternum over second intercostal space	**Stenosis** will tend to be auscultated as a high-pitched systolic murmur with possible radiation to the carotid arteries

- The **atrioventricular bundle** passes through the annulus fibrosus and descends along the posterior border of the membranous part of the interventricular septum to enter the muscular portion of the septum. It transmits electrical activity to the ventricles.

Cardiac Nodal Tissue

Node	Location	Function	Vasculature
Sinoatrial	In myocardium between crista terminalis and opening of superior vena cava	Initiates contractile event with electrical depolarization spreading throughout atrial musculature	Nodal branch of the right coronary artery
Atrioventricular	In right atrial floor near the interatrial septum	Stimulated by atrial depolarization; it leads into the atrioventricular (A-V) bundle to synchronize ventricular depolarization	Branch of right coronary artery near the posterior interventricular branch

- **Autonomic pathways** consist of two motor neurons, a myelinated preganglionic (presynaptic) neuron and an unmyelinated postganglionic (postsynaptic) neuron.

Summary of Autonomic Pathways

Division	Presynaptic Pathway	Postsynaptic Pathway	Effect
Sympathetic	From spinal levels T1-L2 along the ventral root; Reach the chain of sympathetic ganglia via white rami communicantes	1. Fibers that synapse return to the spinal nerve via a gray ramus to mediate cutaneous piloerection, vasoconstriction, and sudomotor activity 2. Fibers that do not synapse pass through the chain as splanchnic nerves to synapse in prevertebral ganglia; from these ganglia, postsynaptic neurons run in perivascular plexuses to innervate visceral target tissues	**Adrenergic neurotransmission** increases heart rate, increases stroke volume, dilates coronary and pulmonary arteries

Division	Presynaptic Pathway	Postsynaptic Pathway	Effect
Para-sympathetic	Presynaptic cell bodies are located in the dorsal vagal nuclei of the brain; The myelinated synaptic axons form cranial nerve X, the vagus nerve	Postganglionic cell bodies lie in numerous ganglia close to the target organ	**Cholinergic neurotransmission** decreases heart rate, decreases stroke volume, and produces bronchoconstriction

Pain Referral from Thoracic Viscera

Organ	Referral Area	Pathway
Pericardial cavity	T1-T5: upper and midthorax	Intercostal nerves T1-T5
Heart	T1-T4: upper thorax, postaxial brachium	Cervical and thoracic splanchnic nerves
Thoracic esophagus	T1-T5: thorax and epigastric region	Thoracic splanchnic nerves
Diaphragm		
Central	C3-C5: neck and shoulder	Phrenic nerve
Marginal	T5-T10: thorax	Intercostal nerves

ABDOMEN

Abdominal Wall

Dermatomal Landmarks

Dermatome	Region
T4	Nipple
T10	Umbilicus
T12	Pubis

- The **abdominal musculature** has three distinct layers that take three different directions. The external oblique muscle, internal oblique muscle, and transverse abdominis muscle may be sequentially split and retracted so that extensive suturing is unnecessary to provide a strong repair (McBurney's incision).

- Because the **linea alba** is relatively avascular, incisions may not heal well and predispose to epigastric herniation.
- **Above the arcuate line,** the anterior leaf of the **rectus sheath** is formed by fusion of the external oblique and internal oblique aponeuroses; the posterior leaf is formed by fusion of the internal oblique and transverse abdominis aponeuroses.
- **Below the arcuate line,** the anterior leaf of the rectus sheath is formed by fusion of all three aponeuroses and there is no posterior leaf.
- The **inferior epigastric artery** passes into the rectus sheath at the arcuate line. This is a potential site for spigelian herniation into the rectus sheath.

Hernia Characteristics

Hernia	Pathway
Direct inguinal	Through the inguinal triangle bounded by inguinal ligament, inferior epigastric artery, and rectus abdominis—therefore, medial to the inferior epigastric artery. Exits through the superficial inguinal ring *adjacent* to the spermatic cord. Usually acquired
Indirect inguinal	Through the deep inguinal ring and along the inguinal canal—therefore, lateral to the inferior epigastric artery. Exits through the superficial ring *within* the spermatic cord. Usually congenital
Femoral	Passes inferior to the inguinal ligament through the femoral ring into the thigh. More prevalent in women

GI Tract

Characterization of Abdominal Structures by Location and Support

Characterization	Organ
Peritoneal (supported by mesentery)	Abdominal esophagus, stomach, superior duodenum, liver, pancreatic tail, jejunum, ileum, a variable portion of the cecum, appendix, transverse colon, and sigmoid colon
Secondarily retroperitoneal (adherent)	Descending and inferior duodenum, pancreatic head and body, ascending colon, and descending colon. These may be surgically mobilized with an intact blood supply
Extraperitoneal	Thoracic esophagus, rectum, kidneys, ureters, and adrenal glands

- **Peptic ulceration** of the lower esophagus, stomach, or superior duodenum is referred along the greater splanchnic nerve to the fifth and sixth dermatomes which include the epigastric region.
- The **hepatic triangle,** bounded by the cystic duct, gallbladder, and common hepatic duct, contains the cystic arteries and right hepatic artery with potential for extensive variation.
- The **duodenal papilla** usually contains the hepatopancreatic ampulla, formed by the joining of the common bile duct and the pancreatic duct. If blocked by a stone, pancreatitis may develop.
- The **tail of the pancreas** contains most of the pancreatic islets (of Langerhans), a consideration in pancreatic resection.
- **Ileal (Meckel's) diverticulum** is found in about 3% of the population, located within 3 ft of the ileocecal junction (on the antimesenteric side of the ileum), and usually less than 3 in. long. Peptic ulceration of adjacent ileal mucosa and volvulus are complications.
- The **hepatic portal vein** directs venous return from the gastrointestinal tract to the liver.
- Because the **hepatic portal system** has no valves, blood need not flow toward the liver. Liver disease (such as cirrhosis) or compression of a vein (as in pregnancy or constipation) results in blood shunting through the anastomotic connections to the systemic venous system.

Portal-Systemic Anastomoses Occur in Several Areas		
Location	**Anastomotic Connections**	**Signs & Symptoms**
Esophagus	Azygos veins with left gastric and short gastric veins	Esophageal varices, intractable hematemesis
Umbilicus	Paraumbilical veins with superior and inferior epigastric veins	Caput medusae
Rectum	Superior rectal vein with middle and inferior rectal veins	Internal and external hemorrhoids

Kidneys, Ureters, and Adrenal Glands

- The **renal fascia** (the false capsule or Gerota's fascia) is a discrete fascial layer that surrounds each kidney. Paranephric fat outside this capsule and perinephric fat inside this fascial layer support the kidney.
- **Minor calyces** receive one or two pyramids before fusing into major calyces. Two to four minor calyces join to form **major calyces** that coalesce to form the renal pelvis.

- The **ureters** narrow at three points—at the renal pelvis, at the pelvic brim, and at the bladder. Kidney stones may lodge at these locations with pain referred, respectively, to the subcostal, inguinal, and perineal regions.
- **Adrenal arteries** arise from the inferior phrenic arteries, the aorta, and the renal arteries. The right adrenal vein usually drains medially into the inferior vena cava; the left adrenal vein usually drains inferiorly into the left renal vein.
- The **superior lumbar trigone** (a posterior approach to the kidneys, suprarenal glands, and upper ureters) is bounded by the quadratus lumborum muscle, superior border of the internal oblique muscle, and the twelfth rib.

Pain Referral from Abdominal Viscera

Organ	Referral Area	Pathway
Diaphragm		
Central	C3-C5: neck and shoulder	Phrenic nerve
Marginal	T5-T10: thorax	Intercostal nerves
Stomach, gallbladder, liver, bile duct, superior duodenum	T5-T9: lower thorax, epigastric region	Celiac plexus to greater splanchnic nerve
Inferior duodenum, jejunum, ileum, appendix, ascending colon, transverse colon	T10-T11: umbilical region	Superior mesenteric plexus to lesser splanchnic nerve
Kidneys, upper ureters, gonads	T12-L1: lumbar and ipsilateral inguinal regions	Aorticorenal plexus to least splanchnic nerve
Descending colon, sigmoid colon, mid ureters	L1-L2: pubic and inguinal regions, anterior scrotum or labia, anterior thigh	Aortic plexus to lumbar splanchnic nerves

PELVIS

Perineum

- The **external anal sphincter,** innervated by the pudendal nerve, provides the brief voluntary contraction necessary to counter the passage of a peristaltic wave.
- The **rectal submucosal venous plexus** forms anastomotic connections between the middle rectal veins that drain directly into the internal iliac veins and the superior rectal veins that drain into the hepatic portal system. This is a site for varices (hemorrhoids).
- The **internal pudendal arteries** are the sole supply of both male and female erectile tissue.

- The **deep dorsal vein** provides venous return from the penis or clitoris by passing through the urogenital diaphragm and draining into the prostatic or vesicle venous plexus, respectively.
- The **cremaster muscle** of the spermatic cord is innervated by the genital branch of the genitofemoral nerve. This provides the efferent limb for the cremaster reflex (L1-L2), the elevation of the testes within the scrotum when the inner thigh is scratched.
- The **cavity of tunica vaginalis** is a potential space that represents the detached portion of the peritoneal cavity that surrounds the testis except at the mesorchium.
- Because the superficial perineal space is limited by fascial attachment to the deep transverse perineal muscle, extravasations of blood or urine will not pass into the anal triangle.

Contents of the Perineal Spaces are Gender Specific		
Gender	**Superficial Perineal Space**	**Deep Perineal Space**
Male	Testes, crura of penis, bulb of penis, penile urethra, superficial transverse perineal muscles	Deep transverse perineal external urethral sphincter, bulbourethral glands, membranous urethra
Female	Crura of the clitoris, vestibular bulbs, superficial transverse perineal muscles, greater vestibular glands	Deep transverse perineal muscle, external urethral sphincter, urethra

- The **male external urethral sphincter** is formed by the deep transverse perineal muscle completely surrounding the membranous urethra. The **female external urethral sphincter** is formed by muscle fascicles of the deep transverse perineal muscle that arch anterior to the urethra but do not pass posterior because the urethra is embedded in the adventitia of the anterior vaginal wall. The arrangement in the female perineum predisposes to urinary stress incontinence.
- A **pudendal block** can be effected by injecting an anesthetic into the vicinity of the pudendal nerve in the pudendal canal close to the ischial spine.

Pelvic Autonomic Function		
Function	**Sympathetic**	**Parasympathetic**
Emission	L1-L2: lumbar splanchnic nerves,	
Erection	hypogastric plexus, pelvic plexus, cavernous plexus	
Ejaculation		S3-S5: pelvic splanchnic nerves

Pelvic viscera

- The **female pelvis** is less massive, the subpubic angle is greater (almost 90°), and the pelvic inlet more ovoid than the male pelvis.
- The **obstetric conjugate** is the least anteroposterior diameter of the pelvic inlet from the sacral promontory to a point a few millimeters below the superior margin of the pubic symphysis.
- The **transverse midplane diameter,** measured between the ischial spines, is the smallest dimension of the pelvic outlet.
- The **levator ani muscle** forms most of the pelvic floor and its puborectalis portion (rectal sling) is the principal mechanism for maintenance of fecal continence when the rectum is full.

Characterization of Pelvic Structures by Location and Support	
Characterization	**Organ**
Peritoneal (supported by mesentery)	Sigmoid colon, uterus, uterine tubes, ovaries, testes
Extraperitoneal	Rectum, anal canal, urinary bladder, cervix, prostate gland, seminal vesicles

- The **rectum** is usually empty because feces are stored in the sigmoid colon. Movement of feces into the rectal ampulla generates the urge to defecate.
- **Metastatic carcinoma of the rectum** may be widely disseminated within the abdomen, pelvis, and inguinal region. The upper rectum drains along the superior rectal lymphatics. The midrectum drains along the middle rectal lymphatics. The lower rectum drains along the inferior rectal lymphatics and then along both internal and external pudendal lymphatic channels.

Urinary Bladder Innervation is by Both Sympathetic and Parasympathetic Routes	
Function	**Pathway**
Sensory awareness of bladder fullness	Hypogastric nerve (sympathetic pathways) to spinal segments T12-L2
Afferent limb of the detrusor (bladder-emptying) reflex	Pelvic plexus and pelvic splanchnic nerves (parasympathetic pathways) to spinal segments S2-S4
Efferent limb of the detrusor reflex	Pelvic splanchnic nerves (parasympathetic pathways) from S3-S5

- **Urinary continence** of the partially full to full urinary bladder is a function of the external urethral sphincter.
- A **patent urachus** (rare) allows reflux of urine through the umbilicus.
- The **testes** develop as retroperitoneal structures, but become peritoneal (supported by mesorchium) in the scrotum. A long **mesorchium** may predispose to testicular torsion with high potential for testicular ischemia and necrosis.
- The testicular **pampiniform plexus** functions as a countercurrent heat exchanger that maintains testicular temperature a few degrees below core body temperature.
- **Compression of the left testicular vein** by a full sigmoid colon produces varices of the pampiniform plexus on the left side; fertility may diminish.
- **In the male, palpable per rectum** are posterior and lateral lobes of the prostate gland, seminal vesicles if enlarged, and bladder when filling.
- Each **uterine artery** crosses immediately superior to a ureter in the transverse cervical ligament—an important surgical consideration.
- **Normal uterine position** is anteflexed (uterus bent forward on itself at the level of the internal os) and anteverted (angled approximately 90° anterior to the vagina), lying on the urinary bladder.
- **In the female, palpable per vagina** are the cervix and ostium of the uterus, the vagina, the body of the uterus if retroverted, the rectouterine fossa, and variably the ovary and uterine tubes.
- The **lymphatic drainage from the vagina** is by three routes: the external and internal iliac nodes from the upper third of the vagina; the internal iliac nodes from the middle third of the vagina; and the internal iliac nodes as well as the superficial inguinal nodes from the lowest third.

Pain Referral from Pelvic Viscera

Organ	Referral Area	Pathway
Testes and ovaries	T10-T12: umbilical and pubic regions	Gonadal nerves to aortic plexus and then to lesser and least splanchnic nerves
Middle ureters, urinary bladder, uterine body, uterine tubes	L1-L2: pubic and inguinal regions, anterior scrotum or labia, anterior thigh	Hypogastric plexus to aortic plexus and then to lumbar splanchnic nerves
Rectum, superior anal canal, pelvic ureters, cervix, epididymis, vas deferens, seminal vesicles, prostate gland	S3-S5: perineum and posterior thigh	Pelvic plexus to pelvic splanchnic nerves

HEAD AND NECK

Somatic Portions

- The scalp layer of loose connective tissue between the epicranial aponeurosis and the periosteum forms the subaponeurotic or "danger" space. Emissary veins connect with the dural sinuses with potential for hematogenous spread of infection through the calvaria.
- Cranial fractures preferentially pass through cranial foramina injuring the contained nerves.

Principal Foramina of the Anterior Cranial Fossa

Foramen	Contents	Result of injury
Olfactory	Olfactory nerves	Anosmia
Foramen cecum	An emissary vein	

Principal Foramina of the Middle Cranial Fossa

Foramen	Contents	Result of injury
Optic canal	CN II	Unilateral blindness
	Ophthalmic artery	Ischemic unilateral blindness
Superior orbital fissure	CN III	Ophthalmoplegia
	CN IV	Inability to look down and out
	CN V$_1$	Unilateral loss of blink reflex
	CN VI	Inability to abduct eye
	Superior ophthalmic vein	Retinal engorgement
Foramen rotundum	CN V$_2$	Loss of sneeze reflex
Foramen ovale	CN V$_3$	Masticatory paralysis, loss of jaw-jerk reflex
Foramen spinosum	Middle meningeal artery	
Foramen lacerum	Nothing (except occasionally the greater superficial petrosal nerve)	
Hiatus of the facial canal	Gr. superficial petrosal n.	Dry eye, loss of submandibular and sublingual secretion

Principal Foramina of the Posterior Cranial Fossa

Foramen	Contents	Result of Injury
Internal auditory meatus	CN VII	Facial paralysis
	CN VIII	Auditory and vestibular deficits
Jugular foramen	CN IX	Loss of gag and carotid reflexes
	CN X	Loss of cough reflex; paralysis of laryngeal muscles and some palatine muscles
	CN XI	Inability to shrug shoulders
	Internal jugular vein	
Anterior condylar canal	CN XII	Paralysis of tongue muscles; lingual deviation toward side of injury upon protrusion

CSF Is Produced by the Choroid Plexuses that Project into the Ventricles of the Brain

CSF Production	Through	Into
Lateral ventricles	Foramina of Monro	Third ventricle
Third ventricle	Iter (cerebral aqueduct)	Fourth ventricle
Fourth ventricle	Foramina of Magendie and Luschka	Cisterna magna of subarachnoid space

From	Through	CSF Uptake
Subarachnoid space	Arachnoid villi	Superior sagittal venous sinus

- The **cerebral aqueduct** is prone to occlusion, leading to hydrocephalus.

Cranial and Cerebral Hematomas

Hematoma	Prognosis	Location	Cause
Epicranial	Resolves	Subaponeurotic space	Superficial vessels
Epidural	Life-threatening	Epidural space	Torn middle meningeal artery
Subdural	Less serious	Subdural space	Torn cerebral vein
Subarachnoid	Lethal	Subarachnoid space	Torn cerebral artery, cerebral aneurysm
Subpial	Usually resolves	Cerebrum	Cerebral contusion

- **Regions of the orbit** that are prone to fracture include the ethmoid lamina papyracea and the maxilla about the infraorbital groove.
- Contraction of the **orbicularis oculi muscle,** innervated by the facial nerve, produces the blink.

Orbital Muscle Function and Innervation

Muscle	Primary Function	Secondary Functions (normally balance)	Innervation
Pupil	Constriction		CN III parasympathetic
	Dilation		Sympathetic chain
Ciliary body	Accommodation		CN III parasympathetic
Superior tarsal muscle	Augment levator palpebrae superioris		Sympathetic chain
Levator palpebrae superioris	Elevate eyelid		CN III (Oculomotor)
Medial rectus	Adduction		CN III (Oculomotor)
Superior rectus	Elevation	Adduction, intorsion	CN III (Oculomotor)
Inferior oblique	Elevation	Abduction, extorsion	CN III (Oculomotor)
Inferior rectus	Depression	Adduction, extorsion	CN III (Oculomotor)
Superior oblique	Depression	Abduction, intorsion	CN IV (Trochlear)
Lateral rectus	Abduction		CN VI (Abducens)

- **Parasympathetic innervation** to the pupil originates in the Edinger-Westphal nucleus and travels with the oculomotor nerve. Temporal lobe herniation (from tumor, hematoma, or edema) compresses the oculomotor nerve within the tentorial notch, causing a dilated pupil that is unresponsive to light.

Special Sensory Tests and Dysfunction

Nerve	Foramen	Dysfunction	Test
CN I (Olfactory)	Cribriform plate	Anosmia	Whiff of clove
CN II (Optic)	Optic canal	Blindness	Optic field tests
CN VIII			
Cochlear	Internal auditory meatus	Deafness	Hearing threshold
Vestibular	Internal auditory meatus	Balance	Nystagmus

- Paralysis of the **stapedius muscle,** as a result of facial nerve palsy, produces hyperacusis.

Visceral Portions

- The **infrahyoid muscles,** innervated by the ansa cervicalis (C1-C3), stabilize the hyoid bone and larynx during deglutition and phonation.
- The **pretracheal space,** deep to the pretracheal fascia, surrounds the trachea and thyroid gland, but is anterior to the esophagus. Infection in this space may track into the superior mediastinum.
- The **retropharyngeal (retrovisceral) space** lies posterior to the oropharynx and esophagus and is defined by septa from the pretracheal fascia. Infection within this space may track into the posterior mediastinum.
- The **mandibular neurovascular bundle** enters the mandibular foramen adjacent to the lingula, the point of minimal movement. It may be anesthetized by directing a needle posteriorly through the buccal wall just lateral to the pterygomandibular raphe.
- The **deep cervical nodes** receive lymph from the anteroinferior portion of the face, the nasal cavities, and the oral cavity.
- The **nasal vestibule** (the most common site for nosebleeds) receives vascular branches from internal and external carotid arteries.
- The **palatine tonsil** receives vascular branches from the maxillary, facial, and lingual arteries.
- **Abduction of the vocal cords** is a function of the posterior cricoarytenoid muscle only, innervated by the recurrent laryngeal nerve.

Branchiomeric Nerve Functions and Tests

Nerve	Course	Sensory	Motor	Test
CN V (trigeminal)				
V1	Superior orbital fissure, supraorbital notch	Forehead	None	Blink reflex
V2	Foramen rotundum, maxillary foramen	Midface	None	Sneeze reflex

Continued

Nerve	Course	Sensory	Motor	Test
V3	Foramen ovale, mandibular foramen, mental foramen	Anterior pinna, jaw	Muscles of mastication, mylohyoid ant. belly of digastric, tensor palatini and tensor tympani	Jaw jerk
CN VII (facial)	Internal auditory meatus, facial canal, stylomastoid foramen	Concha of ear, taste anterior ⅔ of tongue via chorda tympani	Muscles of facial expression, stylohyoid, post. belly of digastric, tensor tympani, parasympathetic to lacrimal, nasal, palatine, lingual and submandibular glands via gr. superficial petrosal nerve	Blink reflex
CN IX (glosso-pharyngeal)	Jugular foramen	External auditory, meatus, oropharynx, carotid body and sinus, taste posterior ⅓ of tongue	Stylopharyngeus muscle, parasym-pathetic to parotid gland via tympanic and lesser super-ficial petrosal nerves	Gag reflex, Carotid reflex
CN X (vagus)	Jugular foramen	External auditory meatus, larynx, taste from epiglottis, aortic body	Palatine muscles, pharyngeal muscles, laryngeal muscles	Phonation

Nerve Functions and Tests				
Nerve	**Foramen**	**Sensory**	**Motor**	**Test**
CN XI (spinal accessory)	Foramen magnum, jugular foramen	None	Sternomastoid Upper trapezius	Turn head to opposite side
CN XII (hypoglossal)	Hypoglossal canal	None	Intrinsic and extrinsic tongue muscles	Protrudes straight

- **Sensory innervation of the face** is by the trigeminal nerve (see figure below).

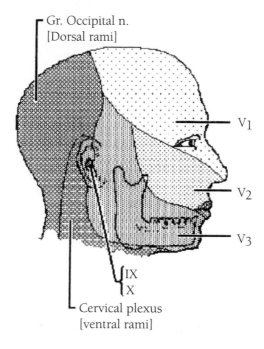

Embryology: Early and General

Questions

DIRECTIONS: Each item below contains a question or incomplete statement followed by suggested responses. Select the **one best** response to each question.

1. The structures shown in the accompanying photomicrograph are derived from

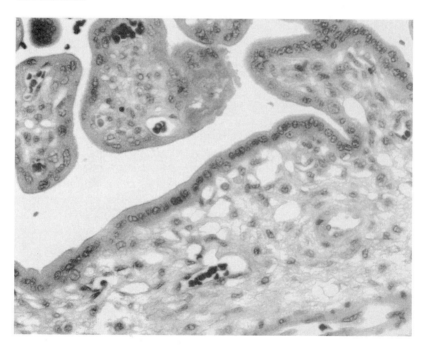

a. A combination of fetal and maternal tissues
b. Endometrial glands
c. Endometrial stroma
d. Fetal tissues
e. Maternal blood vessels

2. The formation of the acrosome involves the

a. Loss of decapacitation factors
b. Release of the developing spermatids from Sertoli cells
c. Maturation of lytic enzymes
d. Mitotic activity
e. Meiotic divisions

3. The secondary oocyte enters the second meiotic division and proceeds as far as metaphase. The stimulus required for continuation of the second meiotic division to produce the haploid ovum is

a. Elevation of progesterone titers
b. The environment of the oviduct and uterus
c. Expulsion from the mature follicle
d. Fertilization by a spermatozoon
e. The presence of human chorionic gonadotropin (hCG)

4. Capacitation requires

a. Initiation immediately after the acrosome reaction
b. Addition of cholesterol to the sperm plasma membrane
c. An increase in the fluidity of the sperm plasma membrane
d. Sequestration of acrosomal enzymes
e. Fusion of the acrosomal membrane with the egg plasma membrane

5. Primary oocytes have developed by the time of birth. From puberty to menopause, these germ cells remain suspended in meiotic prophase. The oocyte of a mature follicle is induced to undergo the first meiotic division just before ovulation as a result of which of the following hormonal stimuli?

a. The cessation of progesterone secretion
b. The gradual elevation of follicle-stimulating hormone (FSH) titers
c. The low estrogen titers associated with the maturing follicle
d. The slow elevation of progesterone produced by luteal cells
e. The surge of luteinizing hormone (LH) initiated by high estrogen titers

6. Which of the following is responsible for the prevention of polyspermy, the fertilization of an oocyte by more than one sperm?

a. Resumption of the first meiotic division
b. Resumption of the second meiotic division
c. Capacitation
d. The zona reaction
e. The release of enzymes from the sperm acrosome

7. Oogonia reach their maximum number at which of the following stages of human development?

a. Five months of fetal life
b. Birth
c. Puberty (12 to 14 years of age)
d. Adolescence (16 to 20 years of age)
e. Early adulthood (21 to 26 years of age)

8. A 26-year-old man contracted viral influenza with an unremitting fever of 39.5°C (103°F) for three days. Because spermatogenesis cannot occur above a scrotal temperature of 35.5°C (96°F), he was left with no viable sperm on his recovery. The time required for spermatogenesis, spermiogenesis, and passage of viable sperm to the epididymis is approximately

a. 3 days
b. 1 week
c. 5 weeks
d. 2 months
e. 4 months

9. Implantation of the conceptus at which site in the accompanying diagram of the female reproductive system could result in excessive, perhaps fatal, vaginal bleeding before parturition?

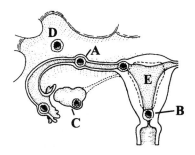

a. A
b. B
c. C
d. D
e. E

10. Cells that form the three primitive germ layers are derived from the

a. Cytotrophoblast
b. Epiblast
c. Syncytiotrophoblast
d. Hypoblast
e. Yolk sac

11. In the developing human embryo, most of the internal organs begin to form in which month?

a. First
b. Second
c. Fourth
d. Sixth
e. Ninth

12. The primitive uteroplacental circulation is established during which period of fetal development?

a. First week
b. Second week
c. Third week
d. End of first month
e. Second trimester

13. The notochord is formed by cells of the

a. Hypoblast
b. Ectoderm
c. Mesoderm
d. Endoderm
e. Nongastrulated epiblast

14. Blood from the placenta is about 80% oxygenated. However, mixture with unoxygenated blood at various points reduces the oxygen content. Which of the following vessels contains blood with the highest oxygen content?

a. Abdominal aorta
b. Common carotid arteries
c. Ductus arteriosus
d. Pulmonary artery
e. Pulmonary vein

15. Which of the following hematopoietic tissues or organs develops from endoderm?

a. Thymus
b. Tonsils
c. Bone marrow
d. Spleen
e. Blood islands

16. Which places the developing heart in the presumptive thoracic region cranial to the septum transversum?

a. Gastrulation
b. Lateral folding
c. Cranial folding
d. Neurulation
e. Fusion of the endocardial heart tubes

17. Which is in direct contact with maternal blood in lacunae of the placenta?

a. Cells of the cytotrophoblast
b. Extraembryonic mesoderm
c. Fetal blood vessels
d. Cells of the syncytiotrophoblast
e. Amniotic cells

18. During which period is the embryo most susceptible to environmental influences that could induce the formation of nonlethal congenital malformations?

a. Fertilization to one week of fetal life
b. The second and third weeks of fetal life
c. The fourth through eighth weeks of fetal life
d. The third month of fetal life
e. The third trimester of fetal life

19. During a visit to her gynecologist, a patient reports she received vitamin A treatment for her acne unknowingly during the first two months of an undetected pregnancy. Which organ systems in the developing fetus are most likely to be affected?

a. The digestive system
b. The endocrine organs
c. The respiratory system
d. The urinary and reproductive systems
e. The skeletal and central nervous systems

20. Polyhydramnios is caused by

a. Duodenal or esophageal atresia
b. Bilateral agenesis of the kidneys
c. Precocious development of the swallowing reflex in the fetus
d. Hypoplasia of the lungs
e. Obstructive uropathy

21. The neural plate forms directly from

a. Ectoderm
b. Endoderm
c. Somatopleuric mesoderm
d. Splanchnopleuric mesoderm
e. Hypoblast

22. Which of the following forms from paraxial mesoderm?

a. Adrenal cortex
b. Adrenal medulla
c. Humerus
d. Biceps brachii
e. Masseter

23. The cerebral cortex forms from

a. Telencephalon
b. Myelencephalon
c. Metencephalon
d. Mesencephalon
e. Diencephalon

24. The primordial germ cells that eventually form the oogonia and spermatogonia originate in the

a. Epiblast
b. Gonadal ridge
c. Endodermal lining of the yolk sac
d. The primary sex cords of the developing gonad
e. Chorion

25. The yolk sac is important in embryonic development of humans as

a. The major site of yolk storage
b. Transfer of nutrients after the uteroplacental circulation has been established
c. The source of blood cells in the third to fourth month of development
d. The source of the amniotic fluid
e. The origin of the primitive gut

26. Monozygotic twins arise by

a. Fusion of the embryonic blastomeres from two zygotes
b. Fertilization of two oocytes by two sperm
c. Fertilization of one oocyte by two sperm
d. Division of the inner cell mass (embryoblast) into two embryonic primordia
e. Extra cleavage divisions of the zygote induced by the presence of a double chorion

27. In the developing embryo, the edge of the ectoderm is continuous with the

a. Chorion
b. Amniotic membrane
c. Yolk sac lining
d. Extraembryonic mesoderm
e. Adventitia of the umbilical vessels

28. Which of the following processes is responsible for fusion of the paired dorsal aortae?

a. Lateral folding
b. Craniocaudal folding
c. Gastrulation
d. Neurulation
e. Looping of the heart tube

Embryology: Early and General

Answers

1. The answer is d. (*Junqueira, 9/e, pp 436–439. Moore, Before We Are Born, 5/e, p 48. Moore, Developing Human, 6/e, p 48. Sweeney, pp 46, 416–419.*) The placental structures shown in the photomicrograph are chorionic villi that are fetal tissues. The mother's contribution to the placenta is the blood that flows past the chorionic villi. A fertilized ovum reaches the uterus about four days after fertilization. At that time, it has developed into a multicellular, hollow sphere referred to as a blastocyst. The blastocyst soon adheres to the secretory endometrium and differentiates into an inner cell mass that will develop into the embryo and a layer of primitive trophoblast. The expanding trophoblast penetrates the surface endometrium and erodes into maternal blood vessels. Eventually, it develops two layers, an inner cytotrophoblast and an outer syncytiotrophoblast. Solid cords of trophoblast form the chorionic villi, which then are invaded by fetal blood vessels.

2. The answer is c. (*Junqueira, 9/e, pp 409–411, Moore, Developing Human, 6/e, pp 22–23, Sweeney, pp 24, 25, 28.*) The formation of the acrosome is one of many maturation events occurring in spermiogenesis (the process by which mature sperm are formed from the spermatids). It involves lytic enzyme maturation and occurs after division of secondary spermatocytes. It involves no mitotic or meiotic activity. The acrosome develops from Golgi vesicles just like any other secretory granules. It contains acrosin, a serine protease, hyaluronidase, and neuraminidase, responsible for the penetration ability of the sperm. The developing cells are in contact with Sertoli cells for all of the stages of spermiogenesis. At the end of spermiogenesis, spermatids are released by Sertoli cells in a process called spermiation. Decapacitation factors are not involved in acrosomal maturation.

3. The answer is d. (*Alberts, 3/e, pp 1022–1024. Junqueira, 9/e, pp 425, 429–430.*) The secondary oocyte enters the second meiotic division just before ovulation and arrests at metaphase. Fertilization by a spermatozoon provides the stimulation for the division of chromatin to the haploid number. By the time the fertilized ovum reaches the uterus, the progesterone produced by the corpus luteum has initiated the secretory phase in the endometrium. Once implantation occurs and the chorion develops, human chorionic gonadotropin (hCG) is synthesized and the corpus luteum is maintained.

4. The answer is c. (*Junqueira, 9/e, p 430. Sweeney, p 25. Moore, Before We Are Born, 5/e, pp 21, 32. Moore, Developing Human, 6/e, pp 22–23, 33–34. Gilbert, 6/e, pp 194–195.*) Capacitation is a process that prepares the sperm for fertilization. Sperm must reside in the female reproductive tract or under appropriate in vitro conditions for about 1 h for capacitation to occur. During this delay phase there is a loss of decapacitation factors that have been added to the sperm by epididymal cells and accessory male reproductive organs. Cholesterol is removed from the plasma membrane during this period, which results in the increased fluidity of the membrane that is required for the fusion of the acrosomal membrane with the sperm plasma membrane. This leads to the release of the acrosomal enzymes, which are required for the breakdown of the corona radiata and the zona pellucida of the oocyte to facilitate sperm penetration. Capacitation does not include the fusion process and release of enzymes that define the acrosome reaction.

5. The answer is e. (*Alberts, 3/e, pp 1022–1024. Junqueira, 9/e, pp 421, 428–429.*) A midcycle surge of luteinizing hormone (LH) triggers the resumption of meiosis and causes the FSH-primed follicle to rupture and discharge the ovum. Under the influence of LH, the ruptured follicle is transformed into a corpus luteum, which produces progesterone. Follicle-stimulating hormone and LH produced in the adenohypophysis result in growth and maturation of the ovarian follicle. Under FSH stimulation, the theca cells proliferate, hypertrophy, and begin to produce estrogen.

6. The answer is d. (*Sweeney, p 28.*) On fusion of the first sperm with the oocyte cell membrane, the contents of secretory granules stored just beneath the oocyte membrane (cortical granules) are released (the zona reaction). Enzymes stored in these granules cause biochemical and electrical changes in the zona pellucida and the oocyte membrane that prevent the binding of additional sperm. Primitive female germ cells (oogonia) enter the first meiotic division during fetal development. This process becomes arrested in the metaphase stage until individual primary oocytes are hormonally induced to resume the first meiotic division during puberty and early adulthood (menarche to menopause). Fusion of the sperm and oocyte membranes initiates the resumption of the second meiotic division, resulting in the formation of a haploid pronucleus in the oocyte and extrusion of the second polar body. Capacitation is a process by which enzymatic secretions of the uterus and oviducts strip glycoproteins from the sperm cell membrane. This is required for penetration of the layer of cells surrounding the oocyte (corona radiata). The release of enzymes from the sperm acrosomal cap (an enlarged lysosome) results in digestion of the zona pellucida surrounding the oocyte, allowing penetration by sperm.

7. The answer is a. *(Moore, Developing Human, 6/e, pp 18–21. Sweeney, pp 26–27.)* Maximum number of oogonia occurs at about the fifth month of development. Differentiation into oogonia begins once the primordial germ cells have arrived in the gonad of a genetic female. After undergoing a number of mitotic divisions, these fetal cells form a cluster in the cortical part of the ovary. Some of these oogonia differentiate into the larger primary oocytes, which by the third month of development are found in the deeper layers of the gonad. The primary oocytes begin meiosis to produce secondary oocytes. At the same time, the number of oogonia continues to increase to about 6,000,000 in the fifth month. At this time, most of the surviving oogonia and some of the oocytes become atretic. However, the surviving secondary oocytes (400,000 to 1,000,000) become surrounded by epithelial cells and form the primordial follicles by the seventh month. During childhood there is continued atresia so that by puberty only about 40,000 secondary oocytes remain.

8. The answer is d. *(Moore, Developing Human, 6/e, pp 22–23.)* In man the time required for the progression from spermatogonium to motile spermatozoon is about two months (61 to 64 days). Spermatogenesis, the process by which spermatogonia undergo mitotic division to produce primary spermatocytes, occurs at 1°C (2°F) below normal body temperature. Subsequent meiotic divisions produce secondary spermatocytes with a bivalent haploid chromosome number and then spermatids with a monovalent haploid chromosome number. The maturation of the spermatid, spermiogenesis, results in spermatozoa. Morphologically adult spermatozoa are moved to the epididymis where they become fully motile.

9. The answer is b. (*Moore, Developing Human, 6/e, pp 24, 44, 55–57. Sweeney, pp 34–35, 414–415.*) Implantation of the conceptus low on the uterine wall near the cervical opening (os) could result in growth of the placenta between the embryo and the cervical os (placenta previa). The placenta could become dislodged from the uterine wall before, as well as during, delivery, resulting in rapidly fatal hemorrhage. Implantation at site A (the uterine tube or oviduct) results in rupture of the oviduct wall, whereas implantation on the ovary (C) would result in destruction of that organ. Implantation could also occur in the wall of the peritoneal cavity (D). Implantation normally occurs in the superior posterior or posterolateral walls of the uterus (E).

10. The answer is b. (*Moore, Developing Human, 6/e, pp 41, 43. Sweeney, pp 32, 36.*) Cells of the inner cell mass (embryoblast) of the blastocyst differentiate into the epiblast and hypoblast. Cells of the epiblast migrate toward the primitive streak during the second week and become internalized, forming the mesodermal and endodermal germ layers. Remaining cells of the epiblast become the ectodermal germ layer. Cells of the hypoblast will contribute to the yolk sac. Cells of the outer cell mass of the blastocyst will differentiate into the cytotrophoblast and syncytiotrophoblast that will contribute to formation of the placenta.

11. The answer is b. (*Sweeney, pp 6, 49. Moore, Developing Human, 6/e, pp 85, 88, 548.*) Formation of most internal organs occurs during the second month, the period of organogenesis. The first month of embryonic development generally is concerned with cleavage, formation of the germ layers, and establishment of the embryonic body. The period from the ninth week to the end of intrauterine life, known as the fetal period, is characterized by maturation of tissues and rapid growth of the fetal body.

12. The answer is b. (*Moore, Developing Human, 6/e, pp 48, 50, 76. Sweeney, pp 42–43.*) During the second week of fetal development, lacunar spaces develop between cells of the syncytiotrophoblast, particularly in the region of the embryonic pole as the conceptus invades the endometrium. Endometrial capillaries in this region become dilated and engorged with blood to form sinusoids. The syncytial cells direct erosion of the endothelium of the maternal capillaries, allowing maternal blood to enter the lacunae and bathe the syncytial cells. This establishes the uteroplacental circulation. During the second week, primary villi consist of projections of syncytial cells surrounding a core of cytotrophoblast cells. During the third week, the villus core is invaded by mesodermal cells to form a secondary villus. Cells of the mesodermal core will then differentiate to form capillaries and blood cells by the end of the third week (tertiary villus). These vessels become connected to the fetal circulation early in the fourth week.

13. The answer is c. *(Sweeney, pp 38, 72. Moore, Developing Human, 6/e, pp 69–71.)* The notochord forms from mesoderm. During the second week of development, the embryoblast gives rise to two primitive germ layers, the epiblast and the underlying hypoblast. At the beginning of the third week, cells from the epiblast migrate toward the midline (primitive streak) and move inward (gastrulation). The migrating epiblast cells may either displace the hypoblast cells to the periphery to form the endodermal lining of the digestive tract or form an intermediate layer of mesoderm that will give rise to muscle, bone, and cartilaginous structures including the notochord. The remaining cells of the epiblast that do not undergo gastrulation form the ectoderm (epidermis and nervous system).

14. The answer is b. *(Moore, Developing Human, 6/e, pp 394–395. Sweeney, pp 282–283.)* Blood from the placenta in the umbilical cord is about 80% oxygenated. Mixture with unoxygenated blood from the vitelline veins and the inferior vena cava reduces the oxygen content somewhat. However, this stream with a relatively high oxygen content is directed by the valve of the inferior vena cava directly through the foramen ovale into the left atrium. This prevents admixture with oxygen-depleted blood entering the right atrium from the superior vena cava. Thus, the oxygen-saturated blood entering the left ventricle and pumped into the aortic arch, subclavian arteries, and common carotid arteries has the highest oxygen content. The oxygen-depleted blood from the superior vena cava is directed into the right ventricle and then to the pulmonary trunk. Although a small portion of this flow passes through the lungs (where any residual oxygen is extracted by the tissue of the nonrespiring lung), most is shunted into the thoracic aorta via the ductus arteriosus and thereby lowers the oxygen content of that vessel. This occurs distal to the origins of the carotid arteries and ensures that the rapidly developing brain has the best oxygen supply.

15. The answer is a. (*Moore, Developing Human, 6/e, pp 223–225. Sweeney, pp 226–227.*) The thymic parenchyma (epithelial cells) develop from endoderm of the third pharyngeal (branchial) pouches. The thymic rudiment is invaded by bone marrow–derived lymphocyte precursors early in the third month of development. The tonsils develop as partially encapsulated lymph nodules. Their parenchymal framework is derived from pharyngeal mesoderm. Bones, of course, whether formed by intramembranous or endochondral ossification, are derived from mesoderm. Their forming marrow cavities are populated by hematopoietic stem cells beginning in the second month of fetal life. The connective tissue capsule and skeletal framework of the spleen develop from splanchnic lateral plate mesoderm during the fifth week and are quickly invaded by hematopoietic cells of the myeloid lineage. It remains an active hematopoietic organ until at least the seventh month in utero. Blood islands develop by differentiation of mesodermal cells in the extraembryonic mesoderm lining the yolk sac during the third week of fetal development. They give rise to vitelline vessels and are the major site of red blood cell formation in the early embryo.

16. The answer is c. (*Moore, Developing Human, 6/e, pp 84–87. Sweeney, pp 79–83.*) Initially, the developing cranial portion of the neural tube lies dorsal and caudal to the oropharyngeal membrane. However, overgrowth of the forebrain causes it to extend past the oropharyngeal membrane and overhang the cardiogenic area. Subsequent growth of the forebrain pushes the developing heart ventrally and caudally to a position in the presumptive thoracic region caudal to the oropharyngeal membrane and cranial to the septum transversum that will form the central tendon of the diaphragm. Gastrulation is the process by which epiblast cells migrate to the primitive streak and become internalized to form the mesodermal and endodermal germ layers. Neurulation refers to formation of the neural tube from surface ectoderm. Lateral folding of the embryo forms the endoderm tube and surrounding concentric layering of mesoderm and ectoderm.

17. The answer is d. (*Moore, Developing Human, 6/e, pp Sweeney, pp 34–35, 42–43, 414–415.*) In the developing fetus, the maternal blood is in direct contact with the syncytiotrophoblast. During implantation, the syncytiotrophoblast invades the endometrium and erodes the maternal blood vessels. Maternal blood and nutrient glandular secretions fill the lacunae and bathe the projections of syncytiotrophoblast. Primary villi consist of syncytiotrophoblast with a core of cytotrophoblast cells. In secondary villi, the cytotrophoblast core is invaded by mesoderm and subsequently by umbilical blood vessels in tertiary villi.

18. The answer is c. (*Sweeney, p 13. Moore, Developing Human, 6/e, pp 181–184.*) Exposure of the embryo to harmful environmental factors (teratogens), such as chemicals, viruses and/or radiation, can occur at any time. During the fourth through eighth weeks of embryonic life, organ systems are developing and are most susceptible to teratogens. During this time, each organ system has its own specific period of peak susceptibility. Exposure of the embryo to teratogens during the first three weeks of fetal life generally induce spontaneous abortion and are, therefore, lethal. After the eighth week of intrauterine development, teratogenic exposure generally results in retardation of organ growth rather than in new structural or functional changes.

19. The answer is e. (*Sweeney, pp 14–15, 91, 108, 122, 154. Moore, Developing Human, 6/e, pp 189, 435.*) Vitamin A is a member of the retinoic acid family. Retinoic acid directs the polarity of development in the central nervous system, the axial skeleton (vertebral column), and probably the appendicular skeleton as well. Retinoic acid turns on various combinations of homeobox genes, depending on tissue type and location (distance and direction from the source of retinoic acid). Exogenous sources of retinoic acid may induce the wrong sequence or combination of homeobox genes, leading to structural abnormalities in the nervous and skeletal systems. The other organ systems listed are not as susceptible to vitamin A.

20. The answer is a. (*Sweeney, pp 16, 298. Moore, Developing Human, 6/e, pp 152, 262, 267, 273, 278, 312.*) Duodenal and/or esophageal atresia result in an inability of the fetus to swallow amniotic fluid. The result is that normal recirculation of amniotic fluid through the embryo is greatly reduced or eliminated, causing an excess of amniotic fluid. Excess is defined as greater than 2000 mL in the third trimester. Low volumes of amniotic fluid (oligohydramnios) are caused by bilateral agenesis of the kidneys or obstructive uropathy (blockage of the calyces or ureters), which prevents urine from being added to the amniotic fluid. Hypoplasia of the lungs and compression of the umbilical cord are associated with oligohydramnios but do not cause it. Apparently, factors in the amniotic fluid are important for lung maturation and the absence of normal amniotic fluid levels inhibits normal lung development.

21. The answer is a. *(Sweeney, pp 62–65. Moore, Developing Human, 6/e, pp 72–74. Alberts, 3/e, pp 1046–1047.)* The first stage of neural tube formation is the induction by notochord and prechordal plate mesoderm of the neural plate that forms from ectoderm. This is known as primary induction and is accompanied by molecular changes in cell adhesion molecules [restriction to neural cell adhesion molecule (N-CAM)]. This first stage of neural tube development is followed by a reshaping phase, neurulation, and neural tube closure. Endoderm is responsible for the formation of the GI tract and respiratory system. The splanchnopleuric mesoderm forms the heart and the muscles of the GI tract and urinary system. The somatopleuric mesoderm makes important contributions to the skin (dermis) and nonmuscle portions of the limbs. The hypoblast is the thin layer of cells ventral to the epiblast and is the precursor to the endoderm.

22. The answer is d. *(Sweeney, pp 88–89.)* The muscles of the extremities form from the somites that are derived from paraxial mesoderm. The intermediate mesoderm is the origin of the urogenital systems and the adrenal cortex. The adrenal medulla forms from neural crest. The humerus forms from somatopleuric mesoderm, but the muscles of the extremities are of somite origin. The masseter is a muscle of mastication formed from the first branchial arch and innervated by branchial visceral efferent (special visceral efferent) fibers from the nucleus ambiguus compared with the general somatic efferent innervation of the biceps and other muscles, not of branchial arch origin.

23. The answer is a. *(Moore, Developing Human, 6/e, pp 465–470, 473. Sweeney, pp 164–167, 174–176, 178–179, 180–181.)* The cerebral cortex forms from the telencephalon. The cortex develops in waves of proliferation forming layers I to VI with the innermost layers forming first and the more superficial layers later. The wall of the developing CNS contains three layers: ventricular, mantle (intermediate), and marginal zones. The cortex, peripheral areas of gray matter, is formed through the migration of cells from the mantle zone to the marginal zone. Segmentation of the cranial neural tube forms the brain vesicles listed in the table below:

Primary Brain Vesicle	Secondary Brain Vesicle	Adult Brain Derivative
Prosencephalon (forebrain)	Telencephalon	Cerebral cortex, corpus striatum
	Diencephalon	Hypothalamus, thalamus
Mesencephalon (midbrain)	Mesencephalon	Superior and inferior colliculi
Rhombencephalon (hindbrain)	Metencephalon	Pons and cerebellum
	Myelencephalon	Medulla

24. The answer is c. *(Moore, Developing Human, 6/e, pp 154, 324. Sweeney, p 352.)* The primordial germ cells are first seen in the endodermal lining of the wall of the yolk sac (derived from the hypoblast) at the end of the third or beginning of the fourth week in the region of the allantois. During embryonic folding, the dorsal part of the yolk sac is incorporated into the embryo as the primitive gut. The primordial germ cells subsequently migrate along the dorsal mesentery of the hindgut and into the gonadal (genital) ridge (by week 6). The primary sex cords grow into the mesenchyme underlying the ridge, and the primordial germ cells become incorporated into the primary sex cords.

25. The answer is e. *(Moore, Developing Human, 6/e, pp 76–77, 154. Sweeney, pp 56, 404–405.)* The endoderm of the yolk sac is incorporated into the embryo as the primitive gut during embryonic folding. There is no yolk storage in human embryos. The transfer of nutrients is an important function of the yolk sac early in development, but once the uteroplacental circulation is established, the placenta takes over that role. The yolk sac is important as a source of blood until the fetal liver replaces this function in about the sixth week of development. The yolk sac produces predominantly hematocytoblasts (stem cells) and primitive erythroblasts from the third week through the second month of gestation. The cells of the amnion form the amniotic fluid with eventual addition of urine from the developing kidneys.

26. The answer is d. *(Moore, Developing Human, 6/e, pp 156–159.)* Monozygotic twins (MZ) arise from divisions of the embryoblast to form two embryos. They also can form from early separation of the blastomeres. Basically, MZ can arise anywhere from the two-cell (blastomere) to the morula stage. MZ may have fused or separate placentae, separate or fused dichorionic sacs or one chorionic sac, and diamniotic sacs. Dizygotic twins (DZ) arise from fertilization of two oocytes by two sperm and are merely womb mates. They differ in genotype and, therefore, may be different sexes.

27. The answer is b. *(Sweeney, pp 46–47. Moore, Developing Human, 6/e, pp 150–154.)* Each of the embryonic germ layers is continuous with an extraembryonic structure. The ectoderm is continuous with the amniotic membrane, the endoderm with the lining of the yolk sac, and the embryonic mesoderm with the extraembryonic mesoderm.

28. The answer is a. *(Moore, Developing Human, 6/e, pp 84–86, 357–358. Sweeney, pp 40–41.)* The fusion of the dorsal aortae occurs through lateral folding. Craniocaudal folding establishes the definitive head and tail regions of the embryo. Fusion is already complete at the time that looping of the heart tube occurs. Fusion of the endocardial heart tube and incorporation of the yolk sac into the primitive gut also occurs as a result of lateral folding. Gastrulation establishes the three germ layers (trilaminar disk), and neurulation establishes the neural groove with two neural folds.

Cell Biology: Membranes

Questions

DIRECTIONS: Each item below contains a question or incomplete statement followed by suggested responses. Select the **one best** response to each question.

29. The region labeled with the arrow in the accompanying electron micrograph of the plasma membrane is responsible for which of the following functions?

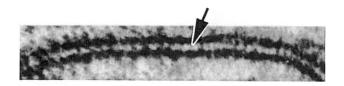

a. Creation of a barrier to water-soluble molecules
b. Specific cellular receptors for ligands
c. Catalyzing membrane-associated activities
d. Transport of small ions
e. Connections to the cytoskeleton

30. Which of the following is primarily responsible for the polyanionic charge on the outer surface of the plasma membrane?

a. Cholesterol
b. Glycoprotein
c. Free saccharide groups
d. Peripheral membrane protein
e. Integrins

31. The face labeled by asterisks in the freeze-fracture preparation shown below may be characterized as

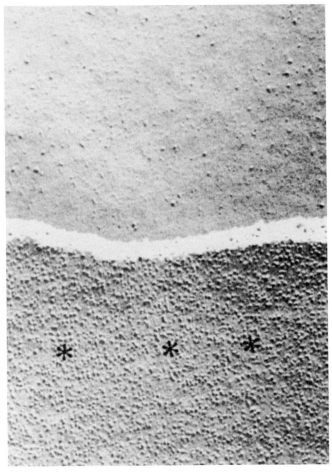

(Reproduced, with permission, from Fawcett DW: The Cell, 2/e, Philadelphia, PA: WB Saunders, 1981)

   a. Containing primarily glycoproteins and glycolipids
   b. Facing away from the cytoplasm
   c. In direct contact with the cytoplasm
   d. Backed by the extracellular space
   e. Generally possessing a paucity of intramembranous particles

32. Glycophorin is a single-pass, transmembrane glycoprotein found in the erythrocyte (RBC). Which of the following is an expected characteristic of this protein?

a. It possesses a hydrophilic portion that spans the lipid bilayer
b. Hydrolysis of carbohydrate will not affect the glycophorin band on an SDS polyacrylamide gel
c. It possesses oligosaccharides on the cytosolic side of the membrane
d. The polypeptide chain crosses the lipid bilayer in an α-helix conformation
e. It may be isolated from the RBC membrane with mild extraction conditions such as altered pH or ionic strength

33. Which of the following increases membrane fluidity under normal conditions?

a. Restriction of rotational movement of proteins and lipids in the membrane
b. Binding of integral membrane proteins with cytoskeletal elements
c. Transbilayer movement of phospholipids in the plasma membrane
d. High cholesterol content of the plasma membrane
e. Binding of an antibody to a cell surface receptor

34. The asymmetry of cell membrane is established primarily by

a. The distribution of cholesterol
b. Membrane synthesis in the endoplasmic reticulum
c. Flipping proteins between the leaflets of the lipid bilayer
d. Presence of carbohydrates on the cytoplasmic surface
e. Membrane modification in the Golgi apparatus

35. Members of the multiple-pass, G protein–linked family of receptors include the muscarinic, cholinergic, and β-adrenergic receptors. Which of the following characterizes these receptors?

a. They possess intrinsic enzyme activity
b. They possess an arrangement of hydrophobic membrane-spanning segments
c. They possess an intracellular ligand-binding domain
d. They possess a single hydrophobic transmembrane segment
e. They are arranged so that both the amino- and carboxy-terminals are located intracellularly

Cell Biology: Membranes

Answers

29. The answer is a. (*McKenzie and Klein, pp 4–5, 30. Junqueira, 9/e, pp 22–24. Alberts, 3/e, pp 478–480.*) The hydrophobic layer of the cell (plasma) membrane is labeled with the arrow. It is responsible for the basic structure of the membrane and provides the barrier to water-soluble molecules in the external milieu. It also provides a two-dimensional solvent for membrane proteins. Other membrane functions are performed primarily by proteins that function as receptors, enzymes (catalysis of membrane-associated activities), and transporters. Connection to the cytoskeleton is performed by members of the spectrin family of proteins.

The membrane consists of a bilayer of phospholipids with the nonpolar, hydrophobic layer in the central portion of the membrane and the hydrophilic polar regions of the phospholipids in contact with the aqueous components at the intra- or extracellular surfaces of the membrane. Proteins are generally dispersed within the lipid bilayer. The polar head groups of the lipid bilayer react with osmium to create the trilaminar appearance observed in electron micrographs of the plasma membrane. Cell membranes range in thickness from 7 to 10 nm [1 nm = 10^{-9} m, 1 μm = 10^{-6} m; the diameter of a red blood cell (erythrocyte) is 7 μm].

30. The answer is b. (*McKenzie and Klein, pp 4–12. Alberts, 3/e, pp 483–485, 502. Junqueira, 9/e, p 22.*) The carbohydrate of biological membranes is found in the form of glycoproteins and glycolipids rather than as free saccharide groups. The polyanionic charge of the membrane is produced by the sugar side chains on the glycoproteins and glycolipids. Glycoproteins often terminate in sialic acid side chains, which impart a negative (polyanionic) charge to the membrane. Similarly, the glycolipids (a/k/a glycosphingolipids), particularly the gangliosides, terminate in sialic acid residues with a strong negative charge. Cholesterol alters membrane fluidity (see answer to question 34). It is amphipathic (hydrophilic and hydrophobic properties). It acts by reducing the packing of lipid acyl groups through its steroid ring structure and hydrocarbon tail and cementing hydrophilic regions of the membrane through interactions with its hydroxyl (OH⁻) region. Peripheral membrane proteins are found on the cytosolic leaflet of the membrane bilayer. Integrins are heterodimeric receptors that bind with extracellular matrix (ECM) molecules such as laminin and fibronectin.

31. The answer is b. *(Alberts, 3/e, pp 153, 494–495. Junqueira, 9/e, p 24.)* The P face of a cell membrane freeze fracture is labeled with the asterisks and faces away from the cytoplasm. Freeze fracture is a procedure in which the tissue is rapidly frozen and fractured with a knife. The fracture plane occurs through the hydrophobic central plane of membranes, which is the plane of least resistance to the cleavage force. The two faces are essentially the two interior faces of the membrane. They are described as the extracellular face (E face) and the protoplasmic face (P face). The cytoplasm is the backing for the P face, which in general contains numerous intramembranous particles (mostly protein). The E face is backed by the extracellular space and in general contains a paucity of intramembranous particles (see upper part of figure) compared with the P face (labeled with asterisks).

32. The answer is d. *(McKenzie and Klein, pp 8–12. Alberts, 3/e, pp 493–494.)* As a transmembrane protein, glycophorin traverses the membrane and crosses the lipid bilayer in a single-pass α-helix conformation. The hydrophobic portion spans the lipid bilayer, and the hydrophilic carboxyl end is exposed to the cytosol, whereas the hydrophilic amino end is exposed to the extracellular surface. The oligosaccharides are found on the hydrophilic amino terminus where the negative surface charge is generated. The oligosaccharides are degraded by carbohydrate hydrolysis. Harsh detergent treatment is required for isolation of transmembrane proteins, such as glycophorin, compared with peripheral proteins, such as spectrin and ankyrin, that can be isolated by mild extraction methods.

33. The answer is e. *(Alberts, 3/e, pp 480–482, 498–499. Junqueira, 9/e, p 23.)* Binding of an antibody to a cell surface receptor results in lateral diffusion of protein in the lipid bilayer, resulting in patching and capping. When such a divalent or multivalent ligand binds to membrane receptors present as intrinsic membrane proteins, initially there is a homogeneous pattern to the binding. Subsequently, the ligand-receptor complexes undergo patching and eventually capping on the cell surface. Rotational and lateral movements of both proteins and lipids contribute to membrane fluidity. Restriction reduces membrane fluidity. Phospholipids are capable of lateral diffusion, rapid rotation around their long axis, and flexion of their hydrocarbon (fatty acyl) tails. They undergo transbilayer movement, known as "flip-flop," between bilayers in the endoplasmic reticulum; however, this is a very rare occurrence in the plasma membrane. Other factors reduce membrane fluidity. Cholesterol at high concentrations decreases membrane fluidity by interacting with the hydrophobic regions near the polar head groups and stiffening this region of the membrane. Association or binding of integral membrane proteins with cytoskeletal elements on the interior of the cell and peripheral membrane proteins on the extracellular surface limit membrane mobility and fluidity.

34. The answer is b. (*Alberts, 3/e, pp 482–485. Junqueira, 9/e, p 22.*) Asymmetry of the lipid bilayer is established during membrane synthesis in the endoplasmic reticulum. One of the best examples is the presence of protein kinase C in the cytoplasmic leaflet of the phospholipid bilayer. Carbohydrates are associated with the N-terminals of transmembrane proteins that extend from the extracellular surface. Cholesterol is different from proteins and phospholipids that are asymmetrically distributed within the bilayer. Cholesterol is found on both sides of the bilayer. The small polar head group structure of cholesterol allows it to flip-flop from leaflet to leaflet and respond to changes in shape. In contrast to cholesterol, most proteins and phospholipids are capable of only rare flip-flop. For example, transbilayer movement of phospholipid is mostly limited to the endoplasmic reticulum.

35. The answer is b. (*McKenzie and Klein, pp 8–11, 18–20. Alberts, 3/e, pp 486–488, 734–735.*) These receptors are all multipass transmembrane proteins consisting specifically of seven hydrophobic spanning segments of the single polypeptide chain. There is a remarkable homology between the cell surface receptors linked to the G proteins. Included in this group are the muscarinic and cholinergic receptors, rhodopsin, and the β-adrenergic receptor. Between the segments, the polypeptide chain loops on both the extracellular and intracellular sides of the membrane. All of these transmembrane proteins show a carboxyl terminus on the cytosolic side and N-linked glycosylation sites on the extracellular surface. Receptors with intrinsic enzyme activity belong to a separate class of single-pass transmembrane proteins. Ligand binding occurs on the extracellular surface.

Cell Biology: Cytoplasm

Questions

DIRECTIONS: Each item below contains a question or incomplete statement followed by suggested responses. Select the **one best** response to each question.

36. The presence of vimentin in immunocytochemical analysis of a metastatic tumor would suggest _____ origin

a. Epithelial
b. Neuronal
c. Skeletal muscular
d. Mesenchymal
e. Endodermal

37. The function of the large subunit of the ribosome is to

a. Bind messenger RNA (mRNA)
b. Bind transfer RNA (tRNA)
c. Catalyze peptide bond formation
d. Link adjacent ribosomes in a polyribosome
e. Initiate protein synthesis

38. The stability and arrangement of actin filaments as well as their properties and functions depend on

a. The structure of the actin filaments
b. Microtubules
c. Intermediate filament proteins
d. Actin-binding proteins
e. Motor molecules, such as kinesin

39. The structures marked with the arrows in the figure shown below are correctly characterized by which of the following statements?

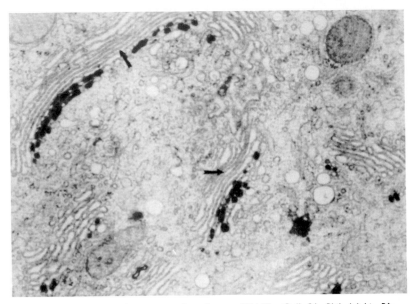

(Reproduced, with permission, from Fawcett DW: The Cell, 2/e. Philadelphia, PA: WB Saunders, 1981.)

a. They present an entry face associated with granule formation
b. They present an exit face associated with transport vesicles
c. They receive proteins but not lipids
d. They are biochemically compartmentalized
e. Topologic organization of the stacks is unrelated to the function of specific enzymes

40. The primary function of intermediate filaments is to

a. Generate movement
b. Provide mechanical stability
c. Carry out nucleation of microtubules
d. Stabilize microtubules against disassembly
e. Transport organelles within the cell

41. The vesicular structures marked throughout the cytoplasm in the electron micrograph below

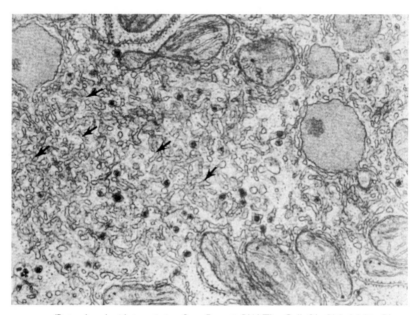

(Reproduced, with permission, from Fawcett DW: The Cell, 2/e. Philadelphia, PA: WB Saunders, 1981.)

a. Cannot be separated by differential centrifugation from other cytoplasmic components
b. Provide energy for muscle contraction
c. Are the primary site of protein synthesis in the cell
d. Are involved in recycling of membrane receptors
e. Are involved in detoxification processes in the liver

42. Which of the following mechanisms is used to establish the mitochondrial electrochemical gradient?

a. The action of ATP synthase
b. Pumping of protons into the mitochondrial matrix by respiratory chain activity
c. Transport of ATP out of the matrix compartment by a specific transporter
d. Proton-translocating activity in the inner membrane
e. Transfer of electrons from NADH to O_2 in the intermembrane space

43. Which of the following events occurs in the rough endoplasmic reticulum?

a. Core glycosylation of proteins
b. O-linked glycosylation
c. Glycogenolysis
d. Sulfation
e. Protein sorting

44. In Zellweger syndrome, tissue shows the presence of empty peroxisomes. Which of the following findings would you expect in patients?

a. Decreased energy production
b. Inability to detoxify alcohol
c. Decreased exocytosis
d. Decreased SER activity
e. Decreased lysosomal activity

45. Inhibition of actin assembly by cytochalasins would interfere with

a. Ciliary movement
b. Vesicular transport between the Golgi apparatus and cell membrane
c. Separation of chromosomes in anaphase of the cell cycle
d. Phagocytic activity by macrophages
e. The structure of centrioles

46. Chloroquine is a weak base that neutralizes acidic organelles. In a pancreatic beta cell, which of the following would be a direct effect of chloroquine treatment?

a. Increased proinsulin content in secretory vesicles
b. Increased release of C peptide
c. Increased number of amylase-containing secretory vesicles
d. Reduced translation of glucagon mRNA
e. Increased stability of insulin mRNA

47. The region in the electron micrograph that is labeled A contains

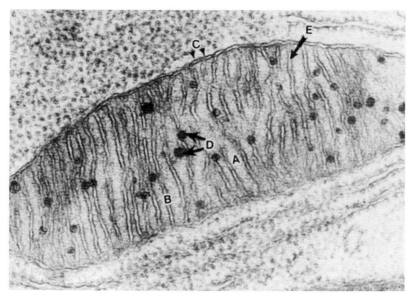

(Reproduced, with permission, from Fawcett DW: The Cell, 2/e. Philadelphia, PA: WB Saunders, 1981.)

a. The mitochondrial genome
b. Enzymes responsible for the oxidative reactions of the electron transport chain
c. ATP synthase complexes
d. Ca²⁺ accumulations
e. Enzymes involved in lipid synthesis and metabolism

48. Movement of vesicles and organelles from the perikaryon of the neuron to the axon terminus occurs along which of the following?

a. Microfilaments (thin filaments)
b. Intermediate filaments
c. Microtubules
d. Thick filaments
e. Spectrin heterodimers

49. Which of the following molecules forms the coating of vesicles involved in endocytosis and exocytosis?

a. Clathrin
b. Spectrin
c. Ankyrin
d. Actin
e. Vimentin

50. Tay-Sachs disease is caused by

a. Absence of mannose-6-phosphate on lysosomal enzymes
b. Absence of mannose-6-phosphate receptor on the *trans*-Golgi
c. A lysosomal enzyme deficiency
d. Overproduction of hydrolases
e. Absence of a signal peptide

51. Which of the following cellular compartments is the sorting and packaging station within the Golgi apparatus?

a. *Trans*-compartment
b. Medial compartment
c. *Cis*-compartment
d. *Trans*-Golgi network
e. Transitional elements

Cell Biology: Cytoplasm

Answers

36. The answer is d. (*McKenzie and Klein, p 35. Alberts, 3/e, pp 798–800.*) Vimentin is the intermediate filament protein that is specific for mesenchymal cells such as fibroblasts, macrophages, endothelial cells, and smooth muscle of the vasculature. The type of intermediate filament protein is relatively specific for cells derived from the three embryonic germ layers. Antibodies to intermediate filament proteins have been used by pathologists to determine the origin of tumors. Cytokeratins (also known as keratins) are specific for epithelial cells; desmin is found in striated and most smooth muscle, except vascular smooth muscle; and glial fibrillary acidic protein (GFAP) is specific for astrocytes, not microglia or oligodendrocytes. Neurofilament proteins (NFL, NFM, NFH) are found in neurons. In Alzheimer's senile dementia syndrome, extensive plaques of neurofilament proteins occur. In addition to the normal structural role of intermediate filaments, they are involved in the anchorage of the proteins that form ion channels. *intermeds= stability*

37. The answer is c. (*McKenzie and Klein, pp 53–57. Alberts, 3/e, pp 231–234, 236, 240–241. Junqueira, 9/e, pp 31–33.*) The large subunit of the ribosome catalyzes peptide bond formation by activation of peptidyl transferase. The small ribosomal subunit contains the peptidyl-tRNA-binding (P) site that binds the tRNA molecule attached to the carboxyl end of the growing end of the polypeptide chain. The small subunit also contains the aminoacyl-tRNA-binding (A) site that holds the incoming tRNA and amino acid. The initiation factors are loaded on the small ribosomal subunit that must locate the AUG (start) codon to initiate protein synthesis. This occurs before binding of the large subunit. In addition, the initiator tRNA containing methionine provides the amino acid necessary to start protein synthesis. The initiator tRNA is also located on the small subunit. It resides at the P site (the normal peptidyl site) even though it is an aminoacyl-tRNA. This occurs before binding to the mRNA. Therefore, the initiation phase of protein synthesis is regulated by the small subunit of the ribosome. Ribosomes are composed of both protein and RNA (predominantly rRNA, but also mRNA and tRNA). Single ribosomes are involved in synthesis of cytosolic proteins.

Polyribosomes (linked by mRNA) synthesize proteins that are translocated into the cisternal space of the rough endoplasmic reticulum (RER) and destined for export or specific organelles.

38. The answer is d. (*McKenzie and Klein, pp 28–29. Alberts, 3/e, pp 834–846.*) The stability, arrangement, and functions of actin filaments depend on the actin-binding proteins. The fundamental structure of the actin molecule is the same no matter what the function or arrangement in a cell. Actin-binding proteins have a variety of functions: (1) tropomyosin strengthens actin filaments, (2) fibrin and villin are actin-bundling proteins, (3) filamin and gelsolin regulate transformation from the sol to the gel state, (4) members of the myosin II family are responsible for sliding filaments, (5) myosin I (minimyosin) is responsible for movement of vesicles on filaments, and (6) spectrin cross-links the sides of actin filaments to the plasma membrane.

39. The answer is d. (*McKenzie and Klein, pp 18–20, 148. Alberts, 3/e, pp 601–603. Junqueira, 9/e, pp 34–37.*) The biochemically compartmentalized organelle, labeled with the arrows in the electron micrograph, is the Golgi apparatus. There is a specific organization to the Golgi stacks related to the function of specific enzymes. Histochemical stains, such as acid phosphatase and nucleoside diphosphates, show that the Golgi apparatus is biochemically compartmentalized. It presents two faces: a *cis* face, which is the point of entry of transport vesicles in transit from the rough endoplasmic reticulum (RER) to the Golgi, and a *trans* face that is the exit point associated with granule formation and the maturation of proteins. Both proteins and lipids are transported from the transitional elements of the ER to the Golgi apparatus. Packaging is not the sole function of the Golgi. This organelle is also involved in the processing of proteins (e.g., addition of oligosaccharide chains) that was initiated in the RER.

40. The answer is b. (*McKenzie and Klein, pp 35–36. Alberts, 3/e, pp 801–803.*) There are differences in the way that intermediate filaments interact with microtubules and microfilaments within the cytoplasm; however, their ropelike arrangement is well suited to providing mechanical stability to the cell and resisting stretch, allowing the cell to respond to tension. The different types of intermediate filaments all have a similar structural pattern: nonhelical head and tail segments with a helical arrangement in the center of the intermediate filament structure. Movement is generated by motor proteins such as myosin, dynein, and kinesin. There is a good mnemonic device for remembering the direction of movement directed by kinesin and dynein. Kinesin *kicks* the molecules out; dynein *drags* them in; also, the *plus* end of the microtubule is oriented toward the *plasma* membrane, so minus end toward nucleus. This works for fibroblasts as well as neurons, to be discussed in a later chapter.

Nucleation of microtubules is conducted by centrosomes. Microtubule-associated proteins (MAPs) stabilize or destabilize microtubules. Microtubules function in organellar transport (e.g., axonal transport).

41. The answer is e. (*McKenzie and Klein, pp 15–16, 148. Alberts, 3/e, pp 577–582. Junqueira, 9/e, pp 33–34.*) The smooth endoplasmic reticulum (SER) is the structure shown in the electron micrograph. It is the portion of the endoplasmic reticulum (ER) that lacks ribosomes. In hepatocytes there is extensive SER, which is involved in detoxification using enzymes such as cytochrome P450. Recycling of membrane receptors involves the shuttling of coated vesicles. SER may be separated from the RER by differential centrifugation using sucrose gradients, a technique in which smooth and rough microsomes are formed. The energy required for muscle contraction is stored in ATP synthesized in the mitochondria. However, SER is involved in the regulation of Ca^{2+} during muscle contraction and, therefore, plays a critical role in this process. The SER arises from the rough endoplasmic reticulum (RER), and most of the membrane components can diffuse freely from RER to SER because they are part of a continuous fluid-mosaic membrane. The enzymes required for SER function are synthesized in ribosomes on the RER, and some enzymes, such as those involved in the degradation of glycogen (e.g., glucose-6-phosphate), are found in both SER and RER.

42. The answer is d. (*McKenzie and Klein, pp 22–24. Alberts, 3/e, pp 653–683. Junqueira, 9/e, pp 29–31.*) The mitochondrial electrochemical gradient is established by a proton pump. The pump is located in the inner membrane, associated with the respiratory chain and ATP synthase. The impermeability of the inner membrane to protons causes an osmotic and electrochemical gradient to develop. Mitochondria produce energy that the cell uses in transport and other energy-dependent processes. Cellular energy is stored as ATP, which is synthesized by the phosphorylation of ADP by ATP synthase. Mitochondria use the electron-transport (respiratory) chain that transfers energy from NADH to O_2. As electrons released by oxidation of substrate in the matrix flow down the respiratory chain, hydrogen ions are pumped into the intermembrane space. Protons in the matrix drive ATP synthase in a mechanism similar to that of a water wheel. ATP synthase, therefore, couples oxidative transport through the electron-transport (respiratory) chain with energy storage (ATP).

43. The answer is a. (*McKenzie and Klein, pp 18–20. Alberts, 3/e, pp 577–579. Junqueira, 9/e, pp 31–37.*) The rough endoplasmic reticulum (RER) is the site of core glycosylation of proteins using the membrane-bound lipid carrier, dolichol, catalyzed by an oligosaccharide transferase. This is N-linked glycosylation, which occurs by an en bloc method in which dolichol is added to the protein. O-linked glycosylation occurs in the Golgi by a mechanism involving oligosaccharide transferases. It does not occur en bloc. N-Linked oligosaccharides are the most common oligosaccharides found in glycoproteins. They contain sugar residues linked to the NH$_2$ amide nitrogen of asparagine. O-linked oligosaccharides have sugar residues linked to hydroxyl groups on the side chains of serine and threonine and are less common than the N-linked species. O-linkage is catalyzed by glycosyltransferase enzymes in the Golgi, not the rough endoplasmic reticulum. However, in both the ER and the Golgi apparatus, the enzymes are located on the luminal side of these cisternal structures. The addition occurs sugar by sugar rather than en bloc as occurs in the rough endoplasmic reticulum for the N-linked oligosaccharides.

The RER is associated with ribosomes involved in the synthesis of proteins for export, but also segregation to the plasma membrane as well as to the membranes of mitochondria and peroxisomes. SER is involved in lipid synthesis and is extensive in cells actively involved in lipid production, such as the cells of the adrenal cortex. An integral membrane protein of SER is also involved in the synthesis and breakdown of glycogen (glycogenolysis). The amount of SER may be increased in cells such as hepatocytes by the systemic administration of drugs such as phenobarbital. Cellular components are degraded in lysosomes. The diversity in oligosaccharides is produced by selective removal of glucose and mannose from the core oligosaccharide. This trimming process begins in the RER before reaching the Golgi, where the final mannose-residue trimming occurs. Protein sorting and sulfation are carried out in the Golgi apparatus.

44. The answer is b. (*Alberts, 3/e, pp 576–577.*) Individuals suffering from Zellweger syndrome are unable to detoxify alcohol because of the absence of alcohol dehydrogenases in the peroxisomes. In this syndrome, peroxisomes are empty because of the failure of the signal system that sorts protein to this organelle. Because the peroxisome lacks a genome or synthetic machinery, it must import all proteins. In the case of Zellweger syndrome, it appears that the defect is in the peroxisomal membrane, but errors or absence of the peroxisomal signal sequence would result in the same symptom. Peroxisomes were first identified in liver and kidney cells, which have large numbers of peroxisomes because of their function in detoxification and waste removal. Peroxisomes protect the cell by removal of H_2O_2 and the detoxification of alcohol. The absence of catalase and other proteins of the peroxisome would result in dramatically reduced detoxification capacity. The SER is the site of barbiturate detoxification, but the process is not dependent on peroxisomes. Lysosomes, mitochondria, and protein synthetic activity should not be affected in Zellweger syndrome.

45. The answer is d. *(Alberts, 3/e, pp 823, 826, 917, 928–932.)* Cytochalasins are potent inhibitors of cell motility and other cellular events that depend on actin assembly: cytokinesis, which is conducted by the actin-containing contractile ring; phagocytosis; and formation of lamellipodia. Cytochalasins bind to the plus end of actin filaments and prevent further polymerization. The movement of chromosomes in anaphase of the cell cycle depends on disassembly of microtubules at the kinetochore (anaphase A) and addition at the plus end of the polar microtubules (anaphase B). Ciliary movement, vesicular transport, and the structure of centrioles depend on microtubules.

46. The answer is a. *(Alberts, 3/e, pp 622, 628–629.)* Chloroquine treatment inhibits the conversion of proinsulin to insulin, resulting in decreased formation of insulin within secretory vesicles. Chloroquine neutralizes acidic compartments such as the secretory vesicles. Acidification causes concentration of the contents of secretory vesicles, facilitates breakdown of the contents of phagosomes and lysosomes, and is involved in the cleavage of prohormones to their active forms (e.g., proinsulin to insulin). The acidification process functions through a vacuolar H^+-proton pump that is present in the membranes of most endocytic and exocytic vesicles, including those of the phagosomes, lysosomes, secretory vesicles, and some compartments of the Golgi. Ribosomes are not dependent on a proton pump mechanism and are, therefore, less sensitive to chloroquine. Gene and message expression and message stability are also not targets for chloroquine. Note that pancreatic beta (β) cells synthesize insulin. Proinsulin is split into

C peptide + insulin in secretory vesicles. In vivo, C-peptide release can be used to measure production of insulin by a patient's pancreatic beta cells. This is particularly useful in patients who are receiving insulin. Glucagon is synthesized by alpha (α) cells, and amylase is an exocrine pancreatic product produced by the acinar cells.

47. The answer is a. (*McKenzie and Klein, pp 35–38, 105–107. Alberts, 3/e, pp 655–658. Junqueira, 9/e, pp 29–31.*) The region labeled A in the electron micrograph of the mitochondrion is the mitochondrial matrix, or intercristal space. The matrix contains the circular DNA of the mitochondrial genome. Most mitochondrial proteins are encoded for by nuclear DNA, but a small proportion are encoded within the mitochondrial DNA and are synthesized on mitochondrial ribosomes. The matrix also contains the enzymes responsible for the Krebs (citric acid) cycle. Matrix granules, which probably consist of accumulations of calcium ions, have been identified (D). The structure labeled B is the inner membrane of the mitochondrion, which is highly impermeable to small ions because of the presence of cardiolipin. The inner membrane contains the proteins required for the oxidative reactions of the respiratory transport chain and a transmembrane complex (ATP synthase) that is responsible for ATP synthesis. This membrane is folded into convolutions called cristae. The number of cristae is directly related to the metabolic activity of the cell. The elementary particles that have been identified on the cristae are composed primarily of ATP synthase complexes. The outer mitochondrial membrane, labeled C, is highly permeable to molecules 10,000 daltons or less because of the presence of porin, a channel-forming protein. This membrane contains enzymes involved in lipid synthesis and lipid metabolism. The outer membrane mediates the movement of fatty acids into the mitochondria for use in the formation of acetyl CoA (also see question 42).

48. The answer is c. (*Alberts, 3/e, pp 796–802, 813–815, 831–832. Junqueira, 9/e, pp 40–47.*) Vesicles and organelles move unidirectionally along microtubules from the perikaryon of a neuron to the axon terminus. This process is driven by the microtubule motor, kinesin, an ATPase that hydrolyzes ATP to ADP, providing the energy required for vesicular movement. Microtubules are composed of tubulin and are involved in motility as the principal protein in the composition of the axoneme (the core of the cilium or flagellum). Microfilaments (thin filaments) are composed of actin, the most abundant protein in cells of eukaryotes. They are involved in cell motility and changes in cell shape. Myosin is the main constituent of the thick filament that binds to actin and functions as an ATPase activated by actin. Intermediate filaments that are "intermediate" in diameter (8 to 10 nm) between thin and thick filaments, are of four different types. Type I is composed of the acidic, neutral, and basic keratins (also known as the cytokeratins) and is found specifically in epithelial cells. Type II intermediate filaments are composed of vimentin, desmin, or glial fibrillary acidic protein. Vimentin is found in cells of mesenchymal origin, desmin in muscle cells, and glial fibrillary acidic protein primarily in astrocytes. Type III intermediate filaments are neurofilament proteins found in neurons. Type IV intermediate filaments consist of nuclear lamins A, B, and C and are associated with nuclear lamina of all cells.

49. The answer is a. (*McKenzie and Klein, pp 22, 30–31, 66–67. Alberts, 3/e, pp 491–495, 620–621, 796–798.*) Clathrin is an important protein that forms the coating of coated pits and vesicles involved in endocytosis and the retrieval of membrane following exocytosis. Intermediate filaments are important cytoskeletal elements with some specificity that depends on the origin of the cells in question. Vimentin is specific for cells of mesenchymal origin, such as fibroblasts and chondrocytes. Actin is the protein found in thin filaments. It is also a cytoskeletal component found in the cytoplasm of red blood cells and other eukaryotic cells. Spectrin heterodimers form tetramers that interact with actin and provide flexibility and support for the membrane. The protein ankyrin "anchors" the band 3 protein to the spectrin-membrane skeleton. This connection is often described as the indirect binding of band 3 protein to the cytoskeleton (spectrin tetramers) of the red blood cell. The band 3 protein is known to be an anion transport protein of the red blood cell.

50. The answer is c. (*McKenzie and Klein, p 21.*) Tay-Sachs disease is one of the lysosomal storage diseases. Lysosomes contain an array of specific hydrolases. In Tay-Sachs disease, hexosaminidase A is deficient, resulting in the buildup of GM2 ganglioside and leading to mental retardation, blindness, and early mortality. The chart below summarizes the enzyme deficiencies and resulting effects in some of the more prominent lysosomal disorders. Mannose-6-phosphate and its receptor are involved in the trafficking of proteins to the lysosomal compartment and are not involved in the lysosomal storage disorders. Overproduction of hydrolases or absence of a signal peptide are also not involved in this disorder.

Lysosomal Storage Disease	Enzyme Deficit	Cellular Site/Accumulation		Organ(s) Most Affected
Tay-Sachs	β-N-hexosaminidase-A	Neurons	Glycolipid	CNS
Gaucher	β-D-glycosidase	Macrophages	Glycolipid	Spleen, liver
Hurler	α-L-iduronidase	Fibroblasts, chondroblasts, osteoblasts	Dermatan sulfate	Skeletal system
Niemann-Pick	Sphingomyelinase	Oligodendrocytes, fibroblasts	Sphingomyelin	CNS
Inclusion (I)-cell	N-acetylglucosamine-phosphotransferase	Fibroblasts, macrophages	Glycoproteins and glycolipids	Nervous and skeletal systems, (liver unaffected)

(Reproduced, with permission, from McKenzie JC and Klein RM: Basic Concepts in Cell Biology and Histology. New York, NY: Mc-Graw-Hill, 2000.)

51. The answer is d. (*McKenzie and Klein, pp 18–20, 69. Alberts, 3/e, pp 601–602.*) The *trans*-Golgi network (TGN) serves as a sorting station for proteins destined for various organelles, including the plasma membrane, and protein for export from the cell. Golgi-derived transport and secretory vesicles bud off from the TGN. Transitional elements are derived from the endoplasmic reticulum (ER) and carry proteins and lipids from the endoplasmic reticulum to the *cis*-face of the Golgi. The Golgi apparatus plays an important role in the processing of proteins for secretion. It is divided into four regions: *cis*-face, medial compartment, *trans*-face, and the *trans*-Golgi network (TGN). The *cis*-face of the Golgi receives the transitional elements and participates in phosphorylation (e.g., in the synthesis of lysosomal oligosaccharides). The medial compartment is responsible for the removal of mannose and the addition of N-acetylglucosamine. The *trans*-face is responsible for the addition of sialic acid and galactose.

Cell Biology: Intracellular Trafficking

Questions

DIRECTIONS: Each item below contains a question or incomplete statement followed by suggested responses. Select the **one best** response to each question.

52. Endocytosis of low-density lipoprotein (LDL) differs from phagocytosis of damaged cells in

a. Use of membrane-enclosed vesicles in the uptake process
b. Coupling with the lysosomal system
c. Dependence on acidification
d. Use of clathrin-coated pits
e. Use of hydrolases

53. In the signal hypothesis, the signal recognition particle (SRP) functions to

a. Bind the docking protein to the ER membrane
b. Bind the N-terminal sequence of the peptide to the ribosome
c. Prevent degradation of newly synthesized peptides by proteases
d. Enzymatically cleave the newly synthesized peptide from the signal sequence
e. Induce an immediate increase in translation rate

54. Chaperonins function to

a. Ensure correct folding of cytosolic proteins
b. Control the docking of the signal peptide with its receptor on the rough endoplasmic reticulum
c. Stabilize microtubules
d. Serve as a start-transfer signal in the membrane of the endoplasmic reticulum
e. Mediate the selective transport of membrane receptors

55. The figure below represents the signal-transduction pathways initiated after ligand binding to the β-adrenergic receptor on the cell membrane. This binding leads to stimulation of secretory granule release from a cell such as a pancreatic or salivary gland acinar cell. Which of the following statements regarding the molecule labeled B is true?

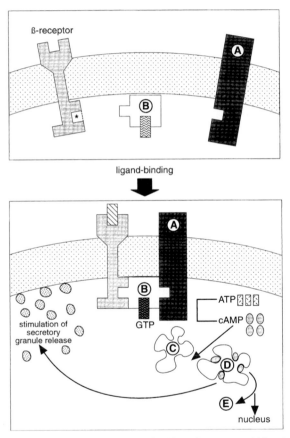

(Modified, with permission, from Avery JK: Oral Development and Histology, 2/e. New York, NY: Thieme Medical, 1994.)

a. It is the inactive cAMP kinase
b. It lacks GTPase activity
c. It inactivates adenylate cyclase
d. It is bound to GTP in the inactive state
e. It is the stimulatory G protein (G$_s$)

56. The figure below is a diagram of the phosphoinositide (PI) cycle and related regulatory processes. The function of molecule A is

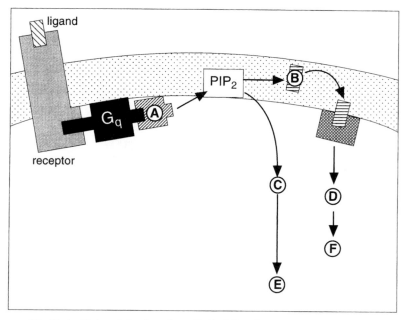

(Modified, with permission, from Avery JK: Oral Development and Histology, 2/e. New York, NY: Thieme Medical, 1994.)

a. Stimulation of G_i activity through phosphorylation of PIP_2
b. Stimulation of G_s activity through phosphorylation of PIP_2
c. Hydrolysis of PIP_2 to form DAG and IP_3
d. Formation of kinase C and PI-phosphate
e. Formation of GTP and ATP

57. The processes illustrated in secretory pathways A → B → C → D (pathway I) and C → E (pathway II) in the diagram differ in

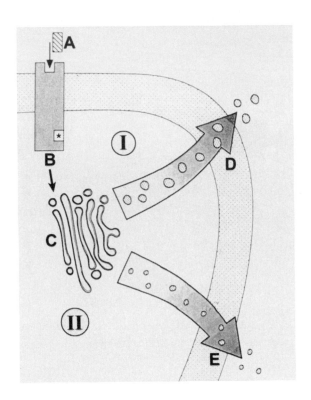

a. Origin of secretory product
b. The requirement for a secretagogue
c. Mechanisms of ER to Golgi transport
d. Passage of vesicular contents through the cell membrane
e. Use of vesicles for transport to the cell membrane

58. Inclusion cell disease is characterized by the absence of lysosomal hydrolytic enzymes. Normal hydrolytic enzymes are uncharacteristically found in the blood. The most likely cause for this defect is

a. Absence of SNARE protein on vesicles
b. Abnormal KDEL sequence on vesicles
c. Upregulation of mannose-6-phosphate receptors
d. Absence of mannose-6-phosphate on lysosomal enzymes
e. Altered gene expression for the lysosomal hydrolases

Cell Biology: Intracellular Trafficking

Answers

52. The answer is d. (*McKenzie and Klein, 21–22, 66–67. Alberts, 3/e, pp 621–624.*) Receptor-mediated endocytosis of ligand-receptor complexes is a selective process that requires invagination of the cell membrane to form clathrin-coated pits and vesicles. Clathrin is not involved in phagocytosis. Phagocytosis of damaged cells occurs by evagination to engulf the IgG-coated surface of the target. Both processes use acidification of compartments and hydrolases to uncouple receptor and ligand (receptor-mediated endocytosis) or destroy engulfed material (phagocytosis). Both processes use membrane-enclosed vesicles and are associated with lysosomal activity.

Low-density lipoprotein (LDL) is the form in which most cholesterol is transported in the blood; cellular uptake of LDL is the classic example of receptor-mediated endocytosis. The receptors are bound to clathrin-coated pits, but the ligand is only directly bound to its cell surface receptor. The LDL-LDL receptor (ligand-receptor) complexes are incorporated into the cell in coated vesicles. The acidic environment of the endosome results in the cleavage of the ligand from its receptor (i.e., LDL from its receptor). The LDL receptors are recycled to the membrane for additional exposure to LDL, and the LDL in the endosome is transferred to lysosomes, where it is broken down to cholesterol.

Other ligands differ in subtle ways from LDL in their endocytic pathways. For example, epidermal growth factor (EGF) binds to its receptor, but the complex is not dissociated at the pH of the endosome; the result is transfer of the complex to the lysosomes with the eventual degradation of EGF receptors and a reduction in the number of EGF receptors on the surface. The decrease in the number of receptors is known as downregulation.

In the case of transferrin, iron-free transferrin (apotransferrin) binds ferrous ions in the blood. The iron-bound molecule (transferrin) attaches to transferrin receptors on the cell surface, initiating the receptor-mediated pathway through coated pits and vesicles. In the endosome, there is dissociation of the iron molecules from the transferrin–transferrin receptor complex. Iron is released into the cytosol for cellular use, and the ligand-receptor complex is recycled to the membrane and subsequently released from the cell. In the neutral pH of the extracellular milieu, the ligand dissociates from its receptor and is ready to bind additional ferrous ions.

53. The answer is c. (*McKenzie and Klein, pp 59–62. Alberts, 3/e, pp 582–586.*) The signal recognition particle (SRP) prevents degradation of newly synthesized peptides because translocation across the ER membrane protects the nascent peptide from proteases. The signal hypothesis is the basis of the targeting of transmembrane, lysosomal, and exportable proteins across the ER membrane. It is the key event in the segregation of non-cytosolic proteins in the ER cisternae. The result of SRP activity is attachment of ribosomes translating the secretory protein to the ER membrane and the translocation of the protein across the ER membrane. The SRP binds to the N-terminus of the signal peptide as the peptide emerges from the ribosome and induces an immediate delay in translation until the ribosome interacts with a docking protein, also known as an SRP receptor, in the ER membrane. In the function of the rough endoplasmic reticulum (RER), a presequence on the 3′ end of the AUG initiation codon is translated as an N-(amino)-terminal presequence [amino-terminal signal leader (prepeptide) sequence] that recognizes the ER membrane and leads to the translocation of the peptide across the ER membrane. This recognition is accomplished through the signal recognition particle (SRP), which cycles between the ER membrane and the cytosol. After the SRP-bound ribosome attaches to the ER membrane via the docking protein, translation continues with displacement of the SRP for subsequent recycling and translocation of the peptide across the ER membrane. Enzymatic cleavage of the signal sequence releases the newly synthesized peptide.

54. The answer is a. (*McKenzie and Klein, p 59. Alberts, 3/e, pp 571–572.*) The chaperonins are proteins that regulate the unfolding of cytosolic proteins. They are members of the heat shock protein family (e.g., hsp 70). The chaperonins assist with the translocation of proteins across internal membranes of the cell (e.g., mitochondria) by maintaining precursor proteins in their unfolded state during movement across the membrane. They do not function in the docking of the signal peptide or as the start-transfer signal in translocation of the internal membrane of the endoplasmic reticulum. Clathrin-coated vesicles are responsible for the selective transport of membrane receptors. Microtubules are stabilized by GTP capping, covalent modifications of tubulins, and microtubule-associated proteins (MAPs). The MAPs regulate disassembly of MTs and provide the linkage between organelles and MTs.

55. The answer is e. (*McKenzie and Klein, pp 109–110. Alberts, 3/e, pp 734–738. Junqueira, 9/e, pp 25–27.*) The structure labeled B is the stimulatory G protein (G_s). The figure illustrates the response of the β-adrenergic receptor to ligand binding. β-Receptors mediate the tissue effects of epinephrine and norepinephrine. They also respond to pharmacologic agents such as isoproterenol, a β-adrenergic agonist. The subsequent signal transduction following ligand binding involves a specific member of the G protein family of cell surface receptors and a chain of intracellular mediators, also known as second messengers. "G protein" is shorthand for guanosine-triphosphate (GTP)-binding regulatory protein. G proteins associated with increasing cAMP levels in the cell are known as stimulatory G proteins (G_s) because of their role in enzyme activation. In the inactive state, G_s is bound to GDP. When isoproterenol or another ligand binds to the β-receptor, a G_s binding site is exposed and the G_s protein (B in the figure) binds to the β-receptor. The resulting complex is capable of binding GTP in exchange for GDP, activating the G protein. A subunit of the activated G_s protein activates adenylate cyclase (A in the figure). Three different polypeptide chains compose G proteins. For this reason they are often called trimeric G proteins. The three subunits are α, β, and γ. The α subunit of the G_s protein exchanges GDP for GTP in response to stimulation in the form of binding to a ligand-activated receptor. This subunit is also responsible for binding to adenylate cyclase and subsequent increase in intracellular cAMP concentration. When this occurs, intrinsic GTPase activity of the α subunit is increased, which results in a short activation time (less than 1 min) for the complex and allows recycling of the subunits to the inactive state. The inactive cAMP-dependent kinase is labeled C in the figure. It is the phosphorylating action of cAMP-dependent protein kinase (kinase A), stimulated by increased intracellular cAMP concentration, that affects many aspects of intracellular metabolism and function. In addition to the effect on phosphorylation (E) that stimulates exocytosis and other cellular events, protein phosphorylation also induces nuclear changes including transcriptional events. The star in the figure delineates the site of ligand-binding-induced conformational change, exposing the G_s-binding site.

56. The answer is c. (*Alberts, 3/e, pp 744–745.*) Molecule A in the figure is phospholipase C that catalyzes the formation of diacylglycerol (DAG) and inositol triphosphate (IP_3) from phosphatidylinositol 4,5-bisphosphate (PIP_2). Phosphoinositides are important intracellular second messengers. The phosphoinositide (PI) cycle illustrated in the figure is based on the formation of PIP_2 in the inner leaflet of the plasma membrane. The break-down of PIP_2 leads to the formation of the key functional agents of the PI cycle. The process begins with the binding of a ligand to its G protein–linked receptor on the cell surface. In this case, the trimeric G pro-tein is known as G_q. It activates a phosphoinositide-specific phospholipase C. PI-specific phospholipase C hydrolyzes PIP_2 to form DAG and IP_3. These two molecules function differently to regulate intracellular function. IP_3 functions in the mobilization of calcium while DAG activates protein kinase C, leading to multiple phosphorylations of cytosolic proteins. DAG (B in the figure) is responsible for activation of protein kinase C (so-called because of its Ca^{2+} dependency), which is labeled D. The protein kinase C phosphory-lates specific serine and threonine residues in the cytosol, and it functions in many cells to alter gene transcription. In contrast, IP_3 functions to mobilize Ca^{2+} (E) by binding to IP_3-gated Ca^{2+}-release channels in the membranes of the endoplasmic reticulum. The two intracellular messenger pathways do interact in that elevated Ca^{2+} translocates protein kinase C from the cytosol to the inner leaflet of the plasma membrane. G_i is the inhibitory G protein that leads to 5'-AMP production through the action of phosphodiesterase instead of cAMP.

57. The answer is b. (*McKenzie and Klein, pp 70–71. Alberts, 3/e, pp 626–628.*) Regulated secretion (A → B → C → D) differs from constitutive secretion (C → E) in several ways. The most important difference is the requirement for a secretagogue in the regulated pathway. Regulated secre-tion shows the recognition of a receptor (B) for its ligand (A), resulting in the release of secretion in response to the stimulus of secretagogue-receptor binding. The synthetic processes are identical until the Golgi. The vesicles that bud from the Golgi (D) in the regulated pathway are clathrin-coated and contain a receptor involved in the concentration of secretory product that normally occurs before release. The constitutive pathway does not require a secretagogue and represents a method for shuttling proteins such as integral membrane proteins and lipids in vesicles to the apical and basolateral membranes. The vesicles are nonclathrin coated in the constitutive pathway. Materials for export in this pathway represent unstimulated release compared with the secretagogue-mediated secretion that occurs in the regulated pathway. Exocytosis requires vesicle fusion with the membrane in both regulated and constitutive pathways.

58. The answer is d. *(Alberts, 3/e, pp 617–618.)* In inclusion (I) cell disease, there is an absence or deficiency of N-acetylglucosamine phosphotransferase and an absence of mannose-6-phosphate receptors on lysosomal enzymes. This results in mis-sorting to the secretory pathway and release from the cell by exocytosis. The absence of mannose 6-phosphate (normally added in the *cis*-Golgi) prohibits segregation of lysosomal enzymes that normally occurs in the *trans*-Golgi through the action of mannose-6-phosphate receptors. Lysosomal enzymes are secreted into the bloodstream, and undigested substrates build up within the cells. There is normal expression of the genes encoding the hydrolases, but a misdirection of the intracellular sorting signal for these hydrolytic enzymes. Loss of the mannose 6-phosphate receptor would have a similar effect in constitutive release of lysosomal enzymes. Overexpression of mannose 6-phosphate receptors could lead to increased shuttling to lysosomes. KDEL is the signal used for retrieval of proteins from the Golgi back to the endoplasmic reticulum. SNAREs [soluble-N-ethylemalemide sensitive factor (NSF) attachment protein receptor] are the receptors for SNAPs [soluble-N-ethylemalemide sensitive factor (NSF) attachment protein] and bind vesicles to membranes. Trafficking to other structures, such as the nucleus and mitochondria, is regulated by nuclear localization signals (NLS) or an N-terminal signal peptide, respectively.

Cell Biology: Nucleus

Questions

DIRECTIONS: Each item below contains a question or incomplete statement followed by suggested responses. Select the **one best** response to each question.

59. The structure labeled in the electron micrograph below is the site of

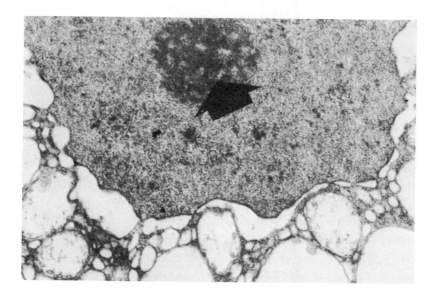

a. Transcription of nuclear proteins
b. Translation of cytosolic proteins
c. Assembly of ribosomal subunits into mature ribosomes
d. Transcription of ribosomal proteins
e. Organelle degradation

60. The dividing cell shown in the electron micrograph is undergoing a specific process that is

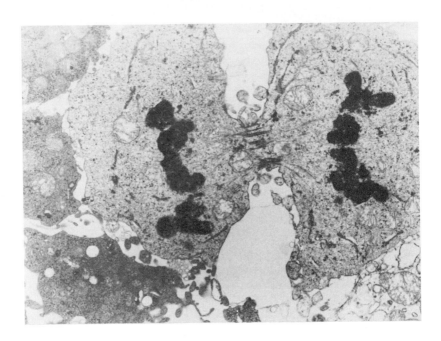

a. Regulated by mitotic promoting factor (MPF)
b. Accomplished by the contraction of a ring composed of cytoskeletal elements
c. Achieved through the lengthening of kinetochore microtubules
d. Achieved through the shortening of polar microtubules
e. Blocked by antitubulin antibodies

61. The function of the nucleosomes is to

a. Package genetic material in a condensed form
b. Transcribe the DNA
c. Form pores for bilateral nuclear-to-cytoplasmic transport
d. Form the nuclear matrix
e. Hold together adjacent chromatids

62. Which of the following proteins binds to membrane proteins and serves as a scaffold to support the nuclear envelope?

a. Lamins
b. Actin
c. Microtubules
d. Chaperonins
e. Porins

63. A metaphase-blocking dose of colchicine works by which of the following mechanisms

a. Depolymerization of actin
b. Depolymerization of myosin
c. Enhancement of tubulin polymerization
d. Inhibition of tubulin polymerization
e. Binding to and stabilizing microtubules

64. The structure labeled A in the electron micrograph is

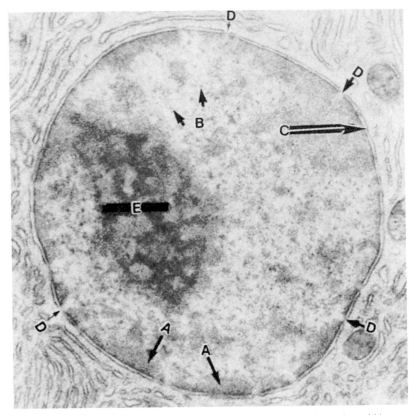

(Reproduced, with permission, from Fawcett DW: A Textbook of Histology, 11/e. Philadelphia, PA: WB Saunders, 1986.)

a. Chromatin that is transcriptionally active during interphase
b. Chromatin that is transcriptionally inactive during interphase
c. The site of ribosomal protein synthesis
d. A shield between the nucleus and cytoplasm in eukaryotic cells
e. The site of aqueous channels for the passage of molecules between the nucleo-plasm and the cytoplasm

65. The figure below summarizes the molecules involved in the cyclin cycle for regulation of entry into the mitotic phase of the cell cycle. The dark stippling in the oval represents inactivation of that component. The molecule labeled D

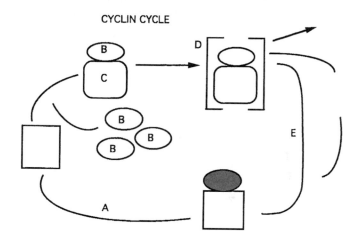

CYCLIN CYCLE

a. Directly phosphorylates lamins
b. Directly phosphorylates the mitotic cyclin
c. Functions as a kinase
d. Is disassembled through the specific action of phosphatase
e. Decreases during the mitotic phase

66. Meiotic crossover occurs in

a. Leptotene
b. Zygotene
c. Pachytene
d. Diplotene
e. Diakinesis

67. An obese 18-year-old male patient presents with small, firm testes, a small penis, little axillary and and facial hair, azoospermia, gynecomastia, and elevated levels of plasma gonadotropins. He has had difficulty in social adjustment throughout high school, but this has worsened and he has been referred for genetic and endocrine screening. The karyotype from peripheral blood leukocytes would most likely show ____ Barr bodies?

a. No
b. One
c. Two
d. Three
e. Four

Cell Biology: Nucleus

Answers

59. The answer is d. (*McKenzie and Klein, pp 39, 45–48. Junqueira, 9/e, pp 21, 52–53.*) The structure labeled in the electron micrograph is the nucleolus, the site of ribosomal protein transcription. It is a highly organized, heterogeneous structure within the nucleus with distinct regions visible by electron microscopy: (1) fibrillar centers, which represent the nucleolar organizer regions where DNA is not being actively transcribed; (2) dense fibrillar components (pars fibrosa) where RNA molecules are being transcribed; and (3) a granular component (pars granulosa) where ribosomal subunits undergo maturation. The nucleolar organizer contains clusters of rRNA genes (DNA). The size and number of nucleoli differ with the metabolic activity of cells.

Ribosomal synthesis occurs in the nucleolus, but the complete assembly and maturation of ribosomes requires transport to the cytoplasm. Ribosomal proteins as well as all proteins that function in the nucleus are synthesized in the cytosol and transported into the nucleus. Nuclear proteins are also synthesized on ribosomes in the cytoplasm and targeted to the nucleus (traveling through the nuclear pores) by specific nuclear localization signals (NLS). Cytosolic proteins are synthesized on isolated ribosomes compared with most protein synthesis that occurs on polyribosomes.

60. The answer is b. (*McKenzie and Klein, pp 123–125, 128–131. Alberts, 3/e, pp 863–866, 917, 934–937. Junqueira, 9/e, pp 56–60.*) The mitotic cell in the micrograph is undergoing cytokinesis, or the cleavage of the cytoplasm to form two cells. Cytokinesis occurs after completion of nuclear division (i.e., nuclear condensation and separation of the chromosomes). It requires the action of the contractile ring composed of actin and myosin. The force for cytokinesis is generated by the action of actin and myosin, which may be inhibited by treatment with antimyosin antibodies in vitro. The contractile ring pulls the plasma membrane of the telophase cell into the cleavage furrow. Kinetochore microtubules, which attach the kinetochores to the spindle apparatus, shorten and pull the chromatids to opposite poles. Growth of polar microtubules results in the separation of the spindle poles. Both of these events occur in anaphase, not cytokinesis. MPF regulates metaphase events through phosphorylation. The stages of the cell cycle and the defining event(s) of each stage is (are) shown in the table below.

Phase of Cell Cycle	Defining Event(s)
Interphase (G₁, S, and G₂ phases)	Duplication of centrioles and DNA synthesis (S phase)
Prophase	Nucleolus disappears
Prometaphase	Nuclear envelope breaks down
Metaphase	Alignment of chromosomes in metaphase plate
Anaphase	Separation of sister chromatids; initiation of cytokinesis
Telophase	Nuclear envelope reforms; completion of cytokinesis

(Reproduced, with permission, from McKenzie JC, Klein, RM: Basic Concepts in Cell Biology and Histology. New York, NY: McGraw-Hill, 2000.)

61. The answer is a. *(McKenzie and Klein, p 41. Alberts, 3/e, pp 342–343, 353–354, 384–385, 561–562. Junqueira, 9/e, p 52.)* Nucleosomes are the basic structural packaging unit of chromatin. Chromatin strands that have been treated to unpack the chromatin structure have the appearance of beads on a string in electron micrographs. The beads are formed by a core of histones as an octamer (i.e., two of each of the four nucleosomal histones: H2A, H2B, H3, and H4) plus two turns of DNA. The nucleosome beads plus the DNA between beads (i.e., linker DNA) constitute the nucleosome. There are additional orders of chromosome packing, including nucleosomal packing. The transcription of DNA is carried out by RNA polymerases I, II, and III, which are responsible for transcription of different types of genes. The nuclear pores are perforations in the nuclear envelope, each composed of a nuclear pore complex. The nuclear matrix is the intranuclear cytoskeleton and forms the scaffolding for nuclear structures. Chromatids are held together at the centromere.

62. The answer is a. *(McKenzie and Klein, 35, 44–45. Alberts, 3/e, pp 569–570, 800–801. Junqueira, 9/e, p 51.)* Lamins are a subclass of intermediate filaments including three nuclear proteins: lamins A, B, and C. The lamins differ from other intermediate filament proteins in some structural respects, but more importantly in the presence of a nuclear import signal.

The lamins form the core of the nuclear lamina, interact with nuclear envelope proteins, and play a role in the maintenance of the shape of the nucleus. Phosphorylation of intermediate filaments leads to disassembly as occurs with the lamins. The disassembly of lamins results in the dissolution of the nuclear envelope in prometaphase of the cell cycle. Dephosphorylation of the lamins is associated with the reassembly of the nuclear envelope in telophase. Porins are transmembrane proteins that form pores in the outer membrane of mitochondria and gram-negative bacteria. Chaperonins are cytosolic protein chaperones essential for the proper unfolding of proteins.

63. The answer is d. (*Alberts, 3/e, pp 924–925, 929–933.*) At a mitosis-inhibiting dose, colchicine functions by binding specifically and irreversibly to tubulin. The colchicine-tubulin complex is added at the positive end of the kinetochore, but it inhibits further addition of tubulin. The result is a biochemical capping of the tubulin at the growth end, preventing further tubulin addition. Cells are blocked in metaphase and cannot escape because microtubule motors are unable to function in generating the forces required for anaphase. At higher doses of colchicine, cytosolic microtubules depolymerize. Actin and myosin are involved in cytokinesis (the division of cytoplasm), whereas tubulin and the microtubules regulate separation of the daughter nuclei and their contents. Taxol, like colchicine, inhibits mitosis, but it uses a different mechanism. Taxol binds and stabilizes microtubules, causing a disruption of microtubule dynamics and inhibition of mitosis. Taxol and colchicine are similar in binding only to α,β-tubulin-dimers and microtubules.

64. The answer is b. (*Junqueira, 9/e, pp 51–53.*) Heterochromatin (A) is visible with the light microscope as condensed basophilic clumps and with the electron microscope as compact, electron-dense material within the nucleus. It is transcriptionally inactive during the interphase stage of the cell cycle, when the genetic material is normally duplicated. Heterochromatin is one of two subclassifications of chromatin on a morphologic basis. Euchromatin (B) is actively transcribed chromatin and is visible only with the use of electron microscopy. Cells with extensive euchromatin are considered metabolically active.

The nucleolus (E) is the site of ribosomal RNA synthesis. ^{3}H-uridine may be localized in the nucleolus by use of autoradiography and is often used as a marker for RNA synthesis because uridine is preferentially incorporated into RNA. RNA is packaged with ribosomal proteins to form ribosomes. The nuclear envelope (C) shields the nucleus from the cytoplasm, which allows the sequestration of the genetic material from mechanical cytoplasmic forces. The separate nuclear compartment also allows for separation of the cellular processes of transcription and translation. The nuclear envelope consists of two concentric unit membranes. The outer membrane is continuous with the rough endoplasmic reticulum. The inner nuclear membrane is associated with a lamina of fibrous proteins including intermediate filament proteins, known as lamins, that regulate the assembly and disassembly of the nuclear membrane during mitosis.

Nuclear pores (D) are interruptions in the nuclear envelope that function as aqueous channels for the passage of soluble molecules from the nucleus to the cytoplasm (ribosomal subunits) and from the cytoplasm to the nucleus (nuclear proteins synthesized in the cytoplasm and transported to the nucleus). The nuclear envelope is highly selective with selection based on pore size, the presence of nuclear import signals, and receptor recognition of RNAs.

65. The answer is a. (*McKenzie and Klein, pp 131–134. Alberts, 3/e, pp 885–890.*) The molecule labeled D in the diagram is mitosis-promoting factor (MPF, a/k/a maturation-promoting-factor). The cell cycle is controlled by a number of regulatory proteins known as the cyclin-dependent kinases (Cdks). One of these proteins, cdc2 kinase (C), combines with the mitotic cyclin (cytoplasmic oscillator) to form MPF. The cdc2 kinase has a similar concentration during all phases of the cycle; however, its enzymatic activity increases during the transition from G_2 to M phase as the cyclin (B) levels increase. The degradation of the cdc2 kinase complex occurs during the M phase (mitosis). Mitosis is controlled because cyclin accumulates during interphase and associates with the cdc2 protein to form pre-MPF, an inactive form of MPF. Then enzymes convert the complex into active MPF that triggers mitosis and a series of phosphorylations, including histones and lamins, and activates enzymes that degrade cyclin. As cyclin is destroyed, MPF disappears, and the cyclin-degrading enzymes are inactivated. At this point, cyclin accumulation begins again. The start (G_1/S) point is regulated in a similar fashion by another Cdk and a different form of cyclin.

66. The answer is c. (*McKenzie and Klein, pp 140–144. Alberts, 3/e, pp 1014–1021.*) Crossover occurs during the pachytene stage of meiosis. Meiosis is the mechanism used by the reproductive organs to generate gametes—cells with the haploid number of chromosomes. DNA synthesis occurs before meiotic prophase I begins and is followed by a G_2 phase. Cells then enter meiotic prophase I. During meiotic prophase I, maternal and paternal chromosomes are precisely paired, and recombination occurs in each pair of homologous chromosomes. The first meiotic prophase consists of five substages: leptotene, zygotene, pachytene, diplotene, and diakinesis. During metaphase I, there is random segregation of maternal and paternal chromosomes. Homologous chromosomes are aligned on the metaphase plate of the meiotic spindle in metaphase I. The second meiotic division is responsible for the reduction in the chromosome content of the cell by 50%. In meiotic division II, metaphase consists of daughter chromatids of single homologous chromosomes aligned on a metaphase plate (metaphase II). Condensation of the chromatids occurs in leptotene. In zygotene the synaptonemal complex begins to form, which initiates the close association between chromosomes known as synapsis. The bivalent is formed between the two sets of homologous chromosomes (one set maternal and one set paternal equals a pair of maternal chromatids and a pair of paternal chromatids). The four chromatids form a tetrad (bivalent). Pachytene begins as soon as the synapsis is complete and includes the period of crossover. The fully formed synaptonemal complex is present during the pachytene stage. At each point where crossover has occurred between two chromatids of the homologous chromosomes, an attachment point known as a chiasma forms. The formation of chiasmata and desynapsing (separation of the axes of the synaptonemal complex) occurs in the diplotene stage. Diakinesis is an intermediate phase between diplotene and metaphase of the first meiotic division.

67. The answer is b. (*Fauci, pp 2041–2042. Moore, Before We are Born, 5/e, pp 155, 157. Moore, Developing Human, 6/e, pp 121–122, 171, 172, 174–175.*) Cells from a patient with the most common form of Klinefelter syndrome (47,XXY genotype) will have one inactive X chromosome and, therefore, one Barr body. The formula is the number of Barr bodies equals the number of X chromosomes minus one. Klinefelter syndrome occurs about 1:500 males and is due to meiotic nondisjunction of the chromosomes. The nondisjunction is more frequent in oogenesis than spermatogenesis, and increased occurrence is directly proportional to increasing maternal age. Klinefelter may occur as 47,XXY, 48,XXYY, 48,XXXY, and

49,XXXXY. A combination of abnormal and normal genotype occurs in mosaic individuals who generally have less severe symptoms. Females have two X chromosomes, one of maternal and the other of paternal origin. Only one of the X chromosomes is active in the somatic, diploid cells of the female; the other X chromosome remains inactive and is visible in appropriately stained interphase cells as a mass of heterochromatin. Detection of the Barr body (sex chromatin) has been an efficient method for the determination of chromosomal sex and abnormalities of X-chromosome number; however, it is not definitive proof of maleness or femaleness. The genotypic sex of Klinefelter syndrome and XXX individuals would be male and female as determined by the presence or absence of the testis-determining Y chromosome. In Turner's syndrome (XO), no Barr bodies would be present. In comparison, "superfemales" (XXX) would possess two inactive X chromosomes (2 Barr bodies) and one active X chromosome. Buccal scrapings for Barr body analysis are being used less—chromosomal analysis is becoming the standard test now.

Epithelium

Questions

DIRECTIONS: Each item below contains a question or incomplete statement followed by suggested responses. Select the **one best** response to each question.

68. The primary function of the structure labeled between the arrows in the photomicrograph is

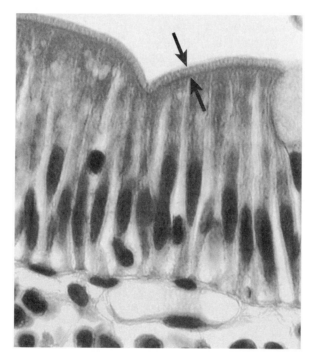

a. Extensive movement of substances over cell surfaces
b. Increase in surface area for absorption
c. Cell motility
d. Transport of intracellular organelles through the cytoplasm
e. Stretch

69. Pemphigus is a disease in which patients make antibodies to one of their own skin desmogleins involved in the formation of the junctional complexes between cells. Which of the following junctional complexes would be most affected in this disease?

a. Macula adherens
b. Hemidesmosomes
c. Zonula occludens
d. Gap junctions
e. Focal contacts

70. The mechanism for tube formation as occurs during development of the neural tube could best be explained by

a. Contraction of microfilament bundles associated with the macula adherens
b. Increased condensation of the transmembrane linkers of the desmosomes
c. Expansion of the sealing strands in the zonulae occludentes
d. Condensation of the gap junctions
e. Contraction of tonofilaments associated with desmosomes

71. In the figure below, A is a transmission electron micrograph, and B is a freeze-fracture preparation of

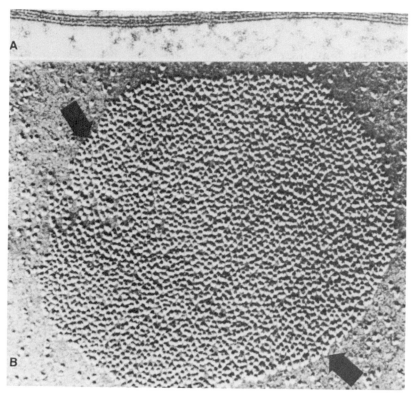

(Reproduced, with permission, from Fawcett DW: The Cell, 2/e, Philadelphia, PA: WB Saunders, 1981.)

a. Macula adherens
b. Zonula adherens
c. Terminal web
d. Terminal bar
e. Gap junction

72. Which of the following is a function of the basement membrane?

a. Molecular filtering
b. Contractility
c. Excitability
d. Modification of secreted protein
e. Active ion transport

73. Which is found only in the lamina densa of the basement membrane?

a. Proteoglycans
b. Adhesion proteins
c. Type IV collagen
d. Fibronectin
e. Laminin

74. Which of the following definitively characterizes the basolateral membrane?

a. The presence of hormone receptors
b. Endocytosis
c. Exocytosis
d. The presence of Na^+/K^+ ATPase
e. The presence of a glycocalyx

75. Which of the following statements best characterizes basal folds in epithelial cells?

a. They are involved in lipid transport
b. They function in absorption
c. They are morphologically associated with large numbers of lysosomes
d. They are associated with cells involved in active transport
e. They are visible at the light microscopic level as the terminal web

76. In Kartagener's syndrome, ciliary immotility is caused by

a. Lack of actin-myosin binding
b. Absence of microtubules
c. Lack of dynein arms
d. Mutations in kinesin
e. Lack of interactions of intermediate filaments with the plasma membrane

77. The structures labeled by the asterisks in the photomicrograph below are

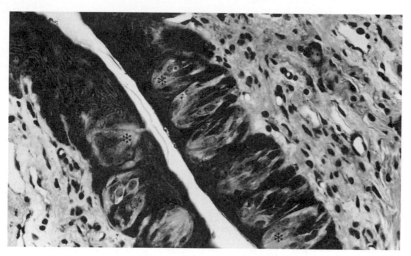

(Courtesy of Dr. John K. Young.)

a. Taste buds
b. Sympathetic ganglia
c. Filiform papillae
d. von Ebner's glands
e. Sebaceous glands

78. In the transmission electron micrograph below the structure labeled D primarily

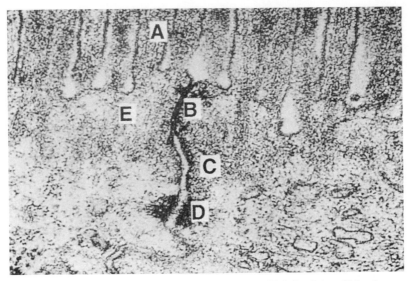

(Reproduced, with permission, from Erlandsen SL, Magney JE: Color Atlas of Histology, St. Louis, MO: CV Mosby, 1992.)

a. Forms a spot weld between cells
b. Interacts with the terminal web
c. Facilitates communication between adjacent cells
d. Seals membranes between cells
e. Moves microvilli

79. The epithelium that typically lines the urinary system is:

a. Simple columnar epithelium
b. Stratified squamous epithelium
c. Transitional epithelium
d. Pseudostratified ciliated epithelium
e. Simple squamous epithelium

80. The figure below represents a cross section of a cilium. The function of the structure labeled C is

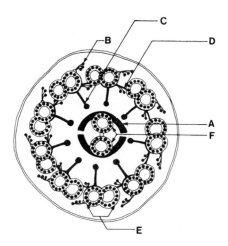

a. The source of ATPase activity
b. Production of bending
c. Inhibition of sliding between doublets
d. Regulation of the ciliary beat
e. Holding neighboring doublets together

81. The structure responsible for the linkage of the intermediate filament network of cells to the basal lamina is

a. Macula adherens
b. Zonula adherens
c. Hemidesmosomes
d. Focal contacts
e. Zonula occludens

82. The triplet arrangement of microtubules is found in

a. Centrioles
b. Cytoplasmic microtubules
c. Flagellae
d. Axonemes
e. Stereocilia

Epithelium

Answers

68. The answer is b. (*McKenzie and Klein, p 294. Young, 4/e, p 91. Junqueira, 9/e, pp 44–45, 71, 72.*) The structure labeled with the arrows in the figure is the brush border, also known as microvilli, which increases surface area for absorption. Microvilli are apical specializations of the epithelia. They are relatively uniform in length and are located on the luminal surface of cells such as small intestinal enterocytes, which are specialized for absorption. Microvilli are supported by a core of microfilaments and are capable of movement; however, cilia function in the movement of substances, such as mucus and foreign material, over the surface. The increased surface area of microvilli facilitates specialized uptake of molecules, which occurs by the processes of pinocytosis, receptor-mediated endocytosis, and phagocytosis, depending on the size and solubility of the molecules. Microtubules facilitate organellar movement within the cytoplasm, whereas cell movement is controlled by interactions between the cytoskeleton and the extracellular matrix. Transitional epithelium characteristic of the urinary system facilitates stretch.

69. The answer is a. (*Alberts, 3/e, p 956. Braunwald, 15/e pp 1841–1843.*) In pemphigus, autoantibodies to desmoglein (a member of the cadherin protein family) result in disruption of the macula adherentes (plural) or desmosomes. The desmogleins are the transmembrane linker proteins of the desmosome. Specific desmogleins are the target of the autoantibodies in different forms of the disease. Cadherins are Ca^{2+}-dependent transmembrane-linker molecules essential for cell-cell contact, so their disruption in pemphigus leads to severe blistering of the skin because of disrupted cell-cell interactions early in the differentiation of the keratinocyte (epidermal cell) and excessive fluid loss. For more details on junctional complexes, see the table in the feedback for question 81.

70. The answer is a. (*Alberts, 3/e, p 1045.*) In the formation of tubular structures from flat sheets, there is contraction of the microfilament bundles associated with the adhesion belt junctions (maculae adherentes). This occurs in neural tube formation, which involves the conversion of the neural plate into the neural tube. In the apical part of the cells, the actin filament bundles contract, narrowing the cells at their apical ends. The position of the zonula adherens, forming a contractile ring around the circumference of the cell, coupled with the contractile nature of the actin microfilament bundles is ideal for regulating morphogenetic changes. Desmosomes are involved in resisting shear forces and are not directly involved in this process. Gap junctions facilitate communication between cells. The zonulae occludentes prevent leakage between cells (see table in feedback for question 81).

71. The answer is e. *(Young, 4/e, p 89. Junqueira, 9/e, pp 67–68, 70. McKenzie and Klein, pp 88–89.)* The transmission and freeze–fracture electron micrographs illustrate the structure of a nexus, or gap junction. Gap junctions are composed of multipass transmembrane proteins that form connexons that traverse the intercellular gap. In the freeze-fracture micrograph, the connexons are seen in circular arrangements on the P face of the membrane. When the connexons of adjacent cells are in alignment, a pore of about 1.5 nm is open, and there is continuity between the interior of the two cells. It is postulated that the channel is formed in a fashion similar to the way a pore is formed by the multipass transmembrane proteins associated with the acetylcholine receptor. The gap junction maintains electrical or chemical coupling or both between cells.

72. The answer is a. *(Alberts, 3/e, pp 992–993. Junqueira, 9/e, pp 64–67.)* Epithelial cells require a basement membrane as a structural support. In most epithelia the basement membrane prevents penetration from the underlying lamina propria into the epithelium. Basement membranes are a pathway for migrating cells during development and repair processes (e.g., healing of skin wounds). In the kidney, the basement membrane of the renal glomerulus forms a selective barrier for the filtration of the plasma. Active ion transport and modification of secretory proteins are characteristics of the epithelia that are positioned on the basement membrane, not of the basement membrane itself. Contractility and excitability are characteristics that are not associated with basement membranes.

73. The answer is c. *(Alberts, 3/e, pp 989–991. Junqueira, 9/e, pp 64–67.)* Type IV collagen forms the electron-dense lamina densa of the basement membrane. At the light microscopic level, a uniform basement membrane is visible under epithelia. Ultrastructurally, basement membranes are composed of one or two electron-lucent areas (laminae rarae), that contain fibronectin, laminin, proteoglycans, and adhesive proteins. Deep to the lamina rara is the lamina densa with its electron-dense type IV collagen. The third layer is the reticular layer that is formed by the underlying connective tissue. This reticular lamina is composed of collagen fibrils formed by the connective tissue below the epithelium (basement membrane = basal lamina + reticular lamina). Fibronectin is found primarily on the connective tissue side of the basement membrane, whereas laminin is found toward the epithelial side.

74. The answer is d. (*Junqueira, 9/e, pp 79, 81–83. McKenzie and Klein, pp 153–154.*) The basolateral membrane is characterized by the ubiquitous presence of the Na^+/K^+-ATPase, responsible for generating the Na^+/K^+ gradient of the cell. Na^+ is pumped out of the cell, and K^+ is pumped into all animal cells by this ATP-dependent pump. Ouabain is a specific inhibitor of the Na^+/K^+ ATPase. Radioactive forms of this inhibitor are used to label Na^+/K^+-ATPase in the membrane in experimental studies. Hormonal receptors are found on both apical and basolateral surfaces. Neurotransmitter receptors are more prevalent on the basolateral surfaces. Exocytosis and endocytosis may occur across both apical and basolateral membranes as does ion transport. The apical surface of cells is covered by a glycocalyx that consists of oligosaccharides linked to glycoproteins and glycolipids and proteoglycans. The presence of these sugars results in a negative (polyanionic) charge on the luminal surface. Polarity of the epithelial cell is based on these apical and basolateral specializations of the cell membrane.

75. The answer is d. (*McKenzie and Klein, p 154.*) Basal folds are modifications of the basal region of the cell. These deep infoldings of the basal plasma membrane increase surface area and compartmentalize numerous mitochondria that provide energy for ionic and water transport. Distal tubule cells of the kidney and striated duct cells of the submandibular glands possess prominent basal infoldings that are observed at the light microscopic level as basal striations.

76. The answer is c. (*Junqueira, 9/e, pp 44–45, 49, 328, 409, 430. McKenzie and Klein, p 276.*) In immotile cilia syndrome, the outer dynein arms may be absent and microtubular arrangements are abnormal. The result is failure of normal ciliary action. Chronic bronchial and sinus infections are common occurrences in these patients because the cilia are unable to remove foreign material. Infertility in the male is due to absence of normal ciliary proteins in the flagella of the spermatozoa. Infertility in the female may be related to problems in movement of the ovum through the oviduct. Many of the patients diagnosed with immotile cilia syndrome are observed to have a lateral transposition of the major organs of the body (situs inversus). Normal ciliary action may be required for normal positioning of organs during development.

77. The answer is a. *(Junqueira, 9/e, pp 446–449.)* The structures shown in the photomicrograph are the taste buds. They are found within the epithelial lining of the circumvalate, foliate, and fungiform papillae of the tongue and open to the surface via a pore. They consist of a barrel-like arrangement of tall supporting and receptive cells in addition to a small population of basal cells that may serve as precursors to the more specialized cells. Receptive cells contain vesicles similar to neuronal synaptic vesicles. The vesicles are found near the base of the cell in close proximity to neuronal dendritic endings near the cell surface. Sympathetic ganglia are characterized by large euchromatic nuclei with prominent nucleoli. They are not found within epithelia. Filiform papillae are rasplike projections of the lingual epithelium. They do not possess taste buds. The von Ebner's glands are present in the connective tissue underlying the lingual epithelium near the circumvallate papillae. Their serous secretions empty via ducts into deep grooves surrounding each papilla. Sebaceous glands are located in the dermis of most regions of the skin and secrete lipids and cholesterol via a holocrine process.

78. The answer is d. *(Young, 4/e, pp 86–89. Junqueira, 9/e, pp 67–70.)* The structure labeled D in the transmission electron micrograph is the macula adherens (desmosome). It forms a spot weld or rivet between the adjacent cells and resists shearing forces on the epithelium. The transmission electron micrograph illustrates a junctional complex between two enterocytes in the small intestine. Label A represents the microvilli, which constitute the brush border. The brush border is covered by the glycocalyx and contains enzymes involved in the degradation of food in the lumen of the small intestine. The structure labeled B is the zonula occludens, which provides a tight seal between the epithelial cells. Label C marks the zonula adherens, which interacts with components of the terminal web (label E).

79. The answer is c. *(Junqueira, 9/e, pp 64–65. McKenzie and Klein, pp 155–159, 397.)* Transitional epithelium is associated with the urinary system including the lining of the renal calyces, ureters, and the bladder, as well as specific portions of the urethrae. The cells of the transitional epithelium increase in size toward the surface, or lumen. This is in contrast to the progressively flattened cells of the stratified squamous epithelium. The cells of the transitional epithelium vary in shape, depending on the degree of stretch of the wall. Epithelia perform a multitude of functions. Simple columnar epithelium is involved in absorption or secretion or both and forms most of the lining of the digestive tract. The stratified squamous epithelium is composed of several layers of cells, which begin with a basal layer of germinative cells where new cells are born and become progressively flattened toward the surface, or lumen. Stratified squamous epithelium provides a protective function and is found in sites such as the skin, where it is keratinized, and in the esophagus and anus, where it is nonkeratinized. The pseudostratified ciliated epithelium is located in the trachea and throughout the respiratory system and in the male reproductive system. As the name implies, the pseudostratified epithelium is not actually stratified. Nuclei at different levels present the appearance of stratification, but all cells reach the basal lamina. A simple squamous epithelium lines blood vessels (endothelium) and mesenteries (mesothelium), and its structure facilitates transport functions. Stratified cuboidal epithelium and stratified columnar epithelium line the sweat ducts and the excretory ducts of the parotid gland, respectively.

80. The answer is d. *(Alberts, 3/e, pp 803–806, 816–817. McKenzie and Klein, pp 105–107. Young, 4/e, p 90. Junqueira, 9/e, pp 44–45, 71–72.)* In the diagram of the cilium, the radial spokes (C) extend from the doublets toward the central pair and are involved in regulation of the ciliary beat. Cilia and the structurally similar flagella produce wavelike bending movements for propulsion of materials over the surface (e.g., movement of mucus in the tracheal epithelium) or cellular movement (e.g., that of sperm). The arrangement of the ciliary axoneme is described as a "9 + 2" structure that consists of nine outer doublets (E) of complete "A" and incomplete "B" tubules that surround a central pair of complete tubules (F). The dynein arms (B) project from the nine doublets and produce interaction between the doublets, which causes bending. Dynein is an ATPase that provides the energy for bending. The nexin links (D) hold neighboring doublets together and inhibit sliding between doublets. The inner or central sheath (A) surrounds the central doublet.

81. The answer is c. *(Alberts, 3/e, pp 950–961. McKenzie and Klein, pp 151–156. Burkitt, 3/e, pp 82–85. Junqueira, 9/e, pp 65–70.)* The hemidesmosome interacts with the extracellular matrix molecules within the basal lamina through intermediate filament proteins. The hemidesmosomes combined with the desmosomes act to distribute tensile forces through the epithelial sheet and the supporting connective tissues. For information on gap junctions see the feedback for question 71.

Junctional complexes are summarized in the table below.

Classification	Type	Function	Interactions
Occluding	Zonula occludens (tight junction)	Prevents passage of luminal substances; confers epithelial tightness or leakiness; maintains apical vs basolateral polarity	Intramembranous sealing strands occlude the space between cells (no. of strands directly proportional to tightness of epithelium)
Anchoring	Zonula adherens	Mechanical stability—cohesive function of cell groups, important during embryonic folding; transmits motile forces across epithelial sheets	Link actin filament network between cells, cadherins are transmembrane linkers
	Focal contacts	Attach cells to the ECM	Link actin filament network of cell to integrins in ECM; actin-binding proteins form link

Continued

Classification	Type	Function	Interactions
Anchoring (*cont.*)	Desmosome (macula adherens)	Spot welds (rivets) provide high tensile strength and resist shearing forces, numerous in stratified squamous epithelia	Link intermediate filaments to transmembrane proteins (cadherins: desmogleins and desmocollins). Linkage through plaque proteins (desmoplakins)
	Hemidesmosome	Increased stability of epithelia on extracellular matrix (ECM)	Link intermediate filaments in the cell to the ECM through integrins rather than cadherins
Communicating	Gap junction (nexus)	Selective communication in the form of diffusible molecules between 1 and 1.5 kD	Connexons in hexameric arrangement with central pores in adjacent cells lined up

82. The answer is a. (*Junqueira, 9/e, pp 44–45, 71–72, 417. McKenzie and Klein, pp 31, 33.*) The centriole consists of nine microtubule triplets arranged together by linking proteins to form a cartwheel arrangement. Microtubules are found in different structural patterns within the cell. The basal body is a centriole-like structure associated with the ciliary axoneme. It too has a nine-triplet arrangement of microtubules. Cytoplasmic microtubules are found in the singlet form and undergo constant association and dissociation of tubulin at their plus ends and minus ends, respectively. The axoneme has the classic "9 + 2" arrangement of microtubules. Flagella have the same "9 + 2" arrangement as cilia but are limited to one per cell and in adult humans are only found in sperm. Stereocilia are large, modified microvilli and are, therefore, not composed of microtubules.

Connective Tissue

Questions

DIRECTIONS: Each item below contains a question or incomplete statement followed by suggested responses. Select the **one best** response to each question.

83. In Marfan syndrome, there are mutations in the fibrillin gene resulting in abnormal structure. Which organ would you expect to be most affected?

a. Middle cerebral artery
b. Basilar artery
c. Aorta
d. Lymphatic vessels
e. Superior vena cava

84. The extracellular matrix and the cytoskeleton communicate across the cell membrane through

a. Proteoglycans
b. Integrins
c. Cadherins
d. Intermediate filaments
e. Microtubules

85. In Alport's syndrome, there is a defect in the α5 chain of type IV collagen. One would expect to see which of the following symptoms?

a. Abnormal bone formation
b. Hematuria
c. Abnormal hyaline cartilage
d. Skin abnormalities
e. Ruptured intervertebral disks

86. The function of fibronectin in the extracellular matrix is

a. Structural support
b. Binding of signaling molecules
c. Selectivity for passage of molecules
d. Elasticity
e. Adhesion and cell attachment

87. Desmosine and isodesmosine are amino acids unique to elastic fibers. They confer elasticity through

a. Cross-linking of microfibrils
b. Cross-linking of tropoelastin
c. Binding of proteoglycans because of the hydrophilic nature of desmosine and isodesmosine
d. Their affinity for elastase, which results in the destabilization of elastic fibers in situ
e. Electrostatic interactions of type IV collagen and elastic fibers

88. In the synthesis of collagen, the hydroxylation of proline and lysine occurs in the

a. Golgi apparatus
b. Secretory vesicles
c. Rough endoplasmic reticulum
d. Smooth endoplasmic reticulum
e. Lysosomes

89. Tropocollagen is not assembled in the cell because of the

a. Action of lysyl oxidase in the Golgi apparatus
b. Acidity of clathrin-coated vesicles
c. Presence of nonhelical registration peptides at the ends of the triple helix
d. Presence of specific collagenases in the RER and Golgi apparatus
e. Presence of specific inhibitors of peptidase activity in the Golgi apparatus

90. The principal proteoglycan with which collagen type IV interacts is

a. Fibronectin
b. Laminin
c. Entactin
d. Heparan sulfate
e. Dermatan sulfate

91. Ehlers-Danlos syndrome occurs in several forms. In type IV disease there is a defect in type III collagen synthesis. Which of the following symptoms would be most expected in a patient with this disorder?

a. Rupture of the intestinal or aortic walls
b. Hyperextensibility of the integument
c. Hypermobility of synovial joints
d. Increased degradation of proteoglycans in articular cartilages
e. Imperfections in dentin formation (dentinogenesis imperfecta)

92. The primary function of brown adipose tissue is

a. To store unilocular energy
b. To provide thermal insulation
c. To mobilize lipid for export as fatty acids
d. To initiate the shivering-induced mobilization of lipid
e. To produce heat

93. The essential role of integrins is

a. Binding of cells to the extracellular matrix
b. Binding of cells to each other
c. Maintaining structural integrity of the basement membrane
d. Binding of Type IV collagen
e. Inhibiting communication between the cytoskeleton and the extracellular matrix

94. Which of the following is necessary for successful tumor metastasis?

a. Increased cellular adhesion molecule expression at the primary site
b. Inhibition of proteolytic enzyme secretion at the primary site
c. Dehydration of the extracellular matrix
d. Maintenance of the basal lamina at the primary site
e. Cell-cell recognition at the site of new metastasis

95. Vitamin C deficiency results in

a. Excessive callus formation in healing fractures
b. Decreased breakdown of collagen
c. Formation of unstable collagen helices
d. Stimulation of prolyl hydroxylase
e. Organ fibrosis

96. Degradation of the extracellular matrix is accomplished by which of the following?

a. Lysyl oxidase
b. Plasmin
c. Plasminogen
d. Serpins
e. TIMPS

97. Which of the following is a major contributor to the tensile strength of collagen?

a. Interactions with the FACIT collagens
b. The double helical arrangement of collagen
c. Electrostatic interactions
d. Intramolecular and intermolecular cross-links
e. Low concentrations of lysine

98. Laminin functions

a. As an integrin
b. In cell-cell adhesion
c. As the insoluble scaffolding of the basal lamina
d. As the filtration molecule in the basement membrane
e. In adherence of epithelia to the basement membrane

99. Which of the following symptoms is most likely to result from systemic mastocytosis?

a. Decreased migration of eosinophils
b. Inhibition of HCl production by parietal cells
c. Decreased vascular permeability
d. Hepatic fibrosis
e. Constipation

100. Wound healing in the skin is mediated by various cytokines and growth factors and results in a series of repair steps. Platelet-derived growth factor (PDGF) is being used effectively to treat poorly healing wounds. Increased levels of PDGF will

a. Inhibit proliferation of fibroblasts at the wound site
b. Inhibit type I collagen synthesis at the wound site
c. Inhibit migration of macrophages to the wound site
d. Stimulate integrins on the surface of platelets
e. Stimulate proliferation of vascular smooth muscle

101. Reticular fibers in lymphoid organs are comprised of which collagen?

a. Collagen type I
b. Collagen type III
c. Collagen type IV
d. Collagen type V
e. Collagen type IX

102. The cells labeled with the arrows in the figure synthesize

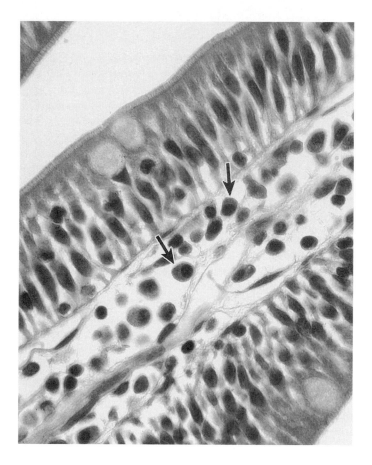

a. Collagen
b. Heparin and histamine
c. Interleukin-1
d. IgE
e. Myeloperoxidase

Connective Tissue

Answers

83. The answer is c. (*McKenzie and Klein, p 163. Alberts, 3/e, p 986. Braunwald, 15/e, pp 1430–1431, 2298–2299.*) The aorta is the most affected organ because of the extensive elastin in the wall, and dissecting aortic aneurysms are common in these patients. Marfan syndrome is an autosomal dominant disease in which persons develop abnormal elastic tissue. Malformations include cardiovascular (valve problems as well as aortic aneurysm), skeletal (abnormal height and severe chest deformities), and ocular systems. The molecular basis of the disease is a mutation in the fibrillin gene. The lens is also often affected in patients with Marfan syndrome. The result is the dislocation of the lens because of loss of elasticity in the suspensory ligament.

84. The answer is b. (*McKenzie and Klein, pp 86, 94–95. Alberts, 3/e, p 997.*) The integrins are transmembrane heterodimers that act as membrane receptors for extracellular matrix components. The best examples are the fibronectin receptor and the laminin receptor. The receptor structure includes an intracytosolic portion that binds to the actin cytoskeleton through the attachment proteins talin or α-actinin. The extracellular portion has specificity for extracellular matrix molecules. The N-cadherins function as transmembrane glycoproteins involved in the formation of parts of the intercellular junctional complexes. Proteoglycans are located on the extracellular surface of the plasma membrane and throughout the extracellular matrix. Cadherins are components of the desmosome and zonula adherens. Microtubules and intermediate filaments are found intracellularly and constitute the cytoskeleton.

85. The answer is b. (*Braunwald, 15/e, p 2300.*) Alport's syndrome results in hematuria from the loss of the normal filtering properties of the glomerular basement membrane, leading to nephritis and eventually renal failure. Alport's is an X-linked syndrome in which there is an absence of the $\alpha5(IV)$ chain, resulting in thickening of the basement membrane with splitting of the lamina densa. The basement membrane is composed primarily of type IV collagen, heparan sulfate proteoglycan, laminin, and entactin. Basement membranes are usually composed of an electron-lucent layer (lamina rara) closest to the epithelial layer and the electron-dense layer (lamina densa) below the lamina rara. Type IV collagen is found in the lamina densa of the basement membrane.

86. The answer is e. *(Alberts, 3/e, pp 986–987. McKenzie and Klein, p 167. Junqueira, 9/e, pp 92, 95.)* Fibronectin is an adhesive glycoprotein that is important for cell attachment. It is important for modulation of cell migration in the adult and during development. Neural crest and other cells appear to be guided along fibronectin-coated pathways in the embryo. Fibronectin is found in three forms: a plasma form that is involved in blood clotting; a cell surface form, which binds to the cell surface transiently; and a matrix form, which is fibrillar in arrangement. Fibronectin contains a cell-binding domain (RGD sequence), a collagen-binding domain, and a heparin-binding domain. Type IV collagen is responsible for providing support. Elastin is responsible for the elasticity of structures such as the pinna of the ear and the wall of the aorta. Proteoglycans are responsible for the selective passage of molecules and the binding of growth factors and other signaling molecules in the extracellular matrix.

87. The answer is b. *(Junqueira, 9/e, pp 103–105.)* The amino acids desmosine and isodesmosine are unique to elastic fibers. They are responsible for the cross-linking of tropoelastin through the lysine residues. Lysyl oxidase is the enzyme that catalyzes this reaction. The microfibrils composed of fibrillin are glycoproteinaceous and facilitate formation of the elastin molecules but are not influenced by lysyl oxidase. Elastase is a serine protease that specifically degrades elastin. Interactions occur between type III collagen and elastic fibers. The collagen may serve to limit the stretch of the elastic components.

88. The answer is c. *(Alberts, 3/e, pp 980–982. Junqueira, 9/e, pp 96–100.)* Prolyl and lysyl oxidase are the two enzymes that carry out hydroxylation of proline and lysine. The process is both co- and posttranslational and, therefore, occurs during, or more often, after the amino acids are inserted into nascent collagen polypeptide chains in the RER. These two amino acids are characteristic of collagen. Hydroxyproline, which constitutes 10% of collagen, is often used to determine the collagen content of various tissues. Hydroxylation of proline stabilizes the triple helix through interchain hydrogen bonds, and hydroxylation of lysine is critical for the cross-linking stage of collagen assembly.

89. The answer is c. (*McKenzie and Klein, pp 163–164. Alberts, 3/e, p 981. Junqueira, 9/e, pp 96–100.*) Nonhelical registration peptides at the ends of the triple helix prevent tropocollagen assembly in the RER, Golgi apparatus, and secretory vesicles. Collagen is synthesized as pro-α-chains, which are assembled into procollagen molecules (triple helix) in the rough endoplasmic reticulum. Procollagen is subsequently transported in transfer vesicles to the Golgi for packaging into secretory vesicles. Transport of secretory vesicles is an energy- and microtubule-dependent process. Outside of the cell, N-terminal and C-terminal specific procollagen peptidases cleave the nonhelical registration peptides, which results in the formation of tropocollagen. Tropocollagen spontaneously assembles in a staggered array to form collagen fibrils. Lysyl oxidase is an extracellular enzyme responsible for the formation of covalent cross-links between tropocollagen molecules. Fibrils form collagen fibers under the influence of other extracellular matrix constituents, such as proteoglycans and glycoproteins. Collagenases specifically cleave tropocollagen in the extracellular matrix.

90. The answer is d. (*McKenzie and Klein, pp 165–167. Alberts, 3/e, pp 972–978. Junqueira, 9/e, pp 90–91.*) Heparan sulfate is primarily associated with type IV collagen in basal laminae. Proteoglycans are large molecules that maintain hydration space in the extracellular matrix. They are composed of glycosaminoglycans such as chondroitin sulfate, dermatan sulfate, heparan sulfate, heparin, and keratan sulfate. Glycosaminoglycans are covalently linked to core proteins to form proteoglycans. The notable exception is hyaluronic acid, which forms the core of proteoglycan aggregates produced by the interaction between proteoglycan subunits and hyaluronic acid. Dermatan sulfate is found predominantly in the skin, blood vessels, and heart. Fibronectin is a fibrillar protein, whereas laminin and entactin are structural glycoproteins found in the extracellular matrix.

91. The answer is a. (*Junqueira, 9/e, p 102–103, 211–212.*) In Ehlers-Danlos disorder type IV there is improperly formed type III collagen, which is responsible for the elasticity of the intestinal and aortic walls. In this form of the disorder there are errors in the transcription of type III collagen mRNA or in translation of this mRNA. Hyperextensible skin occurs in Ehlers-Danlos type VI disorder in which problems with the hydroxylation of the amino acid lysine and subsequent cross-linking result in enhanced elasticity. Type VII Ehlers-Danlos disorder involves a specific deficiency in an amino terminal procollagen peptidase. This results from a genetic mutation that alters the propeptide sequence in such a way that the molecular orientation and cross-linking are adversely affected. The result is hypermobility of synovial joints. Increased degradation of proteoglycans occurs in osteoarthritis. Type I collagen is found in dentin.

92. The answer is e. *(McKenzie and Klein, p 162. Junqueira, 9/e, pp 124–125.)* Brown adipose tissue is multilocular and is found in the human fetus and neonate. Brown fat is involved in nonshivering thermogenesis and generates heat, probably as a protective device for developing organs in the fetus and neonate. Adipose tissue is specialized for lipid storage and functions as a thermal insulator and shock absorber. White adipose tissue is unilocular, and the cells have a single, large lipid droplet in the cytoplasm that provides the "signet-ring" appearance often described for fat cells. Brown adipose tissue has a multilocular appearance and a brown color because of the many mitochondria in these adipocytes. Both types of fat tissue are highly vascularized and function in protection from the cold. Brown fat specifically is involved in heat production, whereas white fat is a true thermal insulator. The former is found in hibernating animals and neonatal humans.

In fat, norepinephrine activates the cyclic AMP cascade through adenylate cyclase. The cyclic AMP activates hormone-sensitive lipase, which removes triglycerides from the stored lipid and hydrolyzes free fatty acids. In white adipocytes, the released fatty acids and glycerol are exported from the cells. In brown adipose tissue the fatty acids are used within the cell. However, the electron transport system is uncoupled from oxidative phosphorylation, which results in the production of heat instead of ATP. Heat is transferred to the blood by the extensive capillary networks found in brown adipose tissue.

Shivering initiates the mobilization of lipid in white adipose tissue because shivering requires energy.

93. The answer is a. *(Alberts, 3/e, pp 995–1000.)* Integrins bind cells to the extracellular matrix (ECM). The fibronectin receptor is the most well-studied member of this class of transmembrane linkers. The integrins recognize RGD cell-binding sequences. Through interactions with talin, the fibronectin receptor links the cytoskeleton with molecules in the extracellular matrix such as fibronectin. Receptors for fibronectin are, therefore, instrumental in regulation of cell motility. Integrins on the surface of blood platelets bind fibrinogen and fibronectin and, therefore, play an important role in blood clotting.

94. The answer is e. *(Alberts, 3/e, pp 1269–1270. Kumar, 6/e, pp 139–140, 161–163. Braunwald, 15/e, pp 521–523.)* Tumor metastasis involves cell-cell recognition as the migrating cells establish a new tumor site, migration, and differentiation. Tumor cells are initially released from adhesion to each other and to the extracellular matrix. Dissolution of basement membrane is required for release of tumor cells from the source and passage through connective tissues and between endothelial cells of the blood or lymphatic vessels. Collagenases and other extracellular proteases are involved in this process. At the site of a new metastasis, there is a reestablishment of cell-cell and cell-matrix interactions. Very few of the tumor cells released into the bloodstream have metastatic capability or are successful in the production of a tumor at a new site.

95. The answer is c. *(Alberts, 3/e, pp 980–981. Junqueira, 9/e, pp 102, 120, 279.)* Scurvy, or vitamin C deficiency, results in an inability to form normal collagen triple helices. In scurvy, the resulting collagen is less stable and is subject to denaturation and proteolytic breakdown. This results partially from slower secretion of collagen from fibroblasts. The collagen formed is not normally hydroxylated at proline and lysine residues because of the absence of vitamin C, which is a specific cofactor for hydroxylation of proline and lysine. Bone growth, development of the dentition, and wound and fracture healing as well as the general stability of adult organs are inhibited because of the importance of collagen in the maintenance of structural support. Periodontal bleeding and ulceration are also common symptoms in scurvy.

96. The answer is b. *(Alberts, 3/e, pp 993–995.)* The extracellular matrix is degraded by plasmin, a protease. It solubilizes fibrin clots and degrades protein fibrinogen and a few coagulation factors. There are two groups of proteases: metalloproteases and serine proteases. Collagenase is one of the metalloproteases. Urokinase-type plasminogen activator (U-PA), a serine protease, converts the inactive molecule plasminogen to the active protease plasmin. Inhibitors of metalloproteases (TIMPs) and serpins are responsible for the inactivation of metalloproteases and serine proteases. Lysyl oxidase is involved in the cross-linking of collagen during synthesis.

97. The answer is d. (*Alberts, 3/e, pp 978–985.*) The fibrillar collagens establish tensile strength at a number of levels including intra- and intermolecular cross-links. Covalent bonding occurs through the OH⁻ groups of hydroxylysine and hydroxyproline and serves to stabilize the triple helix. The triple helix itself functions to resist tensile forces. The degree of cross-linking varies from tissue to tissue. For example, it is highly extensive in tendons. The organization of collagen in tissues also varies, depending on function, from the layered appearance in bone to the axial parallel bundles in tendons and the wickered pattern in skin. The interactions with fibril-associated collagens (with interrupted triple helices) regulate orientation and are also important in establishing tissue organization and flexibility. Electrostatic interactions do not play a significant role in maintenance of collagen tensile strength.

98. The answer is e. (*Alberts, 3/e, pp 990–992. Junqueira, 9/e, pp 64, 66, 92, 95.*) Laminin is a glycoprotein and a major component of all basement membranes that is involved in cell adherence to the basal lamina. Both laminin and fibronectin are found in the basal lamina, but on opposite sides of the lamina densa because laminin appears to bind to epithelial cells and fibronectin to the underlying connective tissue cells. Laminin contains both RGD and YIGSR cell-binding sites as well as binding sites for collagen, entactin, and heparan sulfate proteoglycan. The highly charged glycosaminoglycans are responsible for the filtration characteristics of the basement membrane (e.g., renal glomerular basement membrane).

99. The answer is d. (*Braunwald, 15/e, pp 1918–1920. Junqueira, 9/e, pp 110–113.*) Periportal fibrosis of the liver often occurs in systemic mastocytosis due to the extensive infiltration of mast cells into the liver. Mastocytosis is a disease in which there is an excessive production of mast cells by the bone marrow. The result is an excessive release of the bioactive products contained in mast cell granules: histamine, heparin, eosinophil chemotactic factor of anaphylaxis (ECF-A), slow-reacting substance of anaphylaxis (SRS-A), and leukotrienes. Excessive production of acid by the parietal cells of the stomach occurs because of the overstimulation of histamine receptors on these cells. This can result in peptic ulcers and gastritis. Mastocytosis also induces urticaria pigmentosa, including edema (caused by the increased vascular permeability induced by histamine and SRS-A) and infiltration of eosinophils (attracted by ECF-A), which causes itching. Lower gastrointestinal tract symptoms include increased motility and diarrhea due to the stimulation by mast cell contents.

100. The answer is e. (*Alberts, 3/e, pp 893–894. Kumar, 6/e, pp 51, 55–57.*) Platelet-derived growth factor (PDGF) stimulates proliferation of vascular smooth muscle cells to facilitate blood vessel repair. Wound healing is a complex process initiated by damage to capillaries in the dermis. The clot forms through the interaction of integrins on the surface of blood platelets with fibrinogen and fibronectin. Fibrin is the primary protein that constructs the three-dimensional structure of the clot. Macrophages and fibroblasts are attracted by platelet-derived growth factor (PDGF). In addition to its effect on vascular smooth muscle, PDGF also stimulates proliferation of fibroblasts and extracellular matrix protein synthesis by fibroblasts at the wound site. A scar is formed as a very dense region of type I collagen fibers. Macrophages remove debris at the wound site and are also involved in the remodeling of the scar.

101. The answer is b. (*Alberts, 3/e, p 983. Junqueira, 9/e, pp 95–105. Mayne, pp 94–97, 195–221.*) The reticular fibers form the support for lymphoid organs such as the spleen, bone marrow, and lymph nodes and are composed of type III collagen.

Collagen is a family of extracellular matrix proteins, all of which contain three α chains that vary in structure. There are about 20 defined types. The most important of these are summarized in the table below.

Type	Location	Function and Other Information
I	General C.T., bone, and fibrocartilage	Most abundant type of collagen, 67-nm periodicity, tensile strength
II	Hyaline and elastic cartilage	Thinner fibrils than type I, tensile strength, electrostatic interactions between type II collagen and proteoglycan aggregates form the molecular basis for the rigidity of hyaline cartilage

Type	Location	Function and Other Information
III	Spleen, bone marrow, and lymph nodes	Reticular framework, stains with silver
IV	Basement membrane	Filtration, support, meshwork scaffolding, interacts with heparan sulfate proteoglycan to produce a polyanionic change distribution that facilitates selective filtration; synthesized by epithelia; it retains propeptides that are used to form a meshwork; also interacts with fibronectin
V	Placental basement membrane, muscle basal lamina	Linkage function in basement membrane(?)
VII	Basement membrane of skin and amnion	Anchoring fibers
VIII	Endothelium	Unknown function
IX–XII	Cartilage	Fibril-associated collagens with interrupted triple helices (FACIT) regulate orientation and function of fibrillar collagens

102. The answer is d. (*McKenzie and Klein, p 162. Alberts, 3/e, pp 1198–1199. Young, 4/e, pp 11, 16, 78, 200. Roitt, 5/e, pp 13–29.*) The cells delineated by the arrows in the photomicrograph are plasma cells that are responsible for immunoglobulin (antibody) production. Plasma cells produce all the immunoglobulins: IgG, IgA, IgM, IgD, and IgE and are derived from B lymphocytes. The differentiation of plasma cells requires macrophages (antigen-presenting cells), which phagocytose and present antigen + MHC II and T-helper cells. Plasma cells are characterized by eccentric nuclei with coarse granules of heterochromatin arranged in a radial pattern about the nuclear envelope. Membrane-bound ribosomes are extremely plentiful, providing the cytoplasm with a characteristic intense basophilia. The ribosomes are involved in antibody production, principally immunoglobulin G (IgG). The juxtanuclear region, which does not stain, represents the Golgi complex, in which the antibodies are processed for secretion. The function and origin of the connective tissue cells is summarized in the table below.

Cell Type	Origin	Function
Fibroblast	Mesenchyme	Synthesis of fiber (collagen, elastic, reticular) and ground substance (proteoglycans and glycoproteins of connective tissue matrix
Macrophages (e.g., Kupffer cells, Langerhans cells and microglia)	Monocyte (bone marrow)	Phagocytosis, antigen presentation, produce and respond to cytokines.
Lymphocytes		
T lymphocytes	Bone marrow (thymus-educated)	Cell-mediated immunity (CD_8^+) and helper T cells (CD_4^+)
B lymphocytes	Bone marrow (bone marrow-educated)	Humoral immunity
Plasma cell	B lymphocyte	Immunoglobulin secretion
Neutrophils (PMNs)	Bone marrow	First cells to enter an inflammation site, secrete myeloperoidase, phagocytose bacteria, and die (forming pus)
Eosinophils	Bone marrow	Source of major basic protein, histaminase (breakdown of histamine), arylsulfatases (degradation of leukotrienes), phagocytosis of antigen-antibody complexes and parasites
Basophils	Bone marrow (different stem cell from mast cell)	Blood source of histamine
Mast cells connective tissue mast cells (CTMC) and mucosal mast cells (MMC)	Bone marrow	CTMC are T-lymphocyte independent, MMC are T-lymphocyte dependent, secrete histamine and slow-reacting substance of anaphylaxis [(SRS-A) increase vascular permeability], heparin (anticoagulant), eosinophil chemoattractant factor of anaphylaxis [(ECF-A), chemoattraction of eosinophils], leukotrienes (smooth muscle contraction)

Specialized Connective Tissues: Bone and Cartilage

Questions

DIRECTIONS: Each item below contains a question or incomplete statement followed by suggested responses. Select the **one best** response to each question.

103. Intramembranous ossification differs from endochondral ossification in the

a. Action of osteoblasts
b. Light microscopic appearance of the adult bone
c. Ultrastructural appearance of the adult bone
d. Presence of woven bone early in the ossification process
e. Microenvironment in which ossification occurs

104. After birth, growth in the length of long bones occurs primarily through

a. Increased bone deposition under the periosteum
b. The action of osteoblasts in the primary ossification center
c. The action of osteoblasts in the secondary ossification center
d. Appositional growth from the periphery
e. Interstitial growth of cartilage cells in the epiphyses

105. The molecular basis for shock absorption and resiliency within articular cartilage is the

a. Electrostatic interaction of proteoglycans with type IV collagen
b. Ability of glycosaminoglycans to bind anions
c. Noncovalent binding of glycosaminoglycans to protein cores
d. Sialic acid residues in the glycoproteins
e. Hydration of glycosaminoglycans

106. The cells delineated by the box in the light micrograph of a developing long bone synthesize

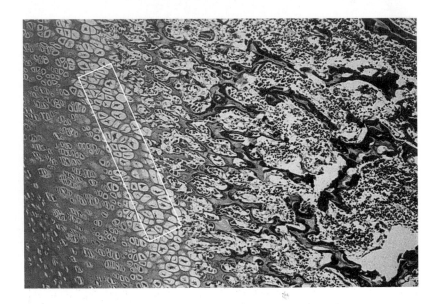

a. Cyclins
b. Acid phosphatase
c. Alkaline phosphatase
d. Type I collagen
e. Osteocalcin

107. The stimulation and activation of the cell in the accompanying electron micrograph (A) and labeled by "C" in the light micrograph (B) is involved in which of the following?

a. Mechanical grinding of the bone matrix
b. Synthesis of alkaline phosphatase
c. Response to vitamin D through receptors on this cell
d. Regulation by PTH receptors on this cell
e. Proton pump activity similar to a parietal cell

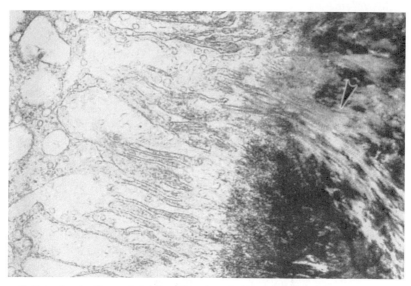

(A. Reproduced, with permission, from Erlandsen SL, Magney JE: Color Atlas of Histology. St. Louis, MO: CV Mosby, 1992.)

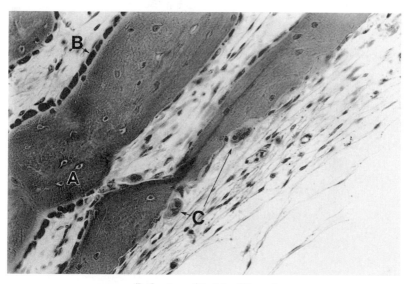

(B. Courtesy of Dr. John K. Young.)

108. A patient with rheumatoid arthritis would exhibit which of the following joint changes?

a. Loss of the proteoglycan matrix and fibrillation in the articular cartilage during the early stages
b. Decreased levels of fibrinogen in the synovial fluid
c. Formation of osteophytes at the articular margins and eburnation of large weight-bearing joints in the later stages
d. Decreased number of leukocytes including PMNs in the synovial fluid
e. Heterologous autoantibodies deposited in joint surface

109. The first step in fracture healing is the formation of the

a. Internal callus
b. External callus
c. Clot
d. Pannus
e. Granulation tissue

110. A 55-year-old woman presents with pain in her right hip and thigh. The pain started approximately six months ago and is a deep ache that worsens when she stands or walks. Your examination reveals increased warmth over the right thigh. The only laboratory abnormalities are alkaline phosphatase 656 IU/L (normal 23 to 110 IU/L), elevated 24-h urine hydroxyproline, and osteocalcin 13 ng/mL (normal 6 ng/mL). X-ray of hips and pelvis shows osteolytic lesions and regions with excessive osteoblastic activity. Bone scan shows significant uptake in the right proximal femur. Which of the following would you include in your differential diagnosis?

a. Paget's disease
b. Multiple myeloma
c. Osteomalacia
d. Osteoporosis
e. Hypoparathyroidism

111. A 66-year-old man with no previous significant illness presents with back pain. The patient had felt well except for an increase in fatigue over the past few months. He suddenly felt severe low back pain while raising his garage door. Physical examination reveals a well-developed white male in acute pain. His pulse is 88 beats per minute and blood pressure is 150/90 mmHg. The conjunctivae are pale. There is marked tenderness to percussion over the lumbar spine. The following laboratory data are obtained: hemoglobin 11.0 g/dL (normal 13 to 16 g/dL), serum calcium 12.3 mg/dL (normal 8.5 to 11 mg/dL), abnormal serum protein electrophoresis with a monoclonal IgG spike, urine positive for Bence Jones protein, and abnormal plasma cells in bone marrow. X-rays reveal lytic lesions of the skull and pelvis and a compression fracture of lumbar vertebrae. Your diagnosis would be

a. Osteoporosis
b. Osteomalacia
c. Multiple myeloma
d. Hypoparathyroidism
e. Paget's disease

112. A 46-year-old woman presents with a pain in the left leg that worsens on weight-bearing. An x-ray shows demineralization and a decalcified (EDTA-treated) biopsy shows reduction in bone quantity. The patient had undergone menopause at age 45 without estrogen replacement. She reports long-standing diarrhea. In addition, laboratory tests show low levels of 25-hydroxyvitamin D, calcium, and phosphorus and elevated alkaline phosphatase. A second bone biopsy, which was not decalcified, shows uncalcified osteoid on all the bone surfaces. On the basis of these data, your diagnosis would be

a. Osteoporosis
b. Osteomalacia
c. Scurvy
d. Paget's disease
e. Hypoparathyroidism

113. Patients with Cushing's syndrome often show osteoporotic changes. Which of the following is involved in the etiology of osteoporosis induced by Cushing's syndrome?

a. Decreased glucocorticoid levels that result in decreased quality of the bone deposited
b. Excess deposition of osteoid
c. Stimulation of intestinal calcium absorption
d. Decreased PTH levels
e. Bone fragility resulting from excess bone resorption

114. DiGeorge syndrome is a congenital malformation in which the embryologic derivatives of the third and fourth branchial pouches fail to form. Which of the following would be expected to occur in children with this syndrome?

a. Absence of the parafollicular cells
b. Increased numbers of cells in the deep cortex of the lymph nodes
c. Tetany
d. Excess activity of osteoclasts
e. Increased Ca^{2+} levels in the blood

115. This electron micrograph is a preparation from bone matrix in close proximity to the cellular components. Which of the following statements is true in regard to these structures?

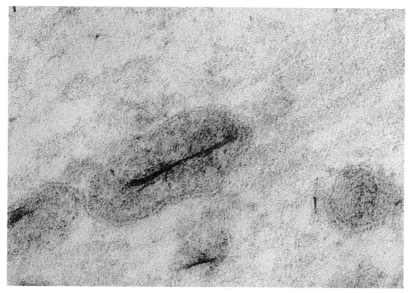

(Courtesy of Dr. H. Clarke Anderson.)

a. They contain type I collagen
b. They are absent during endochondral bone formation
c. They bud off from osteoclasts
d. They may serve a "seed crystal" function in developing bone
e. They contain acid phosphatase

116. The collagenous protein in bone subserves which of the following functions?

a. Growth factor
b. Binding of ionic calcium and physiologic hydroxyapatite
c. Formation of the three-dimensional lattice of the matrix
d. Cell attachment
e. Binding of mineral components to the matrix

117. In the diagram of a joint below, the structure labeled C is the

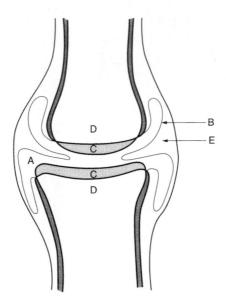

a. Site of macrophage-like cells that phagocytose particles from the synovial fluid
b. Site of cells that synthesize the synovial fluid
c. Structure replaced by the pannus in rheumatoid arthritis
d. Initial site of inflammation in rheumatoid arthritis
e. Perichondrium

Specialized Connective Tissues: Bone and Cartilage

Answers

103. The answer is e. (*McKenzie and Klein, pp 180–181. Junqueira, 9/e, pp 141–145.*) The difference between endochondral and intramembranous ossification is the microenvironment in which bone formation occurs. In both cases, bone development occurs by essentially the same process, the synthesis of collagen and other matrix components by osteoblasts and the calcification of the matrix through the action of alkaline phosphatase from osteoblasts. Bone development occurs in two different locations, which differ in the presence or absence of cartilage models of the bones. For example, in the flat bones of the skull, bone formation occurs through the differentiation of osteoprogenitor cells from mesoderm and is accompanied by vascularization. This is known as intramembranous ossification. In the other form of ossification (endochondral), osteoprogenitor cells differentiate into chondrocytes and establish a cartilage model of the long bone. This method occurs in bones such as the humerus and femur. The cartilage model of each bone is replaced by bone using the cartilage as a scaffolding for bone formation. Bone formed by the two methods cannot be distinguished microscopically or macroscopically. In both endochondral and intramembranous ossification, the first bone formed is woven bone (also known as primary bone). This bone is replaced by adult, lamellar bone through a remodeling process.

104. The answer is e. (*McKenzie and Klein, pp 183–184. Junqueira, 9/e, pp 141–145.*) Growth in the length of long bones after birth (postnatally) occurs through cell proliferation of immature chondrocytes (chondroblasts) in the secondary ossification centers of the epiphyses. Fetal development of long bones occurs by the process of endochondral ossification in which a cartilage model is replaced by bone. Before birth in endochondral ossification, the growth in length of the long bone occurs primarily through the proliferation of chondrocytes in the proliferative zone within the diaphysis of the cartilage model (primary ossification center). Growth in the width of the long bone occurs by the addition of osteoblasts from the periosteum (periosteal collar). This is essentially a form of appositional growth without a cartilage intermediate. It is one of the best examples of intramembranous ossification, even though it occurs in the development of a long bone. The action of osteoblasts is to deposit bone matrix and secrete alkaline phosphatase. The lengthwise expansion of long bones occurs through chondrocyte (chondroblast, cartilage cell) proliferation.

105. The answer is e. (*McKenzie and Klein, pp 169–171. Alberts, 3/e, pp 975–976. Junqueira, 9/e, p 129.*) The hydration of the glycosaminoglycans plays an important role in shock absorption and enhances the resiliency of the cartilage. This role is particularly important in the articular cartilages, which receive pressure during joint movement and are required to resist strong compressive forces. Proteoglycans are the major component of the ground substance of cartilage. They possess a large anionic charge because of the presence of sulfate, hydroxyl, and carboxyl groups within the glycosaminoglycans, which join to form proteoglycan subunits by linking with a core protein. The proteoglycan subunits (monomers) subsequently form an aggregate by linking noncovalently to hyaluronic acid. These aggregates react electrostatically with type II collagen, probably through the sulfate groups of the glycosaminoglycans. The negative charge of the glycosaminoglycans facilitates the binding of cations and the transport of electrolytes and water within the matrix. This is an important aspect of cartilage metabolism because the chondrocytes depend on diffusion to obtain nutrients or to dispose of waste products. Glycoproteins are not a major constituent of the cartilage matrix.

106. The answer is c. (*McKenzie and Klein, pp 181–184. Young, 4/e, pp 184–187.*) The light micrograph illustrates a developing long bone. The zone shown is the region of chondrocyte hypertrophy and the cells synthesize alkaline phosphatase, which calcifies the cartilage matrix. This secretion results in the eventual death of these cells that depend on diffusion to obtain oxygen and nutrients from the matrix. During development of the long bones of the body, specific zones are established as a cartilage model of a long bone is converted to mature bone. The zones from the epiphysis toward the center of the shaft (diaphysis) are as follows: resting zone, proliferative zone, hypertrophy zone, and zone of calcified cartilage that is used as the scaffolding for the deposition of bone. The periosteal bud represents the ingrowth of blood vessels (angiogenesis), bone marrow, and osteoprogenitor cells into the diaphysis. The angiogenesis is required for bone formation. Bone is formed by the action of osteoblasts forming type I collagen, noncollagenous proteins (e.g., osteocalcin, osteopontin, and osteonectin), and alkaline phosphatase, which plays an essential role in mineralization of the osteoid. Cyclins are synthesized by cells passing through the cell cycle (cells in the proliferative zone), acid phosphatase is synthesized by osteoclasts, and type I collagen and osteocalcin are sythesized by osteoblasts.

107. The answer is e. *(McKenzie and Klein, pp 176–178, 186–188. Alberts, 3/e, pp 1182–1184. Guyton, 10/e, pp 904–910. Greenspan, 6/e, pp 274, 278–279, 286–287. Junqueira, 9/e, pp 135–137.)* The cells indicated in the micrographs are osteoclasts that function by releasing lytic enzymes into the calcified matrix and not through a grinding action. The osteoclast acidifies the microenvironment beneath the ruffled border by pumping protons provided in the cytosol from carbonic anhydrase in similar fashion to parietal cells of the stomach. The bone compartment around the ruffled border of the osteoclast is, therefore, analogous to a secondary lysosome in function, albeit an extracellular region. The electron micrograph illustrates the typical ultrastructure of an osteoclast with its distinctive ruffled border. The light micrograph illustrates the position of the osteoclasts (multinucleate cells) in small depressions in the bone (Howship's lacunae). The arrowhead in the electron micrograph indicates collagen within the degraded bone matrix. The plasmalemma of the osteoclast adjacent to the resorbing bone surface is thrown into folds and villous-like processes with tips that reach and even enter the bone surface (ruffled border). The osteoclast is attached to the bone surface, and the resorption area is sealed off by the presence of contractile proteins in the cytoplasm lateral to the site of the ruffled border. The basolateral membrane of the osteoclast possesses a Na^+/K^+-ATPase pump.

Osteoclasts are of hematopoietic origin and arise from the monocytic lineage. They are not the source of monocytes. Osteoclasts are responsive to a number of hormones including parathyroid hormone (PTH), calcitonin, and $1,25(OH)_2$-vitamin D_3. PTH is the major regulator of osteoclastic activity, increasing the number of osteoclasts as well as ruffled border activity. The osteoclasts respond to low serum Ca^{2+} by removing calcium from bone. PTH receptors are located on osteoblasts, not osteoclasts, so PTH affects osteoblasts to release soluble factors that stimulate osteoclasts.

(Vitamin D receptors are also present on osteoblasts and absent from osteoclasts). This indirect receptor effect links the osteoblast and osteoclast in the so-called ARF cycle [(activation of osteoclasts → resorption → formation (of bone)].

Ca^{2+} released by the action of osteoclasts enters the bone fluid, the extracellular fluid, and subsequently the blood. Calcitonin is only responsible for transient changes in bone resorption. In the presence of high Ca^{2+}, calcitonin is synthesized and released from C (interfollicular) cells of the thyroid, which decreases ruffled-border activity. Calcitonin receptors are located on osteoclasts. Long-term responses to elevated Ca^{2+} are mediated by lower PTH levels rather than increased calcitonin production. This is exemplified in patients with an absence of calcitonin secretion (e.g., after thyroidectomy), or with stimulated levels of calcitonin (e.g., in medullary thyroid carcinoma) who exhibit relatively normal bone metabolism. However, calcitonin measurements are an important tool in the diagnosis of medullary thyroid carcinoma, a malignancy of thyroid cells.

108. The answer is e. (*Kumar, 6/e, pp 109–111, 681–682.*) Arthritis involves inflammatory changes in a joint. Rheumatoid arthritis is an autoimmune disease in which a rheumatoid factor composed of heterologous autoantibodies directed against serum γ-globulin (IgG) appears. Rheumatoid factor is present in the serum of 85 to 90% of patients with rheumatoid arthritis. Deposition of rheumatoid factor can be pathogenic and leads to inflammatory destruction of the joint surface. Cell-mediated immunity is also involved in rheumatoid arthritis. Alteration of the synovial membrane results in the formation of a pannus, or inflammatory, hypertrophic synovial villus. The presence of the pannus and release of lysosomal enzymes from the pannus result in degradation of the cartilage. This is followed by hypertrophy and hyperplasia of the articular cartilages, which often leads to bone formation across the joint with welding of the bones together (ankylosis). Because of the inflammation in rheumatoid arthritis, there are elevated numbers of leukocytes, in particular PMNs, in the synovial fluid. During rheumatoid arthritis, fibrinogen, another indicator of inflammatory responses, is elevated. Osteoarthritis begins with loss of hydrated glycosaminoglycans, followed by death of chondrocytes, fibrillation, and development of fissures in the cartilage matrix. The severe wear and tear of osteoarthritis increases with age. During the breakdown of the articular cartilages, the width of the underlying bone increases. Osteoarthritis typically includes the formation of reactive bone spurs called osteophytes, which may break off to form foreign bodies in the joint space (i.e., "joint mice"). In the fingers, osteoarthritis primarily affects distal interphalangeal joints, where it produces painful nodular enlargements called Heberden's nodes. Large weight-bearing joints are also usually involved in osteoarthritis and often exhibit eburnation in the late stages when the articular cartilages have been worn down and result in an osseous articular surface

109. The answer is c. (*McKenzie and Klein, pp 190–192. Junqueira, 9/e, pp 143, 145–146.*) In the healing of fractures, the first step is clotting of extravasated blood. The clot is organized into a callus by granulation tissue that consists of fibroblasts, osteogenic cells, and budding capillaries. An internal (bony) callus forms where local bone factors are most active (i.e., in close proximity to the periosteum and endosteum that retain osteogenic potential). An external (cartilaginous) callus forms bone by endochondral ossification following initial chondrogenesis. These steps involve repetition of the cellular events involved in the histogenesis of bone. A bone graft is more important as a method of forming a temporary bridge in a severe defect than a source of osteoprogenitor cells. Other methods useful in stimulating bone repair include electrical forces and bone morphogenetic protein, a bone growth factor obtained from decalcified bone matrix. This protein stimulates bone formation when implanted at the fracture site.

110. The answer is a. (*Coe, pp 1042–1052. Kumar, 6/e, pp 673–675. Greenspan, 6/e, pp 326–329.*) The correct diagnosis is Paget's disease, also known as osteitis deformans because of its deforming capabilities (e.g., skull or femoral head enlargement). In this disease the serum calcium is normal, but there is an increase in osteoclastic activity (osteolytic lesions and elevated 24-h urine hydroxyproline) and an increase in osteoblastic activity (elevated osteocalcin and alkaline phosphatase). Patients with Paget's disease exhibit a marked increase in osteoid, and the bone actually enlarges. The osteoid is never normally mineralized in this disease. In this patient, the bone scan shows significant uptake of labeled bisphosphonates, which are incorporated into newly formed osteoid during bone formation. Her proximal femur is enlarged and no longer fits properly into the acetabulum, which results in the hip pain.

There are a number of useful biochemical markers of bone metabolism. Osteoclasts synthesize tartrate–resistant acid phosphatase so that increased osteoclastic activity is reflected in increased serum levels of tartrate–resistant acid phosphatase. Bone resorption fragments of type I collagen and noncollagenous proteins increase as bone matrix is resorbed. Hydroxyproline is a good urinary marker of bone metabolism because hydroxyproline is released and excreted in the urine as collagen is broken down. The presence of pyridinoline cross-links, which are involved in the bundling of type I collagen, is used for measurement of bone resorption. These cross-links are released only during degradation of mineralized collagen fibrils as occurs in bone resorption. Usually, pyridinoline cross-links are measured by immunoassay over a 24-h period to detect excess bone resorption and collagen breakdown in disorders such as Paget's disease.

Markers of bone formation include osteocalcin, alkaline phosphatase, and the extension peptides of type I collagen. Osteocalcin is a vitamin K–dependent gla (γ-carboxyglutamic acid) protein that is synthesized by osteoblasts and secreted into the serum in an unchanged state. Serum concentrations of osteocalcin are, therefore, directly related to osteoblastic activity. It is a more specific marker than the marker alkaline phosphatase, because other organs, such as the liver and kidney, produce that enzyme.

Radiologic methods such as conventional x-ray can be used to detect osteoporosis, but only after patients have lost 30 to 50% of their bone mass. Dual-beam photon absorptiometry allows a much more accurate diagnosis of loss of bone mass.

111. The answer is c. (*Alberts, 3/e, p 1216. Coe, pp 803–804. Kumar, 6/e, pp 380–382. Braunwald, 15/e, pp 728–730.*) The patient is suffering from multiple myeloma. In this disease, there are abnormal changes in the bone marrow indicative of altered plasma cell activity and anemia (hemoglobin data and increasing fatigue). These plasma cells produce elevated levels of interleukin 1 (IL-1), which functions as an osteoclast activation factor. The increased IL-1 stimulates osteoclastic activity and results in elevated serum calcium (12.3 mg/dL). The depletion of bone calcium results in lytic lesions of the skull and pelvis as well as the presence of the compression fracture of the spine. The Bence Jones protein represents free–immunoglobulin light chains, which are a diagnostic feature (Bence Jones proteinuria) found in the urine of patients with multiple myeloma.

112. The answer is b. (*Kumar, 6/e, pp 249, 251. Greenspan, 6/e, pp 320–322. Junqueira, 9/e, pp 145–148. Braunwald, 15/e, pp 2201–2204.*) The patient suffers from osteomalacia, a disease related to malnutrition, specifically vitamin D deficiency. On the basis of the first bone biopsy in which the tissue was decalcified, one could make a diagnosis of osteoporosis. The second, nondecalcified bone biopsy indicates that osteoid is being formed but is not undergoing mineralization. This correlates with the low 25-hydroxyvitamin D levels. Vitamin D replacement and calcium supplementation would be prescribed for this patient.

113. The answer is e. (*Coe, pp 831–856. Braunwald, 15/e, pp 2091, 2226–2231, 2236. Greenspan, 6/e, pp 310–320. Kumar, 6/e, pp 669–671.*) Osteoporosis is a major problem of normal aging in both sexes but is particularly prevalent in older women. In this disease, the quality of bone is unchanged, but the balance between bone deposition and bone resorption is lost. The disease is prevalent in postmenopausal women because the protective effect of estrogens is no longer present. Osteoporosis may also be induced by other diseases (e.g., hyperthyroidism) or drugs (e.g., alcohol and caffeine). In addition, excess glucocorticoids induce osteoporosis. For example, in Cushing's syndrome, patients produce high levels of corticosteroids that interfere with bone metabolism. A similar pattern may be seen during prolonged steroid therapy. The result is increased bone resorption compared with bone deposition. Intestinal calcium absorption is inhibited and PTH levels may be increased.

114. The answer is c. (*Junqueira, 9/e, pp 251–252, 262–263, 267, 402–405. Moore, Developing Human, 6/e, pp 229–230.*) DiGeorge syndrome is a congenital malformation that results in the absence of the thymus and parathyroid glands, which arise from the third and fourth pairs of branchial pouches. The absence of the thymus results in a deficiency in T lymphocyte–dependent areas of the immune system. These areas include the deep cortex of the lymph nodes, periarterial lymphatic sheath (PALS) of the spleen, and interfollicular areas of the Peyer's patches. Parathyroid hormone (PTH) stimulates the development of osteoclasts and the formation of ruffled borders in osteoclasts. The absence of PTH results in (1) a drastic reduction in numbers and activity of osteoclasts, (2) reduced Ca^{2+} levels in the blood, (3) denser bone, (4) spastic contractions of muscle called tetany, and (5) excessive excitability of the nervous system. The parafollicular (C) cells arise from the ultimobranchial body that migrates into the developing thyroid gland and should form normally.

115. The answer is d. *(McKenzie and Klein, p 189. Junqueira, 9/e, p 143.)* The electron micrograph includes matrix vesicles that are derivatives of osteoblast, hypertrophied chondrocyte, ameloblast, and odontoblast cell membranes. After budding off from the plasmalemma, matrix vesicles accumulate calcium and phosphate in the form of hydroxyapatite crystals and serve as seed crystals for calcification. Exposure of these crystals to the extracellular fluid leads to seeding of the osteoid between the spaces in the collagen fibrils located in the matrix. Matrix vesicular alkaline phosphatase results in local increases in the Ca^{2+}/PO_4^{2-} ratio. Adult lamellar bone contains very few matrix vesicles, suggesting that mineralization in adult bone occurs by other mechanisms. The three-dimensional arrangement of collagen with the presence of holes or pores where hydroxyapatite crystals form is involved in the mineralization of adult bone.

116. The answer is c. *(McKenzie and Klein, pp 178–179. Junqueira, 9/e, pp 136–137, 143.)* Type I collagen is responsible for the three-dimensional fiber structure of the matrix. It is synthesized by osteoblasts and accounts for 85 to 90% of total bone protein. The noncollagenous bone proteins are primarily synthesized by osteoblasts and constitute 10 to 15% of bone protein. Some plasma proteins are preferentially absorbed by the bone matrix. The noncollagenous proteins include cytokines and growth factors, which are synthesized endogenously and become trapped in the matrix. Also included in the category of noncollagenous proteins are the cell attachment proteins (fibronectin and osteopontin); proteoglycans (e.g., chondroitin 4-sulfate and chondroitin 6-sulfate), which appear to play a role in collagen fibrillogenesis; and the gla proteins, such as osteocalcin (containing γ-carboxyglutamic acid), which binds Ca^{2+} and mineral components to the matrix.

117. The answer is c. *(Young 4/e, pp 189–191. Kumar, 6/e, 109–111, 681–683. Junqueira, 9/e, pp 148–151.)* The structure labeled "C" is the articular cartilage that is the site of pannus formation in rheumatoid arthritis. The ends of the bone (D) are covered by hyaline cartilage that lacks a perichondrium. These cartilaginous structures are called the articular cartilages

(C) and are the primary site of destruction in osteoarthritis. Joints are classified as those that are freely movable (diarthroses) and those with limited or no movement (synarthroses). Synarthroses are subclassified as united by bone (synostoses), united by hyaline cartilage (synchondroses), and united by dense connective tissue of a ligament (syndesmoses).

The joint shown in the figure is a diarthrosis. The joint capsule consists of an epithelium (B) and an external fibrous layer (E). The synovial fluid is formed from the synovial capillary ultrafiltrate as well as mucins, hyaluronic acid, and glycoproteins produced by fibroblast-like cells in the synovial epithelium (B) that lines the fluid-filled synovial cavity (A). Macrophage-like cells in the epithelium perform a phagocytic function. Synovial fluid, which differs from blood serum in its reduced protein content, acts as a lubricant and becomes more viscous with age. It may be used to diagnose joint disorders such as arthritis. Rheumatoid arthritis is an autoimmune disease in which infiltration of cells from the immune system leads to the destruction of the synovial capsule and the articular cartilages. The pannus is a fibrocollagenous structure that replaces the articular cartilage during the onset of rheumatoid arthritis.

Muscle and Cell Motility

Questions

DIRECTIONS: Each item below contains a question or incomplete statement followed by suggested responses. Select the **one best** response to each question.

118. The multinucleate arrangement of skeletal muscle during development is produced by

a. Duplication of DNA in myoblasts without cytokinesis
b. Fusion of mononucleate myoblasts
c. Cell proliferation of myotubes
d. Hypertrophy of myoblasts
e. Satellite cell differentiation

Questions 119 to 120

In a given muscle fiber at rest, the length of the I band is 1.0 mm and the A band is 1.5 mm.

119. What is the length of the sarcomere?

a. 4.0 μm
b. 3.5 μm
c. 2.5 μm
d. 2.0 μm
e. 1.5 μm

120. Contraction of the muscle fiber described above results in a 10% shortening of the sarcomere length. What is the length of the A band after the shortening produced during muscle contraction?

a. 1.50 μm
b. 1.35 μm
c. 1.00 μm
d. 0.90 μm
e. 0.45 μm

121. Alterations of Ca^{2+} are essential to the normal function of skeletal muscle. In the presence of high Ca^{2+}

a. Binding sites for myosin heads on actin are blocked by the troponin-tropomyosin complex
b. Binding of Ca^{2+} to troponin C unmasks the myosin-binding site on the actin filament
c. Troponin C is inactive
d. Troponin T is responsible for the positioning of the troponins at the myosin-binding site
e. Troponin I stimulates the interaction of actin and myosin

122. The sarcoplasmic reticulum of skeletal muscle functions in

a. Cellular calcium storage
b. Cellular glycogen storage
c. Glycogen degradation
d. Transport of Ca^{2+} into the terminal cisternae during muscle contraction
e. Ca^{2+} release from the transverse tubules during muscle relaxation

123. Observation of a histologic preparation of muscle indicates the cross-striations and peripherally located nuclei. The use of histochemistry shows a strong staining reaction for succinic dehydrogenase. The same tissue prepared for electron microscopy shows many mitochondria in rows between myofibrils and underneath the sarcolemma. The best description of this tissue is

a. White muscle fibers
b. Fibers that contract rapidly but are incapable of sustaining continuous heavy work
c. Red muscle fibers
d. Cardiac muscle
e. Smooth muscle

124. In skeletal muscle contraction, the "powerstroke" is initiated by

a. The initial binding of ATP to the myosin heads
b. Release of Pi from the myosin heads
c. Detachment of the myosin head from the actin
d. Phosphorylation of the myosin light chains
e. Release of ADP and subsequent addition of an ATP molecule

125. In muscular dystrophy, the actin-binding protein dystrophin is absent or defective. Dystrophin contains similar actin-binding domains to the spectrins (I and II) and α-actinin and has a similar function. Which of the following is most likely to occur as a result of this deficiency?

a. Deficiency in skeletal muscle actin synthesis
b. Enhanced smooth muscle contractility
c. Loss of binding of the I and M bands to the cell membrane
d. Loss of organelle and vesicle transport throughout the muscle cell
e. Loss of integrity of the desmosomal components of the intercalated discs of cardiac muscle

126. The actin-rich cell cortex is involved in which of the following cell functions?

a. Cytokinesis
b. Chromosomal movements
c. Bidirectional transport of vesicles
d. Fast axoplasmic transport
e. Ciliary movement

127. Which of the following is absent from smooth muscle cells?

a. Troponin
b. Calmodulin
c. Calcium
d. Myosin light chain kinase
e. Actin and tropomyosin interactions similar to skeletal muscle

128. In the accompanying transmission electron micrograph of striated muscle, which of the following is true of the zone labeled "C"?

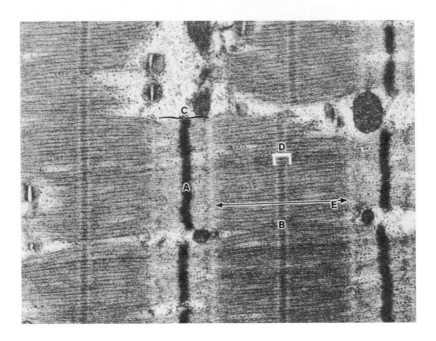

a. The sarcomere is defined as the distance between these two structures
b. Thin filaments are anchored to this structure
c. This structure bisects the H band and is formed predominantly of creatine kinase
d. No overlap of thick and thin filaments occurs in this zone
e. This portion of the A band consists solely of the rodlike portions of myosin

129. The mechanochemical enzyme that can be found on the surfaces of cellular organelles where it mediates movement toward the plus end of microtubules is

a. myosin (myosin II)
b. minimyosin (myosin I)
c. dynein
d. kinesin
e. filamin

Muscle and Cell Motility

Answers

118. The answer is b. (*McKenzie and Klein, p 194. Alberts, 3/e, pp 1176–1178. Junqueira, 9/e, p 181.*) The multinucleate organization of skeletal muscle is derived from the fusion process and not by amitosis (failure of cytokinesis after DNA synthesis). Mitotic activity is terminated after fusion occurs. In the development of skeletal muscle, myoblasts of mesodermal origin undergo cell proliferation. Myocyte cell division ceases soon after birth. Myoblasts, which are mononucleate cells, fuse with each other end to end to form myotubes. This process requires cell recognition between myoblasts, alignment, and subsequent fusion. Satellite cells are supportive cells for maintenance of muscle.

119 to 120. The answers are 119-c, 120-a. (*McKenzie and Klein, pp 99–103. Alberts, 3/e, pp 847–849. Junqueira, 9/e, pp 185–187.*) During contraction, the sarcomere, the distance between adjacent Z lines, decreases in length, and the length of the A band is almost constant. However, as the degree of overlap of thick and thin filaments is altered, the thin filaments, which form the I band and are anchored to the Z line, are pulled toward the center of the sarcomere. As this occurs, the I band decreases in length and the H band is no longer visible. The filaments themselves do not decrease in length; they slide past one another in the sliding-filament model of muscle contraction.

The average length of a sarcomere is 2.5 μm. This distance is measured from one Z line to the next Z line. If the resting length of the A band is 1.5 μm and the length of the I band is 1.0 μm, then the resting length of the sarcomere is determined by adding the length of the I band to the length of the A band. If there is a 20% contraction of the muscle (contraction to 80% of its length), then the sarcomere is reduced in length from 2.5 to 2.0 μm. The size of the A band remains unchanged (whether the contraction is 10 or 20%); therefore, the length of the I band is reduced from 1.0 to 0.5 μm and makes up for the 0.5-μm reduction in length during muscle contraction.

121. The answer is b. (*McKenzie and Klein, p 99. Alberts, 3/e, pp 854–855. Junqueira, 9/e, pp 185–186.*) When calcium levels are elevated (10^{-6} to 10^{-5} M), the myosin-binding site is exposed. This occurs through the binding of calcium to troponin C (named for its calcium-binding activity). The proteins troponin and tropomyosin regulate the interaction of actin and myosin through their response to altered concentrations of calcium. In the resting state, as defined by low-calcium levels (generally below 10^{-8} M), the conformation of the troponin-tropomyosin complex blocks the myosin-binding site. Troponin T (named for its binding to tropomyosin) is responsible for binding of the troponin complex to tropomyosin and the positioning of the troponins at the myosin-binding site during low-calcium conditions. Troponin I (named for its inhibitory function) interferes with the binding of myosin heads to actin. Troponin C is a calmodulin-like molecule required for the calcium dependency of this response.

122. The answer is a. (*McKenzie and Klein, pp 99–103. Alberts, 3/e, pp 853–855. Junqueira, 9/e, pp 184–186.*) The sarcoplasmic reticulum provides a mechanism for the muscle cell to regulate the concentration of cytosolic calcium. It is a modified smooth endoplasmic reticulum that serves alternatively as a storage site and a source of cellular calcium. Calcium is released from the sarcoplasmic reticulum during muscle contraction; it is stored during relaxation. During repolarization, calcium is actively transported from the cytosol to the sarcoplasmic reticulum through the activity of a Ca^{2+}-dependent ATPase. Calsequestrin is a calcium-binding protein found in the sarcoplasmic reticulum. From its name it is clear that it functions in the sequestration of calcium within the sarcoplasmic reticulum. The sarcoplasmic reticulum contains many calcium channels that open in response to depolarization and result in a massive increase in cytosolic calcium. During repolarization of the T system, Ca^{2+} is transported from the cytosol and sequestered in the sarcoplasmic reticulum through the activity of Ca^{2+}-ATPase and calsequestrin, respectively. Glycogen is stored as particles or droplets in the cytoplasm, which contains the enzymes required for the synthesis and breakdown of glycogen.

The transverse tubule system, or T system, is an extension of the plasma membrane of the myofiber (sarcolemma). The T system allows for simultaneous contraction of all myofibrils because the system encircles the A-I bands in each sarcomere of every myofibril. In combination with the paired terminal cisternae, the transverse tubules form a triad. Two triads are found in each sarcomere of skeletal muscle—one at each junction of dark (A) and light (I) bands. Depolarization of the T system during contraction is transmitted to the sarcoplasmic reticulum at the triad. Calcium is responsible for the coupling of excitation and contraction in skeletal muscle. It is important to note that cardiac muscle also has a T system, although it is not as elaborate and well organized as that found in skeletal muscle (e.g., diads are present rather than the triads of skeletal muscle and there are fewer T tubules in the atrial versus ventricular muscle).

123. The answer is c. (*McKenzie and Klein, p 196. Junqueira, 9/e, pp 189–190, 195.*) The histologic sample contains red fibers. The deductive process is based on the fact that the sample must be skeletal or cardiac muscle due to the presence of cross-striations. The presence of peripherally placed nuclei eliminates cardiac muscle as a possibility. Skeletal muscle may be subclassified into three muscle fiber types: red, white, and intermediate fibers. Red muscle fibers have a high content of cytochrome and myoglobin and, beneath the plasmalemma, contain many mitochondria required for the high metabolism of these cells. Mitochondria are also found in a longitudinal array surrounding the myofibrils. The presence of numerous mitochondria provides a strong staining reaction with the use of cytochemical stains such as that for succinic dehydrogenase. Physiologically, red fibers are capable of continuous contraction (high concentrations of myosin ATPase) but are incapable of rapid contraction. The term red (type I) fibers is due to the presence of large concentrations of myoglobin, the colored oxygen-binding protein. White (type IIB) muscle fibers are fast-twitch in function, stain very lightly for succinic dehydrogenase, myosin ATPase, and few mitochondria would be visible at the ultrastructural level. White fibers are capable of rapid contraction but are unable to sustain continuous heavy work. They are larger than red fibers and have more prominent innervation. The white fibers contain relatively little myoglobin. Human skeletal muscle fibers are composed of red, white, and intermediate-type fibers. The intermediate (type IIA) fibers possess characteristics including a size and innervation pattern intermediate between red and white muscle fibers. The intermediate fibers contain a concentration of myoglobin between white and red muscle fibers.

124. The answer is b. (*McKenzie and Klein, pp 96–99. Alberts, 3/e, pp 851–853. Junqueira, 9/e, pp 185–190.*) The "powerstroke" is initiated by the release of Pi from the myosin heads, leading to the tight binding of actin and myosin. The tight binding induces a conformational change in the myosin head. The myosin head subsequently pulls against the actin filament to cause the "powerstroke" of the myosin head walking along the actin filament. This walking process is unidirectional and is based on the polarity of the actin filament (i.e., walking occurs from the minus to the plus end of the actin filament). The cycle of ATP-actin-myosin interactions during contraction begins with the resting state. In the quiescent period, ATP binds to myosin heads; however, hydrolysis occurs slowly and only allows the weak binding of myosin heads to the actin filaments. Tight binding occurs only when Pi is released from myosin heads, leading to the "powerstroke." Recycling occurs through the release of ADP and the subsequent addition of an ATP molecule and detachment of the myosin head from actin. Rigor results from the lack of ATP because one ATP molecule is required for each myosin molecule present in the muscle. *Rigor mortis* occurs from the total absence of ATP.

Myosin is composed of two coiled heavy chains and four light chains. It may be separated into heavy and light meromyosin by enzymatic treatment. Heavy meromyosin has two segments: S1 (the globular head region) and S2. The S1 subfragment includes the light chains that are associated with the globular head regions. This region is significant because it is the site of the actin binding that activates ATPase activity. S2 is a dimeric portion of the myosin molecule that connects the two S1 segments to the coiled light meromyosin subunit. The P light chain is one of the two light chains associated with the globular heads and is phosphorylated by myosin light chain kinase. In skeletal muscle, phosphorylation of the light chain is not required for binding to actin.

125. The answer is c. (*Alberts, 3/e, p 855. Braunwald, 15/e pp 2529–2531. Kumar, 6/e, pp 689–690.*) Dystrophin, like these other actin-binding proteins, binds actin to the skeletal muscle membrane and, therefore, binds the I and M bands to the cell membrane. The inability to bind actin to the plasma membrane of skeletal muscle leads to disruption of the contraction process, weakness of muscle, and abnormal running, hopping, and jumping. Gowers' maneuver is the method used by persons suffering from muscular dystrophy to stand from a sitting position. Respiratory failure occurs in these persons because of disruption of diaphragmatic function. Dystrophin is found in muscle of all types and is part of a complex that regulates interactions of the sarcolemma with the extracellular matrix through associated glycoproteins (dystrophin-glycoprotein complex). Therefore, loss of dystrophin causes a destabilization of the sarcolemma.

Muscular dystrophy refers to a group of progressive hereditary disorders (1/3500 male births) that involve mutations in the dystrophin gene. Dystrophin is similar in structure to spectrins I and II and α-actinin. Dystrophin is absent in Duchenne muscular dystrophy. Becker muscular dystrophy is a less severe dystrophy in which dystrophin is defective. Synthesis of actin is not reduced in skeletal muscle from these patients; in fact, hypertrophy and pseudohypertrophy (replacement of muscle with connective tissue and fat) occurs. Microtubules perform vesicular and organelle transport functions, and intermediate filaments not actin from the intracellular connection in desmosomes.

126. The answer is a. (*McKenzie and Klein, pp 26, 96–99, 105. Alberts, 3/e, pp 813–814, 834.*) The cell cortex is an area of the cell immediately underneath the plasma membrane and is rich in actin, which is required for cytokinesis. This region is important in maintaining the mechanical strength of the cytoplasm of the cell. It is also essential for cellular functions that require surface motility. These functions include phagocytosis, cytokinesis, and cell locomotion. Although movement of vesicles along filaments is regulated by minimyosins (myosin I), movement of vesicles and organelles is predominantly a function of microtubules under the influence of the unidirectional motors kinesin and dynein. The movements of cilia and flagella are driven by dynein and chromosomal movements occur through microtubular kinetics.

127. The answer is a. (*McKenzie and Klein, pp 99–105. Alberts, 3/e, pp 856–857. Junqueira, 9/e, pp 194–200.*) Smooth muscle is the least specialized type of muscle and contains no troponin. The contractile process is similar to the actin-myosin interactions that occur in motility of nonmuscle cells. In the smooth muscle cell, actin and myosin are attached to intermediate filaments at dense bodies in the sarcolemma and cytoplasm. Dense bodies contain α-actinin and, therefore, resemble the Z lines of skeletal muscle. Contraction causes cell shortening and a change in shape from elongate to globular. Contraction occurs by a sliding filament action analogous to the mechanism used by thick and thin filaments in striated muscle. The connections to the plasma membrane allow all the smooth muscle cells in the same region to act as a functional unit. Sarcoplasmic reticulum is not as well developed as that in the striated muscles. There are no T tubules present; however, endocytic vesicles called caveolae are believed to function in a fashion similar to the T tubule system of skeletal muscle.

When intracellular calcium levels increase, the calcium is bound to the calcium-binding protein calmodulin. Ca^{2+}-calmodulin is required and is bound to myosin light chain kinase to form a Ca^{2+}-calmodulin-kinase complex. This complex catalyzes the phosphorylation of one of the two myosin light chains on the myosin heads. This phosphorylation allows the binding of actin to myosin. A specific phosphatase dephosphorylates the myosin light chain, which returns the actin and myosin to the inactive, resting state. The actin-tropomyosin interactions are similar in smooth and skeletal muscle.

Smooth muscle cells (e.g., vascular smooth muscle cells) also differ from skeletal muscle cells in that they are capable of collagen, elastin, and proteoglycan synthesis, which is usually associated with fibroblasts.

128. The answer is d. (*McKenzie and Klein, pp 99–103. Junqueira, 9/e, pp 181–184, 186–187.*) Myofibrils are composed of sarcomeres, which are repeating units that extend from Z disk ("A" on the TEM) to Z disk in the transmission electron micrograph (TEM). With the use of polarizing microscopy the A (anisotropic) bands ("E" on the TEM) are visible as dark, birefringent structures, and the I (isotropic) bands are visible as light-staining bands ("C" on the TEM). The I band (labeled "C") consists of thin filaments without overlap of thick filaments. At the center of the myofibril and consisting of thick filaments is the A band, which interdigitates with the I band. Each I band is bisected by the Z disk. The Z disk is composed mostly of the intermediate filament protein desmin and other proteins such as α-actinin, filamin, and amorphin, as well as Z protein. In the center of the A band is a lighter staining area that consists only of thick (rodlike portions of myosin) filaments and is known as the H band ("D" on the TEM). Lateral connections occur between adjacent thick filaments in the region of the M line ("B" on the TEM), which bisects the H zone and is composed primarily of creatine kinase, an enzyme that catalyzes the formation of ATP.

129. The answer is d. (*McKenzie and Klein, pp 26–29. Alberts, 3/e, pp 813–814, 816–818, 836.*) Kinesin moves vesicles unidirectionally from the minus end to the plus end of the microtubule, e.g., from the cell body to the axon terminus in fast axonal transport. Myosin, minimyosin, dynein, dynamin, and kinesin are all mechanochemical enzymes or molecular "motors" that hydrolyze ATP and undergo conformational changes that are converted into movement. Cytoplasmic dynein is responsible for movement toward the minus end of the microtubules. Remember *k*inesin *k*icks out and dyne*in* drags them *in* (see feedback question 40). Ciliary and flagellar bending is the classic model for microtubule-based motility. The motor is dynein, which causes the relative sliding between microtubules in the axoneme.

Structural constraints within the axoneme as a whole convert sliding into ciliary bending.

Dynamin is another ATPase motor that mediates sliding between adjacent cytoplasmic microtubules.

Filamin or other actin cross-linking proteins form a gel network in the cell cortex (the area just beneath the cell membrane). The presence of the actin gel in the cell cortex contributes to the rigidity of the cell and is also involved in changes in cell shape.

Nervous System

Questions

DIRECTIONS: Each item below contains a question or an incomplete statement followed by suggested responses. Select the **one best** response to each question.

130. In the histogenesis of the neural tube, which zone will become the white matter of the adult CNS?

a. Ventricular zone
b. Marginal zone
c. Mantle zone
d. Ependymal zone
e. Intermediate zone

131. The cells responsible for the entry of human immunodeficiency virus (HIV) into the CNS are

a. Microglia/macrophages
b. Astrocytes (astroglia)
c. Oligodendrocytes (oligodendroglia)
d. Endothelial cells
e. Schwann cells

132. The action potential in the neuron results from

a. Hyperpolarization
b. The opening of K^+ channels
c. The opening of Na^+ channels
d. Entrance of Na^+ ions into the neuron
e. Inward flux of K^+

133. Toxins or viruses reach the perikaryon by endocytosis followed by

a. Slow anterograde transport
b. Slow retrograde transport
c. Rapid anterograde transport
d. Dendritic transport
e. Rapid retrograde transport

134. Myelination in the central nervous system differs from myelination in the peripheral nervous system in

a. Its formation only during fetal development
b. The function of myelin
c. Its ultrastructural appearance
d. The involvement of oligodendrocytes
e. The involvement of astrocytes

135. The light micrograph below

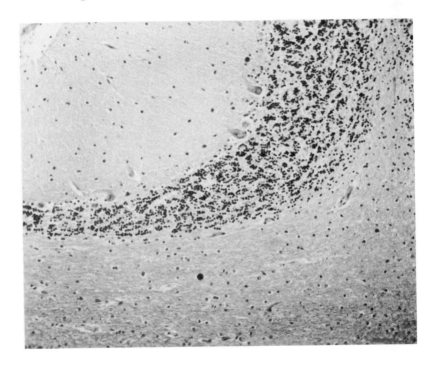

a. Is a cross section of the spinal cord
b. Contains pyramidal cells that in different layers of the cortex project to different parts of the nervous system
c. Contains a central area of gray matter
d. Contains vertical columns that are perpendicular to the surface and subserve one sensory modality
e. Contains glia and basket cell axons situated in the vicinity of Purkinje cells

136. The neurons shown in the accompanying photomicrograph of a dorsal root ganglion have which of the following functions?

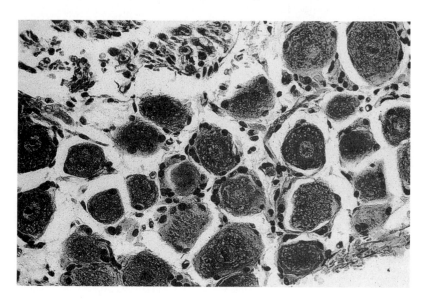

a. Transmission of autonomic information
b. Transmission of proprioceptive information
c. Innervation of striated muscle
d. Transmission of dental pain
e. Transmission of visual stimuli

137. Regeneration of axons

a. Occurs in the segment distal to the damage
b. Is independent of the survival of the perikaryon
c. Includes a decrease in the volume of the perikaryon
d. Is dependent on proliferation of Schwann cells
e. Is initiated with an increase in production of Nissl substance

138. The nodes of Ranvier

a. Occur only in the CNS
b. Contain few Na^+-gated channels
c. Represent the midpoints of myelination segments
d. Are completely covered by myelin
e. Increase the efficiency of nerve conduction

139. The blood-brain barrier is formed by

a. Fenestrations between brain capillary endothelial cells
b. Occluding junctions between brain capillary endothelial cells
c. Astrocytic foot processes surrounding blood vessels entering the brain parenchyma
d. The basement membrane associated with the glia limitans
e. Microglial activity

140. At the neuromuscular junction, action potentials are coupled to neurotransmitter release by voltage-gated

a. Ca^{2+} channels
b. Na^+ channels
c. K^+ channels
d. Cl^- channels
e. Gap junctions between the presynaptic terminal and the muscle cell

141. In the photomicrograph below of tissue taken from the central nervous system, the predominant cells are

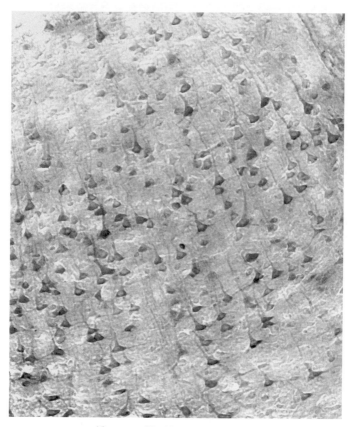

(Courtesy of Dr. Nancy E. J. Berman.)

a. Basket cells
b. Granule cells
c. Glial cells
d. Pyramidal cells
e. Purkinje cells

142. In the accompanying photomicrograph, the structure labeled C is

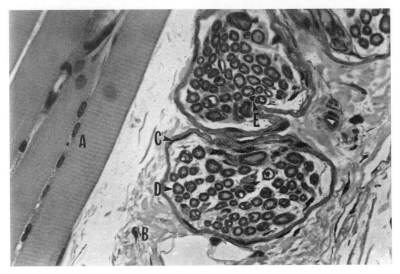

(Courtesy of Dr. John K. Young.)

a. Perineurium
b. Epineurium
c. Endomysium
d. Myelin sheath
e. Tunica media

143. The neural crest gives rise to which of the following?

a. Zona glomerulosa of the adrenal gland
b. Pyramidal cells
c. Ventral horn cells
d. Astrocytes
e. Sensory neurons of the cranial ganglia

144. The structure indicated by the arrow is

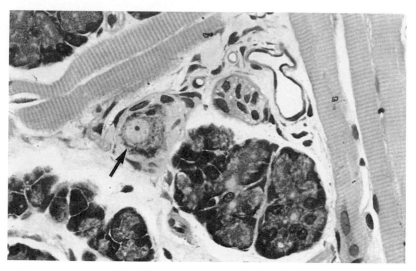

(Courtesy of Dr. John K. Young.)

a. An artery
b. A vein
c. A peripheral nerve
d. A ganglion cell
e. A serous acinar cell

145. The cells labeled by the arrows in the accompanying figure

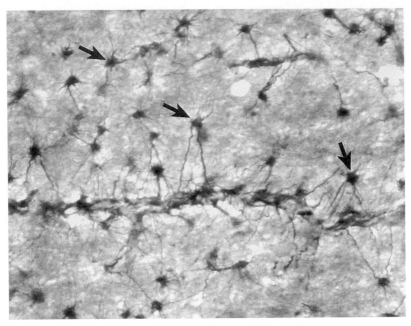

(Reproduced, with permission, from Fawcett DW: The Cell, 2/e. Philadelphia, PA: WB Saunders, 1981.)

a. Form synaptic contacts with neurons
b. Are derived from the bone marrow monocyte lineage
c. Form the blood-brain barrier
d. Are responsible for gliosis following damage in the CNS
e. Form myelin in the CNS

146. The structure labeled C in the accompanying electron micrograph of a synapse is the site of

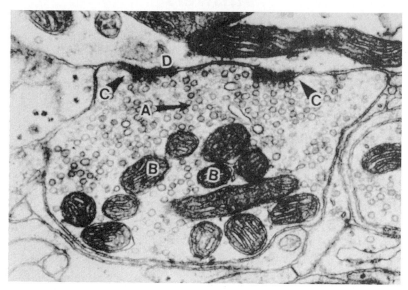

(Reproduced, with permission, from Kandel ER, Schwartz JH, Jessell TM: Principles of Neural Science, 4 ed. New York, NY: 2000.)

a. Neurotransmitter uptake in synaptic vesicles by endocytosis
b. Postsynaptic receptors
c. Neurotransmitter-induced alteration of membrane permeability
d. Membrane continuity between adjacent neurons
e. Recycling of synaptic vesicle membranes by endocytosis

147. The venous sinuses are located in the

a. Epidural space
b. Dura mater
c. Subdural space
d. Arachnoid
e. Pia mater

Nervous System

Answers

130. The answer is b. (*McKenzie and Klein, p 206. Junqueira, 9/e, p 152. Moore, Before We Are Born, 5/e, pp 70–72, 424–425, 428–429. Moore, Developing Human, 6/e, pp 72–74, 453–456, 475–477.*) The white matter of the adult CNS is derived from the marginal zone of the developing neural tube. The other layers of the neural tube are the mantle zone, which forms the gray matter, and the ventricular zone from which astrocytes, oligodendrocytes, and neurons differentiate. Ultimately, the cells that remain in the ventricular zone become the ependymal cells that line the central canal.

The first stage of neural tube development involves cell proliferation and occurs before neural tube closure. The second stage involves the differentiation of neurons from the germinal (ventricular) layer of the epithelium and is initiated after closure of the neural tube. Differentiation of three distinct layers of the wall is observed. Mitotic activity occurs in the ventricular zone, closest to the lumen. The next zone is the mantle (intermediate) zone, where cell bodies of differentiating motor neurons are located. The most peripheral zone is the marginal zone, which contains the myelinated axons of the developing motor neurons (adult white matter).

In the central nervous system, neural tissue is separated into two types. White matter contains a predominance of myelinated fibers. The gray matter contains mostly cell bodies of neurons. The formation of three layers in the developing neural tube results in the pattern of peripheral white matter with a central H-shaped region of gray matter, which is seen in the spinal cord. Astrocytes and oligodendrocytes, the macroglia, arise from the neural epithelium and not from neural crest cells. Microglia (the macrophages of the brain) are bone marrow-derived arising from monocytes.

It is important to note that the cerebral and cerebellar cortex are areas of peripheral gray matter. CNS cortex is formed through a second wave of cell proliferation. In the cerebellum this occurs from the external granular layer that is present during development. In the cerebral cortex, the layers (I to VI) are formed by waves of proliferation and migration from deep to superficial layers.

131. The answer is a. *(Kandel, 4/e, p 20. Braunwald, 15/e, pp 1873, 1890–1891.)* Microglia are the macrophages of the brain. They become infected with HIV and carry the virus into the CNS. The virus remains latent until a stimulus activates viral production. These cells are the most conspicuous elements of HIV-induced CNS pathology. Infection, proliferation, and fusion of microglia/macrophages appear to be involved in the development of giant cell encephalitis of acquired immune deficiency syndrome (AIDS) and other pathologies associated with neuronal damage in AIDS dementia. The CNS effects of AIDS are extensive as indicated by the fact that 90% of AIDS patients show abnormalities in the cerebrospinal fluid (CSF), even in asymptomatic stages of the disease.

132. The answer is c. *(McKenzie and Klein, p 210. Alberts, 3/e, p 531. Junqueira, 9/e, pp 152. Kandel, 4/e, pp 29–39, 147–148.)* The action potential in a neuron results from depolarization following the opening of Na^+ channels. In the resting state, sodium and potassium pumps build up high ionic gradients across the axolemma. The resting potential is about 290 mV and is displaced toward 0 volts. When the threshold voltage is reached, sodium channels open and sodium ions enter the neuron. K^+ channels also open in response to changes in membrane potential but bring the membrane to a hyperpolarized state. Inward flux of K^+, combined with the closing of Na^+ channels, is important in the return to the resting membrane potential. The action potential is an all-or-none phenomenon and occurs with constant amplitude and duration for a given axon. Myelination results in a much more rapid conduction of the action potential.

133. The answer is e. *(McKenzie and Klein, p 205. Alberts, 3/e, p 814. Junqueira, 9/e, p 157. Kandel, 4/e, pp 99–103.)* Extracellular materials, such as tetanus toxin and viruses, may be endocytosed by a receptor-mediated process and subsequently transported to the perikarya by rapid retrograde transport. Axonal transport occurs by several different mechanisms. Slow axonal transport involves the movement of cytoskeletal elements such as actin, tubulin, and neurofilaments from the perikaryon down the axon. Slow transport occurs at a velocity of 1 to 5 mm/d. Dendritic transport occurs in a manner similar to that of slow axonal transport. In contrast to slow axonal transport, rapid anterograde (away from the perikaryon) transport and retrograde (toward the perikaryon) transport occur at rates of 200 to 300 mm/d. Membrane-bound organelles, such as newly formed secretory vesicles and mitochondria, are transported rapidly in an anterograde direction. Receptors, recycled membranes, and worn-out organelles are transported following a retrograde mechanism. Retrograde transport is also used experimentally by neuroanatomists to map connections in the CNS.

Colchicine and other microtubule toxins block fast axonal transport. The molecular motors for rapid retrograde and anterograde transport differ. Kinesin is a microtubule motor that hydrolyzes ATP and in so doing moves organelles along microtubules in an anterograde direction (toward the plus ends of the microtubules). Dynein is also an ATPase and a microtubule-based motor that moves organelles along microtubules in a retrograde direction (toward the minus ends of the microtubules).

134. The answer is d. (*McKenzie and Klein, pp 207–208. Young, 4/e, pp 121, 123–125, 137. Junqueira, 9/e, pp 161, 164, 170–173. Kandel, 4/e, pp 20, 147–148.*) Myelination in the central (CNS) and peripheral (PNS) nervous systems occurs by similar methods, although there are differences in the supportive cells responsible. In the CNS, the oligodendrocytes myelinate axons, whereas the Schwann cells conduct myelination in the PNS. Oligodendrocytes myelinate several axons at one time, whereas the Schwann cells myelinate only one axon. Myelin is similar in both locations but different in the presence of Schmidt-Lanterman clefts, which only appear in the PNS and represent the presence of Schwann cell cytoplasm that is not displaced toward the periphery. This provides a continuous cytoplasmic pathway from the exterior to the interior of the myelin sheath. Myelin is an insulator and also decreases membrane capacitance. White matter is high in myelin content and is named by the presence of tracts of axons that appear white (myelinated). Gray matter represents neuron-rich areas low in myelin (e.g., cell bodies).

In the PNS, formation of myelin is initiated by the invagination of an axon into a Schwann cell. A mesaxon is formed as the outer leaflets of the cell membrane fuse. Subsequently, the mesaxon of the Schwann cell wraps itself around the fiber. In the CNS, oligodendrocytes form myelin around several axon segments compared with the 1:1 relationship between Schwann cells and axon segments in the PNS. Myelination occurs in both pre- and postnatal development. For example, the extrapyramidal system is myelinated postnatally, and its maturation may be assessed by use of the Babinski reflex. CNS myelin is the target for attack by components of the immune system in multiple sclerosis.

135. The answer is e. *(McKenzie and Klein, p 364. Young, 4/e, pp 376. Junqueira, 9/e, pp 164–167.)* The photomicrograph is from the cerebellum containing three layers from the outside to the inside: molecular, internal granule layer, and Purkinje cell layer. The white matter is inside of the three layers of gray matter. Basket cells, Purkinje cells, and granule cells are located in the cerebellar cortex. The basket cells make profuse dendritic contact with the Purkinje cells, which have a very characteristic flask shape. The granule cells are small neurons located in the vicinity of the Purkinje cells. Multipolar neurons contain prominent Nissl substance (RER and attached ribosomes) when using appropriate stain. Large, multipolar neurons in the cerebral cortex are pyramidal cells. Forming the stroma of the brain, the glia, which are small compared with the motor neurons, are located along the dendrites, axons, and soma of the neurons.

136. The answer is b. *(Young, 4/e, p 133. Junqueira, 9/e, pp 171, 174, 177.)* The cell bodies (perikarya) of neurons carrying sensory information, such as pain and proprioception, from the body wall, are found in the dorsal root ganglia of spinal nerves. They are pseudounipolar neurons, in contrast to the large multipolar neurons with eccentric nuclei and coarse granular Nissl bodies that characterize neurons of the autonomic ganglia. Large pyramidal neurons that innervate skeletal muscle are found in the ventral horns of the spinal cord. Pain from facial structures, including the teeth, is carried in the fifth cranial (trigeminal) nerve. Visual stimuli are carried in the second cranial (optic) nerve. Satellite cells can be observed surrounding the neuronal perikarya and are similar to Schwann cells in function (e.g., insulation and metabolic regulation) but do not produce a myelin sheath.

137. The answer is d. *(McKenzie and Klein, p 210. Junqueira, 9/e, pp 176–180. Kandel, 4/e, p 1108–1109.)* Regeneration depends on the proliferation of Schwann cells, which guide sprouting axons from the proximal segment toward the target organ. This process is referred to as Wallerian regeneration. Axonal regeneration occurs in neurons if the perikarya survive following damage. The segment distal to the wound, including the myelin, is phagocytosed and removed by macrophages. The proximal segment is capable of regeneration because it remains in continuity with the perikaryon. Chromatolysis is the first step in the regeneration process in which there is breakdown of the Nissl substance, swelling of the perikaryon, and migration of the nucleus peripherally. Degeneration of perikarya and neuronal processes occurs when there is extensive neuronal damage. Transneuronal degeneration occurs only when there are synapses with a single damaged neuron. In the presence of inputs from multiple neurons, transneuronal degeneration does not occur.

138. The answer is e. *(McKenzie and Klein, p 208. Junqueira, 9/e, pp 170, 171, 174. Kandel, 4/e, pp 21–22, 148, 160.)* The nodes of Ranvier increase the efficiency of nodal conduction because of restriction of energy–dependent Na^+ influx to the node. The nodes of Ranvier represent the space between adjacent units of myelination. This area is bare in the CNS, whereas in the PNS the axons in the nodes are partially covered by the cytoplasmic tongues of adjacent Schwann cells. Most of the Na^+-gated channels are located in the bare areas. Therefore, spread of depolarization from the nodal region along the axon occurs until it reaches the next node. This is often described as a series of jumps from node to node, or saltatory conduction.

139. The answer is b. *(McKenzie and Klein, pp 235, 366–367. Junqueira, 9/e, pp 169, 205, 208–209. Kandel, 4/e, pp 1288–1295.)* The blood-brain barrier is formed primarily by occluding junctions (zonulae occludentes) between endothelial cells that compose the lining of brain capillaries. The capillary endothelium is nonfenestrated, which also adds to the barrier. In addition, astrocytes form foot processes around the brain capillaries. Surrounding the CNS is a basement membrane with a lining of astrocyte foot processes; this forms the glia limitans, which also contributes to the integrity of the blood-brain barrier. Oligodendrocytes function in myelination of CNS axons. Microglia function as brain macrophages and are involved in antigen presentation and phagocytosis.

140. The answer is a. *(McKenzie and Klein, p 196. Alberts, 3/e, pp 540–541. Junqueira, 9/e, pp 157–159, 186, 194. Kandel, 4/e, pp 43, 175–177, 183, 210–211.)* Ca^{2+} entry through specific channels results in fusion of acetylcholine-containing synaptic vesicles with the presynaptic membrane and ultimately the release of neurotransmitter. Neuromuscular, or myoneural, junctions represent the site at which end feet (boutons terminaux) come in close proximity to the surface of muscle cells. The arrangement is similar to that found in a synapse, and a neuromuscular junction can be considered the best-studied synapse. Na$^+$, K$^+$, and Cl$^-$ voltage–gated channels are involved in the transmission of a nerve impulse but are not involved in the coupling of the action potential (an electrical signal) to neurotransmitter release (a chemical alteration). Ca^{2+} influx into the end feet may have a direct effect on phosphorylation of synapsin I, a vesicular membrane protein, which in its nonphosphorylated state blocks vesicle fusion with the presynaptic membrane.

141. The answer is d. (*McKenzie and Klein, pp 363–364. Junqueira, 9/e, pp 153–157.*) Pyramidal neurons are labeled with the arrows in the photomicrograph. Axons are evident in the histologic section accompanying the question. The axon arises from the axon hillock. Neither the axon nor axon hillock contains Nissl substance (rough ER), which is dispersed throughout the soma and dendrites. Dendrites generally are wider than axons, are of nonuniform diameter, and taper to a point. Motor neurons, such as the one illustrated, usually display large amounts of euchromatin and a distinct nucleolus characteristic of high synthetic activity.

142. The answer is a. (*McKenzie and Klein, p 368. Junqueira, 9/e, pp 171, 175–176.*) In this high–magnification light micrograph, several cross sections through small peripheral nerves are visible. "C" indicates the perineurium, a layer of two to three fibroblast-like cells with contractile properties that surround individual fascicles. Cells of the perineurium are joined by tight junctions and form a barrier to macromolecules. "B" indicates dense irregular connective tissue surrounding the small nerves. They contain numerous nerve fibers surrounded by myelin sheaths (D) produced by Schwann cells (nucleus visible at E). Other nuclei visible within the fascicle include (1) those of fibroblasts, which secrete the reticular connective tissue elements forming the endoneurium surrounding the individual neuronal fibers and (2) nuclei of capillary endothelial cells. Neuronal perikarya are not present in peripheral nerves. "A" indicates skeletal muscle, identifiable by its striations and peripherally located nuclei.

143. The answer is e. (*McKenzie and Klein, p 322. Junqueira, 9/e, p 152. Kandel, 4/e, pp 880, 883, 1027, 1046–1048. Moore, Before We Are Born, 5/e, pp 70, 424–425. Moore, Developing Human, 6/e, pp 72, 217, 219, 236, 319, 322, 369, 440, 483–484, 486, 522.*) The neural crest forms most of the peripheral nervous system, in contrast to the neural tube, which is the embryonic source of the central nervous system. The sensory neurons of the cranial and spinal sensory ganglia (e.g., dorsal root ganglia), sympathetic chain ganglia, postganglionic sympathetic and parasympathetic fibers of the autonomic nervous system, cells of the pia and arachnoid, Schwann cells, and satellite cells of the dorsal root ganglia are neural elements derived from neural crest. Nonneuronal structures formed from neural crest include melanocytes of the skin, odontoblasts in teeth, derivatives of the branchial arch cartilages (e.g., pinnae of ear), and the adrenal medulla (not the adrenal cortex, e.g., zona granulosa). The adrenal medulla represents postganglionic sympathetic fibers that respond to inputs from preganglionic sympathetic fibers in splanchnic nerves. Ventral horn cells are derived from the neuroepithelium of the neural tube.

144. The answer is d. (*Junqueira, 9/e, pp 171, 174, 176.*) The arrow indicates a single intramural parasympathetic ganglion cell distinctly characterized by its large, euchromatic nucleus and prominent nucleolus. Several small satellite cells surround the ganglion cell. Other structures within the field include serous acini from an exocrine gland, a small peripheral nerve, a venule, and several skeletal muscle fibers.

145. The answer is d. (*McKenzie and Klein, p 206. Junqueira, 9/e, pp 161–162.*) Astrocytes (delineated with arrows in the photomicrograph) are large stellate cells that undergo cell proliferation and form the glial scar (gliosis) following CNS injury. Astrocytes stain positively for the intermediate filament protein, glial fibrillary acidic protein (GFAP). They form from the neuroepithelium, and they have important functions in the developing and adult nervous systems. Astrocytes occur in two subtypes: protoplasmic and fibrous astrocytes. These subtypes differ in morphology and location. Fibrous astrocytes are found in the white matter, whereas protoplasmic astrocytes are located in the gray matter of the CNS. The astrocytes may function as a potassium sink during prolonged neuronal activity; however, they have several better-defined functions. The astrocytes form a scaffolding for the migration of developing neurons during the differentiation of the embryonic nervous system. Astrocytes also form a scaffolding for neuronal elements in the adult brain. Many astrocytes in the adult CNS have extended foot processes called vascular end feet, which contact brain vascular elements. The function of the end feet is probably associated with ion transport from the area surrounding the neurons to the blood vessels and induction of the blood-brain barrier. The CNS is surrounded by the glia limitans found beneath the pial surface; it is a basement membrane lined by astrocytes. Astrocytes are also the source of the most common glioma, astrocytoma.

146. The answer is e. *(McKenzie and Klein, pp 209–210. Junqueira, 9/e, pp 157–160. Kandel, 4/e, pp 265–269.)* The electron micrograph of the synapse shows the presynaptic membrane (C), postsynaptic membrane (D), mitochondria (B), and synaptic vesicles (A). Recycling of synaptic vesicle membrane occurs at the presynaptic membrane in conjunction with neurotransmitter release by exocytosis. Neurotransmitter release is induced by membrane depolarization, leading to transient opening of calcium channels followed by calcium influx. There is no cytoplasmic continuity between adjacent neurons. Transmission from neuron to neuron occurs by chemical transmission in the form of neurotransmitter release. The neurotransmitter (from the synaptic vesicles) crosses the synaptic cleft (between the pre- and postsynaptic membranes) and interacts with receptors on the postsynaptic membrane, which results in changes in the permeability of this membrane. Numerous mitochondria and synaptic vesicles are typically found on the presynaptic side of the synapse. The postsynaptic surface typically is more dense than the presynaptic membrane.

147. The answer is b. *(McKenzie and Klein, p 365. Junqueira, 9/e, pp 166–169.)* The dura mater ("tough mother") contains the venous sinuses and is composed of dense connective tissue and possesses very limited osteogenic potential. The dura mater is one of the three protective layers that comprise the meninges surrounding the brain and spinal cord. In the spinal cord, the dura is separated from the periosteum by the epidural space. The thin subdural space lies between the dura mater and the arachnoid. The arachnoid is composed of a weblike avascular connective tissue that forms villi for the reabsorption of cerebrospinal fluid (CSF) into the venous sinuses found in the dura. The subarachnoid space contains the CSF, which is formed both by ultrafiltration of the blood and transport across the epithelial lining of the choroid plexuses. The pia covers the brain and spinal cord as a delicate, vascular connective tissue. It lines the perivascular spaces through which blood vessels penetrate the CNS. The periosteum is an important connective tissue layer surrounding the bone of the skull. This layer retains osteogenic potential even in the adult.

Cardiovascular System, Blood, and Bone Marrow

Questions

DIRECTIONS: Each item below contains a question or incomplete statement followed by suggested responses. Select the **one best** response to each question.

148. Vasa vasorum provide a function analogous to that of

a. Valves
b. Basal lamina
c. Coronary arteries
d. Endothelial diaphragms
e. Arterioles

149. Glanzmann's disease (also known as thrombasthenia) is a disease in which there is a defect in the glycoprotein IIb-IIIa complex, resulting in a defect in β_3-integrin structure on platelets. In these patients, platelets

a. Are reduced in size
b. Have limited ability to secrete platelet-derived growth factor (PDGF)
c. Are unable to undergo normal shape changes
d. Demonstrate poor aggregation
e. Demonstrate accelerated hemostasis

Questions 150 to 153 refer to the diagram below.

150. The cell labeled A is best described as a

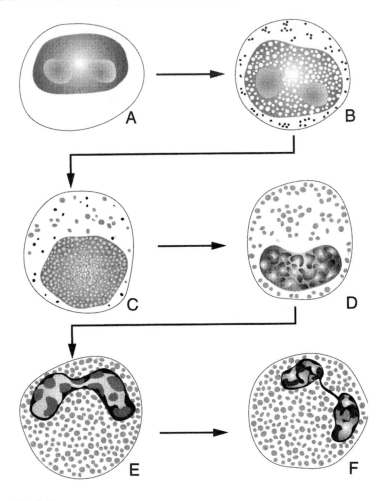

a. Myeloblast
b. Proerythroblast
c. Metamyelocyte
d. Myelocyte
e. Promyelocyte

151. The granules that develop during differentiation of this cell type contain

a. Heparin
b. Histamine
c. Histaminase
d. Platelet-derived growth factor (PDGF)
e. Thymosin

152. In the human fetus, the predominant site of this process in gestational months 5 to 9 is the

a. Liver
b. Yolk sac
c. Spleen
d. Thymus
e. Bone marrow

153. In the adult, the best place to sample for cells of this lineage would be

a. Sternum
b. Fibula
c. Humerus
d. Tibia
e. Scapula

154. Which of the following structures best represents the large endothelial pores defined in physiologic studies?

a. Zonulae occludentes
b. Gap junctions
c. Pinocytotic vesicles
d. Zonula adherens
e. Coatomer-coated vesicles

155. Anionic proteins, such as insulin and transferrin, cross capillary endothelial cells primarily via

a. Diffusion through the membrane
b. Intercellular space
c. Fenestrated diaphragms
d. Gap junctions
e. Vesicular and channel pathways

156. Organs such as the brain and thymus have a more effective blood barrier because their blood capillaries are of the

a. Continuous type with few vesicles
b. Fenestrated type with diaphragms
c. Fenestrated type without diaphragms
d. Discontinuous type with diaphragms
e. Discontinuous type without diaphragms

157. Atherosclerosis is usually initiated by

a. Proliferation of smooth muscle cells
b. Formation of an intimal plaque
c. Attraction of platelets to collagen microfibrils
d. Adventitial proliferation
e. Injury to the endothelium

158. The blood vessel in the accompanying electron micrograph is involved primarily in

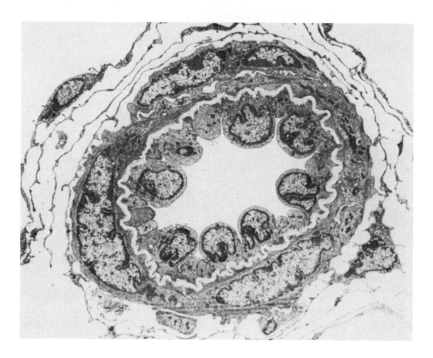

a. Adaptation to systolic pressure
b. Distribution of blood within an organ
c. Blood flow from the aorta to specific organs
d. Return of lymphocytes to the blood
e. Return of venous blood to the heart

159. If fresh human blood is centrifuged in the presence of an anticoagulant such as heparin to obtain a hematocrit, the resulting fractions are

a. Serum, packed erythrocytes, and leukocytes
b. Leukocytes, erythrocytes, and serum proteins
c. Plasma, buffy coat, and packed erythrocytes
d. Fibrinogen, platelets, buffy coat, and erythrocytes
e. Albumin, plasma lipoproteins, and erythrocytes

160. Thrombocytopenia is a reduction in the number of circulating blood platelets. Which of the following would most likely occur in thrombocytopenia?

a. Decreased vascular permeability
b. Failure of initiation of the blood-clotting cascade
c. Failure of conversion of fibrinogen to fibrin
d. Absence of plasmin
e. Absence of thrombin

161. The structure labeled A in the photomicrograph below is

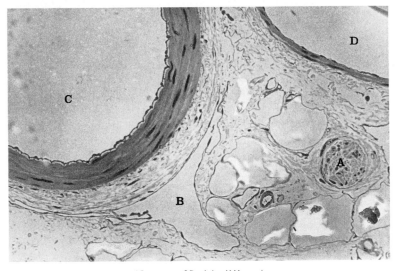

(Courtesy of Dr. John K. Young.)

a. A Pacinian corpuscle
b. Peripheral nerve
c. Smooth muscle bundle
d. Skeletal muscle bundle
e. A venule

162. Erythrocytes may have abnormal shapes and sizes in certain diseases. In iron deficiency you would expect to see

a. Microcytic, hypochromatic anemia with smaller mature erythrocytes
b. Macrocytic, hyperchromatic anemia with fewer, larger mature erythrocytes
c. Poikilocytosis (shape change) and more fragile erythrocytes
d. Spherical rather than biconcave erythrocytes
e. No change in erythrocyte size or shape, but a substantial drop in the hematocrit

163. A 43-year-old woman who has suffered from diabetes for 30 years comes into the clinic. She is anemic with a hematocrit of 22. Which of the following would most likely explain her condition?

a. Decreased hepatic production of erythropoietin, leading to decreased numbers of circulating reticulocytes in the bloodstream
b. Increased erythropoietin production by the liver, resulting in increased numbers of reticulocytes
c. Decreased renal erythropoietin production, leading to reduced numbers of red blood cells
d. Decreased estrogen levels, stimulating hepatic production of erythropoietin
e. Decreased estrogen levels, inhibiting renal production of erythropoietin

164. Which of the following is a metabolic function of endothelial cells?

a. Formation of angiotensinogen
b. Activation of bradykinin
c. Production of type III collagen
d. Synthesis of plasminogen activator
e. Production of thromboxane

165. The cell shown in drawing D below functions

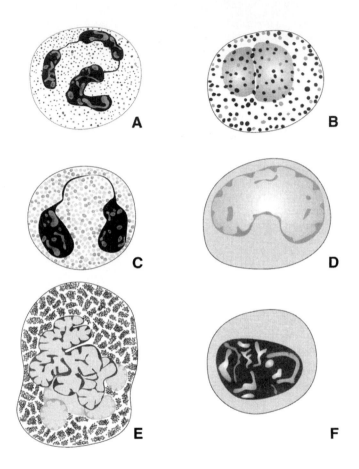

a. In the formation of pus
b. As the precursor of Langerhans cells
c. As a specific phagocyte for parasites
d. As a specific phagocyte for bacteria
e. In immediate hypersensitivity reactions

Cardiovascular System, Blood, and Bone Marrow

Answers

148. The answer is c. (*McKenzie and Klein, p 240. Junqueira, 9/e, pp 202–204.*) Vasa vasorum are vessels within a vessel and are found primarily in the adventitia of large arteries and veins. They provide nutrition and oxygenated blood to the thick media and adventitia of these vessels, which are unable to obtain nutrition by diffusion from the lumen. Coronary arteries fulfill a similar function for the myocardium.

149. The answer is d. (*Alberts, 3/e, p 996. Braunwald, 15/e, p 748.*) Glanzmann's disease, or thrombasthenia, is caused by a defect in the β_3-integrins. The result is the loss of normal binding to fibrinogen and loss of normal aggregation of platelets. The effect on the patient is delayed clotting time, reduced hemostasis, and therefore excessive bleeding following injury. Hemostasis is the term used for the body's response to endothelial disruption leading to the entrance of blood into the subendothelial connective tissue. It is often divided into two phases: (1) primary, which is the formation of a platelet plug, and (2) secondary, which results in the formation of the clot, composed of fibrin. Granule release, platelet-derived growth factor (PDGF) secretion, size, and normal shape changes do not appear to be affected in Glanzmann's disease.

150 to 153. The answers are 150-a, 151-c, 152-e, 153-a. (*McKenzie and Klein, pp 224–225. Moore, 6/e, Developing Human, pp 115, 279. Sweeney, pp 398, 404–405. Junqueira, 9/e, pp 218–219, 222, 224–228, 234–235, 241–242, 246.*) The first stage in granulopoiesis is the myeloblast (A), a large cell with prominent light-staining nucleoli with only a little cytoplasm, generally without granules. The lineage shown in the figure illustrates eosinophilic development in the bone marrow. The promyelocyte (B) is the next cell in the lineage. It is larger than the myeloblast, nucleoli are less visible, and primary granules are present in the cytoplasm. In the next stage, myelocyte-specific granules are seen in the cytoplasm with flattening of the nucleus. The eosinophilic myelocyte (C) differentiates into the eosinophilic metamyelocyte (D) when invagination of the nucleus begins. Further invagination leads to the formation of an eosinophilic band (E) and ultimately a mature eosinophil (F). An eosinophil has a bilobed nucleus and plays an important role in allergic and parasitic infections. The granules stain with eosinophilic dyes and contain major basic protein, histaminase, peroxidase, and some hydrolytic enzymes. This cell has an affinity for antigen-antibody complexes and, although phagocytic, it is not as active against bacteria as neutrophils. The histaminase secreted by eosinophils counteracts the release of histamine from basophils and mast cells, essential in hypersensitivity reactions. B lymphocytes differentiate into antibody-producing plasma cells; T lymphocytes are primarily responsible for graft rejection; and neutrophils are responsible for phagocytosis of bacteria.

Hematopoiesis occurs in the flat bones of the skull and other bones in the adult human. Although most bones in the body are involved in hematopoiesis during growth, the marrow of the sternum, ribs, vertebrae, iliac crest, skull, and proximal femora are the primary sites of blood cell development by the time that skeletal maturity is achieved. It also occurs in the long bones during development, but many of these areas become dominated by yellow marrow that contains many fat cells (adipose tissue). The inactive yellow marrow can be reactivated on exposure to the proper stimulus (e.g., severe blood loss).

During prenatal development the first site of blood cell development (hematopoiesis) is extraembryonic, in the yolk sac. The yolk sac produces hematocytoblasts and primitive erythroblasts from the third week through the second month of gestation. Hepatic erythropoiesis begins during the sixth week, reaches its maximum in the third month, and then ceases about the seventh month. The bone marrow begins to function in the second month and becomes the predominant hematopoietic site during months 5 to 9 of gestation, whereas the spleen is involved specifically in the production of red blood cells (erythropoiesis) from months 2 to 5 of gestation with some activity continuing until shortly after birth. Although erythropoiesis ceases in the spleen, this organ continues to produce monocytes and lymphocytes throughout life. In addition, from the second month the lymph nodes produce lymphocytes, and the thymus is responsible for the education of T cells after the second month of gestation. These T lymphocytes seed to T-dependent areas, such as the deep cortex of the lymph node.

The kidney produces erythropoietin, a growth factor that stimulates red cell development, but it is not considered a site of blood cell development.

154. The answer is c. (*Junqueira, 9/e, pp 206–208.*) The large pores (50 to 70 nm in diameter) are represented by the pinocytotic vesicles. Endothelial cells are joined together by tight junctions (zonula occludens) with a rare desmosome (macula adherens) observed between the cells. Gap junctions may be present between adjacent endothelial cells and permit transfer of information between adjoining cells. Intercellular junctions, particularly the tight junctions, function as the small endothelial pores (approximately 10 nm in diameter) observed in physiologic studies. Coatomer-coated vesicles shuttle material between the rough ER and *cis-*Golgi.

155. The answer is e. (*Junqueira 9/e, pp 206–208.*) Plasmalemmal vesicles and channels are neutrally charged and rich in galactose and N-acetylglucosamine. Vesicular and channel pathways are required for transport of anionic proteins such as insulin, transferrin, albumin, and low-density lipoprotein (LDL).

Capillary endothelia are continuous, fenestrated, or discontinuous (sinusoids). Transcellular openings known as fenestrae occur in many of the visceral capillaries. In hematopoietic organs, there are large gaps in the endothelium, and the capillaries are classified as discontinuous. Diaphragms contain proteoglycans with particularly high concentrations of heparan sulfate. This results in numerous anionic sites that repel anionic proteins. The diaphragms facilitate the passage of water and small molecules dissolved in fluid. Fenestrations do not permit the passage of cells. Except under pathologic conditions, intercellular junctions do not allow the passage of large proteins. The paracellular pathway through the intercellular junctions is a mechanism for passage of water and small dissolved molecules.

156. The answer is a. (*McKenzie and Klein, pp 235, 366–367. Young, 4/e, pp 139, 203. Junqueira, 9/e, pp 169, 204–209, 255.*) The capillary endothelia in the brain and thymus are continuous, as is the basal lamina. The blood-thymus barrier provides the appropriate microenvironment for education of T cells without exposure to self. The capillary is further surrounded by perivascular connective tissue and epithelial cells and their basement membrane. In the blood-brain barrier, there is also a continuous endothelium with a basal lamina and an absence of fenestrations. Surrounding the basal lamina in the brain are the foot processes of astrocytes, which form the glia limitans; however, it is important to note that the blood-brain barrier is formed specifically by endothelial cell occluding junctions with many sealing strands. Other capillary endothelia in the body are fenestrated or discontinuous (sinusoids). The fenestrae are transcellular openings that occur in many of the visceral capillaries. In hematopoietic organs, there are large gaps in the endothelium, and the capillaries are classified as discontinuous. Diaphragms (thinner cell membrane) are present in some fenestrated capillaries and produce an intermediate level of molecular transit.

157. The answer is e. (*Junqueira, 8/e, pp 212.*) Atherosclerosis is initiated by damage to the endothelial cells, which exposes the subjacent connective tissue (subendothelium). The loss of the antithrombogenic endothelium results in aggregation of platelets. Atherosclerosis is one form of arteriosclerosis (hardening of the arteries) that involves deposition of fatty material primarily in the walls of the conducting arteries. The intima and media become infiltrated with lipid. Intimal thickening occurs through the addition of collagen and elastin with an abnormal pattern of elastin cross-linking. Platelets release mitogenic substances that stimulate proliferation of smooth muscle cells. The thickening of the intima is also called an atheromatous plaque and worsens with repeated damage to the endothelium. It is most dangerous in small vessels, particularly the coronary arteries, where occlusion can result in a myocardial infarction. Atherosclerotic plaques also lead to thrombi and aneurysms.

158. The answer is a. (*McKenzie and Klein, p 234. Young, 4/e, pp 147, 149. Junqueira, 9/e, pp 204, 209–211, 213.*) The blood vessel in the electron micrograph is an arteriole (small artery) involved in intra-organ blood flow. There is only one layer of smooth muscle, but a distinct internal elastic membrane is present. Muscular (medium) arteries contain more smooth muscle and distribute blood to organs. Elastic (large) arteries contain extensive elastic tissue for adaptation to systolic pressure. Large veins contain smooth muscle in the adventitia. There is no visible internal elastic membrane in a venule. A capillary lacks smooth muscle and is composed only of a single layer of endothelial cells.

The large arteries, such as the aorta, contain extensive elastic fibers that permit rapid arterial wall stretch and relaxation and maintenance of arterial blood pressure. The conducting arteries are required to adjust to the force of ventricular contraction during systole (120 to 160 mmHg) followed by sudden relaxation (60 to 90 mmHg) during diastole. Blood is ejected from the left ventricle into the large arteries only during systole; however, blood flow is uniform because of the elasticity of the large, conducting arteries.

The muscular (distributing) arteries regulate blood flow to organs. Contraction of muscular arteries is regulated by local factors as well as sympathetic innervation. The degree of contraction regulates blood flow between organs. When the tunica media of the muscular artery is contracted, less blood flow occurs to the organ. In a more relaxed state, there is increased blood flow to the same organ.

The thoracic duct returns lymphocytes from the lymphoid compartment to the circulation. The thoracic duct shows complete disorganization in the wall with no distinct media or adventitia. The large veins, such as the vena cava, that return blood to the heart contain smooth muscle bundles in the adventitia and are also the only vessel in which one sees both cross sections and longitudinal sections of smooth muscle in the same vessel.

159. The answer is c. (*McKenzie and Klein, pp 211–212. Junqueira, 9/e, pp 218–219.*) When centrifuged with anticoagulants, blood separates into three layers: plasma, buffy coat (a thin white layer consisting of leukocytes found immediately above the lowest layer), and the packed erythrocyte layer at the bottom of the tube. After blood is removed from the body, it forms a clot that contains platelets, erythrocytes, leukocytes, and a clear, yellow fluid known as serum. Hematocrit is the volume of erythrocytes per unit volume of blood (e.g., 40 to 50% in adult human males).

160. The answer is c. (*McKenzie and Klein, pp 212, 217–218. Junqueira, 9/e, pp 229–232.*) Platelets (thrombocytes) are involved in the conversion of fibrinogen to fibrin through the action of phospholipids. In thrombocytopenia, fibrinogen will not be converted to fibrin in sufficient quantity to allow normal clotting. The absence of platelet aggregation interferes with normal endothelial maintenance and repair after injury. The endothelium becomes increasingly leaky and eventually may permit thrombocytopenia purpura with seepage of blood from the vessel.

Platelets (thrombocytes) are fragments of megakaryocytes that function in aggregation, coagulation, clot retraction, and removal. The cytoskeleton of the platelet is extensive and facilitates changes in shape of the platelet as well as contractions, which assist in the release of secretory granules. Platelet-derived growth factor (PDGF) is released by platelets and stimulates the proliferation of endothelial cells, vascular smooth muscle cells, and fibroblasts. Thrombin is involved in conversion of fibrinogen to fibrin, but it is a plasma protein, not a platelet secretory factor. Platelets are not required for the initiation of the blood-clotting cascade, but they are required for the adherence and normal formation of a clot. Plasmin is not secreted by platelets but is formed by the conversion of plasma-derived plasminogen under the influence of plasminogen activator secreted by endothelial cells. Plasmin is involved in dissolution, not formation, of blood clots.

161. The answer is b. (*Junqueira, 9/e, pp 170–171, 209–213, 216–217.*) The photomicrograph shows several types of blood or lymphatic vessels. Frequently, peripheral nerves are found in association with blood vessels (neurovascular bundle). In this section, a small peripheral nerve is labeled "A." It is characterized by an outer covering of perineurium consisting of two or three layers of fibroblast-like cells. The dark nuclei visible within the cross section belong to either Schwann cells or fibroblasts. Neuronal cell bodies (perikarya) are not found within peripheral nerves. The structure labeled "B" is a small lymphatic vessel. Small lymphatic vessels are characterized by a wall consisting only of an exceedingly thin, single layer of endothelium. The lumen is usually larger than that of comparable venules. As observed in the photomicrograph, valves are also present in lymphatic vessels. A small muscular artery (C) and comparable vein (D) are also present in the field.

162. The answer is a. (*Junqueira, 9/e, p 219, 221. Braunwald, 15/e, pp 349–352.*) In iron deficiency, anemia results with the presence of smaller, pale-staining erythrocytes (microcytic, hypochromatic). In hemolytic anemia, there is excessive destruction of red blood cells in the spleen. Hyperchromic, macrocytic anemia results from vitamin B_{12} deficiency. The presence of spherical rather than biconcave erythrocytes is associated with spherocytosis, which often results in hemolysis. The membrane undergoes deformation due to the inability of ankyrin to bind spectrin.

163. The answer is c. *(Braunwald, 15/e pp 348, 656, 658, 1574, 1590. McKenzie and Klein, p 223. Junqueira, 9/e, pp 234–237.)* The most likely cause of the anemia is renal failure, leading to decreased production of the kidney–derived red blood cell growth factor, erythropoietin. In the initial stages of renal failure the kidneys will increase their production of erythropoietin, but as renal damage continues the cells that produce this factor are destroyed. Therefore, there are initially increased levels of reticulocytes (immature red blood cells) in the bloodstream, but as in the anemia of renal disease, low production of reticulocytes is a hallmark of the disease. Although the patient may have decreased estrogen levels, estrogen decreases hematocrit. Also, women who are pregnant (third trimester) can have slightly decreased hematocrits [37 ± 6 (third trimester pregnant women) vs. 40 ± 6 (adult women) and 42 ± 6 (postmenopausal women)]. Administration of recombinant erythropoietin (EPO) is the preferred treatment for anemia caused by advanced renal disease. Generally, EPO is administered if the hematocrit is less than 30% and whether the patient is on dialysis.

Erythropoietin is synthesized by the peritubular (interstitial) cells of the kidney cortex, stimulates the differentiation of cells from the erythrocyte colony–forming units (E-CFUs) and stimulates the differentiation and release of reticulocytes from the bone marrow. Colony-forming units (CFUs) are distinct cell lineages derived from pluripotential stem cells in the bone marrow.

164. The answer is d. *(McKenzie and Klein, pp 218, 236. Kumar, 6/e, pp 27–28, 53–54, 65–67, 69, 101, 469–470. Junqueira, 9/e, pp 209, 230, 231–232. Braunwald, 15/e, pp 1826, 1939, 1958.)* Endothelial cells synthesize a number of antithrombogenic factors including plasminogen activator and prostacyclin. Prostacyclin functions through cyclic AMP to inhibit thromboxane production by platelets. Endothelial cells synthesize the basal lamina including types IV, V, and VIII collagens, fibronectin, and laminin. Secretion of A and B blood group antigens also occurs in endothelial cells. Angiotensin converting enzyme on the endothelial cell surface converts angiotensin I to angiotensin II (a potent vasoconstrictor), but also serves as an inactivation enzyme (bradykininase) for bradykinin, a vasodilator. The endothelium produces nitric oxide, also known as endothelium–derived relaxing factor (EDRF), and endothelin, the most potent vasoconstrictor in the body. Endothelial cells also synthesize plasminogen inhibitor, a coagulant and von Willebrand factor (factor VIII) which is found in Weibel-Palade granules in endothelial cells of vessels larger than capillaries. A deficiency of factor VIII leads to decreased platelet aggregation and hemophilia.

165. The answer is b. (*Young, 4/e, pp 47–57. McKenzie and Klein, p 214. Junqueira, 9/e, pp 107–113, 222–232, 243, 246–247.*) The cell labeled "D" is a monocyte. The monocyte (D) contains an eccentric nucleus, which is often kidney-shaped. The chromatin generally has a ropelike appearance and, therefore, is less condensed than the chromatin of the lymphocyte (F). The monocyte has some phagocytic activity in the blood, but its major role is as a source of macrophages throughout the body including Langerhans cells (skin), microglia (brain), and Kupffer cells (liver). Unlike neutrophils, eosinophils, and basophils, monocytes are agranular. The basophil (B) is about the same size as the neutrophil (A) and contains granules of variable size that may obscure the nucleus. The nucleus of the basophil is irregularly lobed with condensed chromatin. The eosinophil (C) is bilobed with more regular granules than the basophil. The megakaryocyte (E) is a large cell with a multilobular appearance and is the source of platelets. The lymphocyte (F) is considered an agranular cell with an ovoid nucleus and scanty cytoplasm. The shape and the arrangement of chromatin vary, depending on the classification of the lymphocyte: small, medium, or large. Small and medium are involved in chronic inflammation, whereas large lymphocytes are the source of T and B cells. The functions of the major blood cells are as follows.

Neutrophils are involved in the acute phase of inflammation and are responsible for the phagocytosis of invading bacteria. Neutrophils contain lysozyme and alkaline phosphatase within their granules. They die soon after phagocytosing bacteria and are added to the pus, which consists of dead neutrophils, serum, and tissue fluids.

Eosinophils have less phagocytic ability than neutrophils and may kill parasites by either phagocytosis or exocytotic release of granules. Eosinophils contain major basic protein, histaminase, acid phosphatase, and other lysosomal enzymes. Eosinophils are essential for the destruction of parasites such as trichinae and schistosomes.

Basophils appear to be involved in the very early stages of parasitic infection, and they are involved in the attraction of eosinophils to the site of infection. This also occurs in nonparasitic infections and involves chemoattraction by histamine and eosinophil-chemoattractant factor of anaphylaxis (ECF-A). They are similar in structure and function to the connective tissue mast cell. Basophils are also phagocytic granulocytes but are involved in inflammation through the release of histamine and heparin. Immunoglobulin E (IgE) produced by plasma cells becomes bound to the cell surface of mast cells and basophils on first exposure. At the time of secondary exposure, the antigen binds to the IgE and stimulates the degranulation of mast cell and basophil granules that contain histamine and heparin. Basophils and mast cells are involved in anaphylactic and immediate hypersensitivity reactions.

Lymphocytes are either T cells or B cells based on their education in the thymus or bone marrow. Plasma cells differentiate from B lymphocytes that undergo mitosis and form a plasma cell and a memory cell after exposure to appropriate antigen. An antigen-presenting cell and a specific subtype of T lymphocyte called a helper T cell are required for B cell differentiation into antibody-producing plasma cells.

Megakaryocytes fragment to form the platelets which are key elements of the blood (see question 165 for structure of megakaryocytes).

Lymphoid System and Cellular Immunology

Questions

DIRECTIONS: Each item below contains a question or incomplete statement followed by suggested responses. Select the **one best** response to each question.

166. Clonal selection functions to

a. Increase the antigen specificity of the immune system
b. Stimulate immunoglobulin class switching
c. Stimulate the production of self-reacting lymphocytes
d. Form specific colony-forming units for erythropoiesis and granulopoiesis in the bone marrow
e. Choose the appropriate homing receptors for lymphocytes

167. Antigen-specific cell-mediated immunity, as occurs in graft rejection, results directly from the activity of

a. T lymphocytes
b. Plasma cells
c. Monocytes
d. Eosinophils
e. Mast cells

168. Anaphylactic shock is primarily due to the action of

a. Macrophages
b. Mast cells
c. T lymphocytes
d. B lymphocytes
e. Eosinophils

169. This organ, shown at low (top) and high (bottom) magnification, is

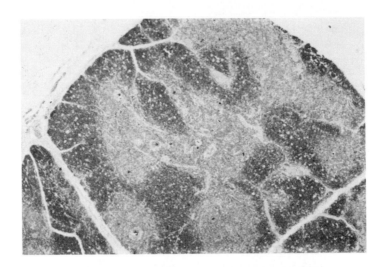

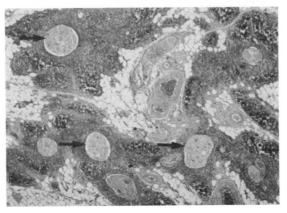

a. A site of antibody production
b. The site of filtration of the lymph and blood
c. Derived embryologically from the third branchial arch
d. The site of production of CD_4^+ and CD_8^+ cells
e. A major site of red blood cell degradation and bilirubin recycling

170. Gene rearrangement of cytotoxic T cells occurs primarily in the

a. Bone marrow
b. Spleen
c. Germinal centers
d. Thymus
e. Mesenteric lymph nodes

171. Gene products of class II major histocompatibility complex (MHC) present antigenic peptides primarily to

a. Helper T cells
b. Cytotoxic T cells
c. Antigen-presenting cells
d. B cells
e. Plasma cells

172. Expression of antigen associated with class I major histocompatibility complex (MHC) molecules is recognized primarily by

a. B cells
b. CD_4^+ T lymphocytes
c. CD_8^+ T lymphocytes
d. Plasma cells
e. Macrophages

173. Interleukin 2 is made by

a. Plasma cells
b. Natural killer cells
c. CD_4^+ T lymphocytes
d. CD_8^+ T lymphocytes
e. Macrophages

174. The tissue immediately surrounding the structure labeled with the arrow functions primarily as a

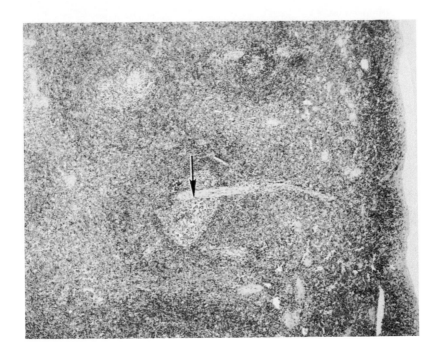

a. T cell-dependent area
b. B cell-dependent area
c. Region specialized for phagocytosis
d. Region specialized for T cell education
e. Region specialized for erythrocyte destruction

175. The cell shown in the accompanying photomicrograph was treated with fluorescein-labeled antihuman immunoglobulin. This cell would most likely be found in the

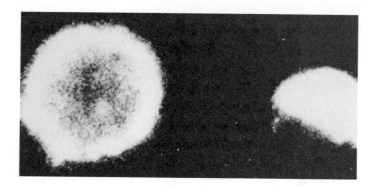

a. Cortex of the thymus
b. Medulla of the thymus
c. Deep cortex (paracortex) of the lymph node
d. Germinal centers in the spleen
e. Periarterial lymphoid sheath in the white pulp of the spleen

176. Immunoglobulin switching from IgM to IgG occurs primarily in the

a. Bone marrow
b. Peripheral blood
c. Germinal centers
d. Thymus
e. Splenic red pulp

177. In a positive tuberculin skin test, helper T cells assist in which of the following ways?

a. Autocrine-mediated inhibition of proliferation of helper T cells
b. The downregulation of IL-2 receptors on helper T cells
c. Secretion of interleukins that promote T cell proliferation
d. Secretion of IL-1
e. Inactivation of macrophages by release of γ-interferon

178. Which of the following would occur during a viral infection?

a. Phagocytosis of virus by $CD_4{}^+$ T cells
b. Presentation of antigen by $CD_4{}^+$ T cells
c. Killing of virus-infected cells by $CD_4{}^+$ T cells
d. Formation of memory B and memory T cells
e. Killing of virus-infected cells by $CD_4{}^+$ T cells

179. The mechanism for lymphocyte circulation from the lymphoid compartment in the region marked with the asterisk to the blood involves which of the following?

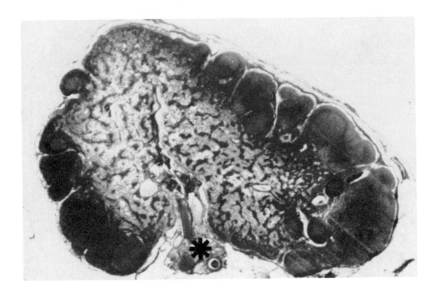

a. Homing receptors on lymphocytes that recognize vascular addressins on high endothelial venule cells
b. Lymphocyte binding to endothelial integrins followed by passage through endothelial cells lining the high endothelial postcapillary venules
c. Lymphocyte passage through the zonulae occludentes by diapedesis after dissolution of the junctions by proteolytic enzyme release
d. Lymphocyte passage from the efferent lymphatic vessel to the thoracic duct and subsequently the venous system
e. Passage of lymphocytes through the discontinuous sinusoidal wall into the blood

180. Macrophages are directly involved in immune responses in which of the following ways?

a.   Production of IL-2
b.   Presentation of antigen
c.   Specific killing of tumor cells
d.   Production of antibodies
e.   Inactivation of helper T cells

181. In comparison with the primary immune response, which of the following is true of the secondary response?

a.   It has a longer lag period
b.   It has a shorter duration
c.   It is of diminished intensity
d.   It lacks specificity
e.   It is due to the presence of memory B and T cells

Lymphoid System and Cellular Immunology

Answers

166. The answer is a. (*McKenzie and Klein, p 266. Alberts, 3/e, pp 1199–1200. Roitt, 5/e, p 8. Male, 3/e, p 6.*) Clonal selection is the method by which B and T cells develop specificity for antigens they have not yet seen. B cells function through humoral immunity (i.e., secretion of antibodies specific for the antigen that generated them); T cells are involved in cell-mediated immunity (e.g., the cytotoxic action of CD_8^+ T cells). In clonal selection a clone of lymphocytes is committed to respond to a particular antigen. The antigenic determinants, which consist of specific amino acids or monosaccharides, actually induce many clones and a wide variety of humoral and cell-mediated responses. This occurs during the development and maturation of the immune system and is responsible for the specificity of lymphocyte cell surface receptors for antigens. Immunoglobulin class switching occurs during the education (maturation) of B cells. Homing receptor differentiation is an important part of T and B cell education in the thymus and bone marrow, respectively.

167. The answer is a. (*McKenzie and Klein, pp 257–260. Male, 3/e, pp 19, 51, 97. Roitt, 5/e, pp 353–365.*) Transplant (graft) rejection is mediated by the action of T cells. Helper T (TH) cells recognize peptides associated with MHC antigens from the donor tissue and become activated. Activated TH cells release interleukin 2 (IL-2) and interferon-γ (IFN-γ), which activate cytotoxic T (TC) cells, B cells, and macrophages. Although all of these cells are involved in the rejection process, T cells are the primary agents of transplant rejection. This has been confirmed by animal studies: animals deficient in T cells are incapable of rejecting grafts.

168. The answer is b. (*McKenzie and Klein, p 162. Braunwald, 15/e, pp 1805, 1811–1218, 1818, 1827, 1914, 1916. Junqueira, 9/e, p 110–112, 250. Male, 3/e, p 107. Roitt, 5/e, pp 302, 309. Alberts, 3/e, pp 1208–1211.*) Mast cells and basophils are the key cells in the development of anaphylactic shock, a type of hypersensitivity reaction. In this allergic response, a person who has been sensitized to a particular antigen on first exposure responds with release of secretions (heparin and histamine) from both mast cells and basophils, resulting in smooth muscle contraction (e.g., constriction of bronchioles), increased vascular permeability (dilation of blood vessels), and a reduction in blood pressure. In severe cases, circulatory or respiratory failure may occur.

On an initial exposure to an antigen, IgE binds to receptors on the mast cell and basophil surfaces. On second exposure, this bound IgE functions as an antigen receptor. Presence of antigen-antibody complexes on the cell surface induces release of secretion, including release of eosinophil-chemoattractant factor of anaphylaxis (ECF-A), histamine, heparin, and slow-reacting substance of anaphylaxis (SRS-A). In the presence of allergens, allergy symptoms are induced by histamine and heparin, which increase vascular permeability and dilate blood vessels.

169. The answer is d. (*McKenzie and Klein, pp 247–250. Male, 3/e, p 18. Roitt, 5/e, pp 31–36. Alberts, 3/e, pp 158–161.*) The organ in the photomicrograph is the thymus, which produces CD_4^+ (helper) and CD_8^+ (cytotoxic) T cells. It functions in the generation of self/nonself discrimination because self-reactive T cells are deleted and self-MHC-restricted cells are expanded during their education within the thymus. T cell receptors for antigen develop during the education of T cells in the thymus. These T cells also develop homing receptors for subsequent seeding to T-dependent areas of lymph nodes, spleen, and other lymphoid tissues throughout the body. The thymus can be identified at low magnification (top) from the lobulation with cortex and medulla in each lobule and the absence of germinal centers. At high magnification (bottom) the presence of Hassall's (thymic) corpuscles is an identifying characteristic. Hassall's corpuscles contain degenerating epithelial cells in concentric arrays that increase with age. Their precise function is unknown. The thymus is derived from the third and fourth branchial pouches not the third branchial arch. Production of memory B cells as well as effector and memory T cells occurs in the secondary lymphoid organs. Production of antibodies is the responsibility of plasma cells, which arise from B lymphocytes and are found in germinal centers in lymph nodes throughout the body as well as in the spleen and tonsils. The lymph nodes filter the lymph and blood. The spleen is the site of erythrocyte degradation and bilirubin recycling.

170. The answer is d. *(McKenzie and Klein, p 251, 265–266. Alberts, 3/e, pp 1228–1229. Roitt, 5/e, pp 158–161.)* T cell gene rearrangement occurs during the education of T cells in the thymus in fetal and early neonatal development. The T cell receptor (TCR) is composed of α and β chains. Each chain contains a variable amino-terminal portion and a constant carboxyl-terminal portion. These chains are encoded for by V, D, J, and C gene segments, which undergo rearrangement during development in the thymus. There are three types of T cells: cytotoxic T cells, suppressor T cells, and helper T cells. Helper T cells possess a specific cell membrane marker and are known as CD_4^+ cells, whereas CD_8^+ cells have a different cell surface marker and include the suppressor and cytotoxic subgroups. T cells require close contact with other cells to perform their cell-mediated function. This is quite different from B cells, where antibodies are secreted into the bloodstream. B cell gene rearrangement occurs in the bone marrow during B cell education by a similar process. It must be remembered that T cell receptors are antibody-like heterodimers. Gene rearrangement in B and T cell education involves similar V(D)J recombinations.

171. The answer is a. *(McKenzie and Klein, pp 260–261. Alberts, 3/e, pp 1238–1240. Junqueira, 9/e, pp 229, 253.)* Fragments of antigen associated with class II MHC glycoproteins are recognized by helper T cells. Activation of helper T cells is required as an early step in the immune response. For B cells to respond to most antigens, helper T cells are an absolute requirement. However, in the case of some bacterial polysaccharides, B cells respond to the antigens in the absence of helper T cells. The primary cell type for expression of class II MHC is the macrophage that serves as an antigen-presenting cell, but thymic epithelial cells and B cells can also present antigen under appropriate conditions.

172. The answer is c. *(McKenzie and Klein, pp 244–245, 257–259. Alberts, 3/e, pp 1235–1238.)* Cytotoxic T cells possess the CD_8 cell surface marker. CD_8+ T cells recognize foreign antigen in association with class I MHC molecules. Cytotoxic T cells are effective in killing virus-infected cells because these cells express fragments of virus combined with MHC I molecules on their surfaces. In contrast, helper T (CD_4^+) cells recognize antigen in association with class II MHC molecules. MHC class I is present on the surface of most cells, whereas antigen-presenting cells (including B lymphocytes) and thymic epithelial cells possess MHC class II.

173. The answer is c. (*McKenzie and Klein, pp 258–259. Junqueira, 9/e, pp 229, 251–52.*) Interleukin 2 (IL-2) is produced by helper T cells (cell surface marker CD₄). IL-2 stimulates proliferation of activated T cells and B cells. IL-2 is a lymphokine, a subtype of cytokine, that affects the proliferation and differentiation of other cells. Antigen-presenting cells make IL-1 with helper T cells as the primary target. Helper T cells are greatly diminished during the immunodeficiency that follows AIDS infection. Natural killer cells comprise about 10 to 15% of circulating lymphocytes. They produce products that kill tumor cells.

174. The answer is a. (*McKenzie and Klein, pp 250, 261–62. Young, 4/e, pp 203, 207–221. Junqueira, 9/e, pp 263–269.*) The region shown is a T-dependent region of the spleen. The photomicrograph is a medium-magnification view of the spleen. The region shown is an area of white pulp with a central artery. The sheath surrounding the central artery is known as the periarterial lymphoid sheath (PALS) and is analogous to the deep cortex (paracortex) of the lymph node or the interfollicular zone of Peyer's patches, the other T-dependent regions within lymphoid tissue. The histologic structure of the spleen includes the presence of a connective tissue capsule with extensions into the parenchyma, forming trabeculae. The parenchyma consists of red pulp, which represents areas of red blood cells, many of which are undergoing degradation and phagocytosis by macrophages lining the sinusoids of the red pulp, and white pulp, which represents lymphocytes involved in the filtration of the blood. The germinal centers within the white pulp are the B-dependent regions of the spleen.

175. The answer is d. (*McKenzie and Klein, pp 256, 264. Roitt, 5/e, pp 14–19.*) Immunoglobulin-producing cells would be found in the germinal centers of the white pulp of the spleen and other secondary lymphoid organs (i.e., germinal centers in the cortex of the spleen and in the tonsils and lymphoid follicles in the MALT). Lymphocytes that are the equivalent of the bursa-dependent B lymphocytes of the chicken can be identified by the presence of immunoglobulin on their surface membranes. These are the cells that ultimately differentiate into antibody-secreting plasma cells under the appropriate conditions. T lymphocytes, on the other hand, do not have readily detectable cell membrane immunoglobulin. The thymus and the periarterial lymphoid sheath would contain T cells.

176. The answer is c. (*McKenzie and Klein, pp 255–257. Alberts, 3/e, pp 1226–1227. Roitt, 5/e, pp 102–103, 166–168.*) Immunoglobulin switching normally occurs in the germinal centers during the maturation of B cells. Synthesis of B cell antibody begins as IgM inserted into the cell membrane and then switches to membrane-bound IgM and IgD. After antigen stimulation, a switch to surface IgM, IgA, IgG, or IgE occurs, and these antibodies are secreted. Most antibody production occurs in the germinal centers of the lymph nodes, tonsils, and spleen. It occurs to a lesser extent in the bone marrow, but the bone marrow functions in the education of B cells as well as representing the major site of hematopoiesis in the adult. The thymus is responsible for the education of T cells. The splenic red pulp is the site of red blood cell breakdown.

Recognition of antigen by B cells is accomplished by the expression of IgM molecules on the cell surface. Some investigators use the term pre-B cell, or virgin B cell, to distinguish those B cells that have not yet synthesized IgM from those that have synthesized and inserted IgM into their cell membranes. IgD, which is produced later by maturing B cells, also serves as an antigen receptor.

177. The answer is c. (*Alberts, 3/e, pp 1242–1245. Kumar, 6/e, pp 94, 421. Paul, 4/e, pp 1360–1361. Junqueira, 9/e, pp 229, 251–252.*) In a tuberculin skin test, T cell proliferation is increased by secretion of interleukins. An extract of tuberculin (an antigen of lipoprotein composition obtained from the tubercle bacillus) is injected into the skin of a person who has had tuberculosis or has been immunized against tuberculosis. Memory helper T cells react to the tuberculin and secrete IL-2, which upregulates IL-2 receptors. IL-2 binding to IL-2 receptors on the same cell is an example of autocrine regulation in which a cell secretes a ligand for a receptor on its own surface. The result of this upregulation and ligand-receptor binding is an increase in T cell proliferation. T cell–derived cytokines such as tumor necrosis factor-alpha and beta (TNFα and β) induce leukocyte recruitment. Production of gamma-(γ)-interferon by helper T cells attracts and activates macrophages (monocytes comprise most of the cellular infiltrate). γ-Interferon also converts other cells (such as endothelial cells) to antigen-presenting cells by induction of class II MHC expression, which further augments the response. The result of the activity of helper T cells is a dramatic increase in the number of lymphocytes and macrophages at the test site, which produces swelling. IL-1 is only synthesized by antigen-presenting cells and helper T cells are the targets.

178. The answer is d. *(McKenzie and Klein, pp 257–259. Alberts, 3/e, pp 1197, 1202–1204, 1238–1240.)* During a viral infection, both cell-mediated and humoral responses are stimulated. Therefore, both memory T and memory B cells will be formed. B cells will divide to form a plasma cell and a memory B cell. Activated T cells also enlarge to form large lymphocytes and subsequently undergo cell proliferation to form T cells and memory T cells. In these responses, macrophages phagocytose virus. Cells that become infected with virus can be killed by CD_8^+ cytotoxic T cells, which can react to the antigen in the presence of MHC class I molecules. T and B cell areas of the spleen and lymph nodes will be involved in the filtration of the blood and lymph, respectively. B cell differentiation requires the presence of CD_4^+ helper T cells and an antigen-presenting cell. The antigen-presenting cell will phagocytose the virus and present it to helper T cells in the presence of MHC class II molecules. The B cell also presents antigen during viral infections.

179. The answer is d. *(McKenzie and Klein, pp 252, 301. Junqueira, 9/e, pp 262–264. Paul, 4/e, pp 495–497.)* Passage of lymphocytes from the lymphoid compartment of the lymph node to the bloodstream involves passage from the efferent lymphatic vessel to the thoracic duct and eventually into the venous system (at the juncture of the left brachiocephalic and subclavian veins). The region of the lymph node marked with the asterisk in the photomicrograph is the hilus of the lymph node. Passage from the blood to the lymphoid compartment involves specific homing receptors on lymphocytes, which are complementary to addressins on the postcapillary high endothelial venules (HEVs) and explains the specificity of lymphocyte homing. The cells that line the HEVs permit the selective passage of lymphocytes by diapedesis through the intercellular junctions. Lymphocytes have specific homing receptors on their cell surfaces that provide entry for mucosal (versus lymph node) seeding. High endothelial venules (HEVs) provide a mechanism for lymphocytes to leave the bloodstream and enter specific areas of the lymph nodes. HEVs are also found in Peyer's patches and during inflammation of tissues (e.g., the synovium in rheumatoid arthritis). Under normal conditions, HEVs are found in the T-dependent areas, i.e., the deep cortex (paracortex) of the lymph nodes and the interfollicular regions of the Peyer's patches. T cells home to T-dependent areas of the lymph nodes, spleen, and Peyer's patches. The circulation and recirculation of lymphocytes is a constant process that allows lymphocytes to continuously monitor the presence of antigen. The circulation process also allows augmentation of the immune response to infection. Plasma cells never enter the bloodstream under normal conditions but secrete antibodies into the circulation from the medulla of the lymph nodes or the marginal zone of the spleen. Lymphocytes and other cells (e.g., monocytes and neutrophils) that leave the blood never pass through the endothelial cells.

In the histologic section of a lymph node, there is a distinctive cortex and medulla with a connective tissue capsule. The organ possesses the classic bean shape with a hilus (marked by an asterisk in the figure). Afferent lymphatics enter the lymph node on the convex side, and lymph percolates through the subcapsular, cortical, and medullary sinuses. The medullary sinuses converge on the hilus, where the efferent lymphatic vessel drains the node. The hilus also contains an artery and a vein.

180. The answer is b. (*McKenzie and Klein, p 260–261. Alberts, 3/e, pp 1238–1240. Junqueira, 9/e, pp 252–253.*) Macrophages are a group of monocyte-derived phagocytic cells that present antigen and synthesize IL-1. Macrophages arise from the bone marrow (monocytes) and include the Kupffer cells of the liver, Langerhans cells of the skin, and microglia of the central nervous system. Antigen presentation is the process by which macrophages and dendritic cells (antigen-presenting cells) phagocytose antigen and partially degrade the antigen in the endosomal system. Certain portions of the antigen are returned to the cell surface. IL-1 is a lymphokine (i.e., cytokine) that activates the helper T cell. Although in many cases macrophages are required for the differentiation of plasma cells from B cells, they are not directly involved in antibody production.

181. The answer is e. (*McKenzie and Klein, p 267. Alberts, 3/e, pp 1202–1204.*) A secondary immune response is more rapid, of longer duration, and more intense than the primary immune response and involves memory cells. Humoral immunity and cell-mediated immunity involve retention of immunologic memory through memory B and T cells, respectively. A secondary immune response may involve memory T cells, helper cells, macrophages, and memory B cells. The proliferation of either T or B cells during the first exposure to antigen results in the production of memory cells. Specificity is retained. For example, the introduction of a different (new) antigen induces a primary rather than a secondary response.

Respiratory System

Questions

DIRECTIONS: Each item below contains a question or incomplete statement followed by suggested responses. Select the **one best** response to each question.

182. A 52-year-old male patient, who has smoked two packs of cigarettes per day for the past 38 years, presents with diminished breath sounds detected by auscultation accompanied by faint high-pitched rhonchi at the end of each expiration and a hyperresonant percussion note. In addition, he shows discomfort during breathing and is using extra effort to involve accessory muscles to lift the sternum. The diminished lung sounds in this patient are primarily due to which cellular events?

a.   Monocytic infiltration leading to collagenase destruction of bronchiolar connective tissue support
b.   Neutrophilic infiltration leading to destruction of bronchiolar and septal elastic fibers
c.   Monocytic infiltration leading to breakdown of the bronchiolar smooth muscle
d.   Neutrophilic infiltration leading to excess production of antiprotease activity in the lung parenchyma
e.   Monocytic infiltration leading to excess production of antiprotease activity in the lung parenchyma

183. The smallest active functional unit (including conduction and air exchange) of the lung is

a.   An alveolus
b.   A respiratory bronchiolar unit
c.   A bronchopulmonary segment
d.   Segmental bronchi
e.   An intrapulmonary bronchus

184. The lung cells known as "congestive heart failure cells" are

a. Type I pneumocytes
b. Type II pneumocytes
c. Macrophages
d. Erythrocytes
e. Fibroblasts

185. Cystic fibrosis (CF) is an important genetic pediatric disorder in which there is a defect in the cystic fibrosis transmembrane conductance regulator (CFTR), a protein that functions as a chloride channel. Abnormalities of CF include

a. A decreased concentration of chloride in the sweat
b. Increased chloride secretion into the airways
c. Decreased water reabsorption from the lumen of the airways
d. Decreased active sodium absorption
e. Accumulation of mucus in airways

186. In a premature infant the cell labeled with the arrows in the electron micrograph fails to

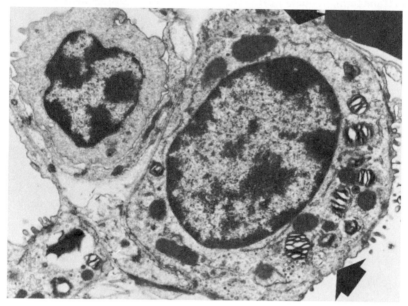

(Courtesy of Dr. Kuen-Shan Hung.)

a. Form during gestation
b. Proliferate sufficiently during gestation
c. Differentiate sufficiently during gestation
d. Produce sufficient amniotic fluid
e. Form its basal lamina resulting in an incomplete blood-air barrier

187. A teenage girl presents in the emergency room with paroxysms of dyspnea, cough, and wheezing. Her parents indicate that she has had these "attacks" during the past winter, and that they have worsened and become more frequent during the spring allergy season. Which of the following cell types is correctly matched to a function it may perform in this patient's disease?

a. Alveolar macrophages, enhanced mucociliary transport
b. Plasma cells, bronchoconstriction
c. Eosinophils, bronchodilation
d. Goblet cells, hyposecretion
e. Mast cells, edema

188. Signal transduction in the epithelium lining the region with the arrow differs from that in rod cells stimulated by light in which of the following ways?

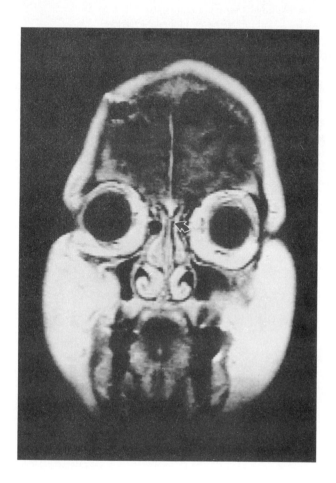

a. Sodium influx into receptor cells
b. Involvement of specific G proteins
c. Stimulation of a cyclic nucleotide
d. Stimulation leading to depolarization
e. Bypass of the protein kinase system

189. Major defense mechanisms of the respiratory system include which of the following?

a. Phagocytic activity of type II pneumocytes
b. Specific cell killing by type I pneumocytes
c. Mucociliary action for tracheobronchial clearance
d. The pores of Kohn
e. Phagocytic activity by Clara cells

190. Which of the following is part of the minimal blood-air barrier in the lungs?

a. Fused laminae of epithelial and endothelial cells
b. Surfactant pores of Kohn
c. Alveolar macrophages
d. Type II pneumocytes
e. Smooth muscle cells of the pulmonary vessels

Respiratory System

Answers

182. The answer is b. (*McKenzie and Klein, p 281. Junqueira, 9/e, pp 335, 341. Kumar, 6/e, 398–402, Fauci, 14/e, p 1455.*) The patient suffers from emphysema, in which neutrophils enter the lung parenchyma and secrete elevated levels of elastase, leading to the destruction of the bronchiolar and alveolar septal elastic tissue support. The destruction of the elasticity in emphysema leads to diminished breath sounds. This is coupled with faint high-pitched rhonchi at the end of expiration and a hyperresonant percussion note. The rhonchi are adventitious (not normally present) sounds that may be high pitched, generally because of bronchospasm, or low pitched, generally because of the presence of airway secretions. Emphysema is a disease characterized by parenchymal tissue destruction and, therefore, is not associated with adventitious breath sounds. However, because most emphysema is due to cigarette smoking, there is almost always some degree of chronic bronchitis, and therefore, rhonchi can be auscultated.

There are genetic and environmental causes of emphysema. The environmental causes include smoking and air pollution, whereas deficiency in α_1-antitrypsin (antiprotease) activity is the genetic cause of the disease. The balance between normal elastase-elastin production and protease-antiprotease activity is altered in emphysema. Persons with a deficiency in α_1-antitrypsin activity lack sufficient antiprotease activity to counteract neutrophil-derived elastase. When there is an increase in the entry and activation of neutrophils in the alveolar space, more elastase is released, and elastic structures are destroyed. In smoking there is an increase in the number of neutrophils and macrophages in alveoli and increased elastase activity from neutrophils and macrophages. These changes are coupled with a decrease in antielastase activity because of oxidants in cigarette smoke and antioxidants released from the increased numbers of neutrophils. The increased protease activity causes breakdown of the alveolar walls and dissolution of elastin in the bronchiolar walls. The loss of tethering of the bronchioles to the lung parenchyma leads to their collapse. The bronchioles, unlike the trachea and bronchi, do not contain hyaline cartilage. A relatively thick layer of smooth muscle is found in the bronchioles, but the bronchioles are tethered to the lung parenchyma by elastic tissue, which plays a key role in the stretch and recoil of the lungs during inhalation and exhalation.

183. The answer is b. *(Moore, Anatomy, 4/e, pp 104, 106, 108.)* The smallest functional unit of the lung is the respiratory bronchiolar unit, which contains a respiratory bronchiole and the alveoli associated with it. This unit allows for air conduction and gas exchange. The alveolus is only associated with gas exchange, and the bronchi form part of the conduction system. The bronchopulmonary segment is a functional unit of lung structure, but it is not the smallest unit. Bronchopulmonary segments are particularly important in surgical resections of the lung because they represent functional units with connective tissue boundaries and individualized vasculature, including pulmonary and bronchial arteries, pulmonary lymphatics, and pulmonary nerves, all of which follow the air-conducting system of the bronchial tree and its branches.

184. The answer is c. *(McKenzie and Klein, pp 280–281. Kumar, 6/e, pp 309–310. Junqueira, 9/e, p 341.)* The alveolar macrophage (containing hemosiderin) has been called the "congestive heart failure cell." The presence of these cells is an indicator of edematous lung changes. During congestive heart failure, edema results in leakage of erythrocytes into the alveoli. Transferrin and hemoglobin are also present in the edematous fluid released from the capillaries. These two products are phagocytosed by alveolar macrophages, which convert these products to hemosiderin.

185. The answer is e. *(McKenzie and Klein, pp 277, 315–316. Kumar, 6/e, pp 207–209. Braunwald, 15/e, pp 1487–1490.)* Accumulation of mucus in the airways is a common finding in children with cystic fibrosis (CF). CF is a frequent occurrence in white children (1 in 200 births). It is a genetic disease in which the defect has been determined to occur in the CFTR protein that functions as a chloride channel. In the sweat glands, a decrease in sodium transport results in increased chloride levels in the sweat (the original detection test for CF). In the airways, decreased chloride secretion occurs in conjunction with active sodium absorption, resulting in loss of water from the lumen as water follows sodium. The result is increased viscosity of mucous secretions and obstruction of the airways and other organs. The pancreas and salivary gland secretions are affected in a similar way, although these abnormalities do not occur in all cases. In the case of the lungs, the loss of the mucociliary escalator action results in susceptibility to opportunistic lung infections.

186. The answer is c. *(McKenzie and Klein, pp 279–280. Junqueira, 9/e, pp 338–340, 343, 344. Kumar, 6/e, pp 204–205. Moore, Developing Human, 6/e, pp 114, 263–264.)* Differentiation of type II pneumocytes (shown in the electron micrograph) occurs late in gestation and is, therefore, incomplete at birth in premature infants. These newborn "premies" have a deficiency of surfactant because of the immaturity of the type II pneumocytes. The deficiency of surfactant inhibits normal expansion of the alveoli and results in idiopathic respiratory distress syndrome [(RDS); hyaline membrane disease]. The lecithin/sphingomyelin ratio is a test that can be performed on a sample of amniotic fluid obtained by amniocentesis. It is used to determine whether the type II pneumocytes are mature and are synthesizing and secreting surfactant. Maternally administered glucocorticoids may be used to induce surfactant production prior to birth, and surfactant may be given intratracheally to premature infants to reduce the severity of RDS.

The surfactant is produced by type II pneumocytes in the lung and is stored in the form of lamellar bodies (the whorls seen in the electron micrograph). Surfactant consists of an aqueous layer, or hypophase, that contains proteins and mucopolysaccharides. That layer is covered by a functional layer of phospholipid that consists predominantly of dipalmitoyl phosphatidylcholine (lecithin). The release of lamellar bodies by exocytosis is followed by their general unraveling to form tubulomyelin figures. The tubulomyelin consists of a crisscross lipid bilayer that covers the type II pneumocytes. Surfactant-associated proteins (SAP) stabilize surfactant, activate surfactant recycling, enhance surfactant-induced reduction of surface tension, and possess antiviral and antibacterial activities. Turnover occurs by both endocytosis (type I and II pneumocytes) and phagocytosis (macrophages); 90% of surfactant is recycled.

The blood-air barrier is formed by the type I pneumocyte, the capillary endothelial cell, and their fused basal laminae.

187. The answer is e. *(Kumar, 6/e, pp 395–398. Braunwald, 15/e, pp 1456–1460. Junqueira, 9/e, pp 335–336, 344.)* The teenage patient is suffering from an asthmatic attack, probably allergen-induced. Mast cells are a key player in this airway disease. Mast cells in the bronchioles are stimulated to release histamine and heparin that induce the contraction of smooth bronchiolar muscle and edema in the wall. If the bronchoconstriction is chronic, the long-term result is thickening of the bronchiolar musculature. Other cells involved in asthma include eosinophils, neutrophils, macrophages, and lymphocytes, which signal to each other through a complex cytokine network. Mediators released include bradykinin, leukotrienes, and prostaglandins, which enhance bronchoconstriction, vascular congestion, and edema. The airway epithelium also is involved in response to and release of mediators. These muscle changes are usually accompanied by goblet cell hypersecretion of a viscous mucus, which can obstruct the airway. Eosinophils release proteins that destroy the airway epithelium (releasing Creola bodies). T lymphocytes are also present in more severe "attacks" and, along with B lymphocytes, may play a role in the initiation of allergic asthma. T lymphocytes also release cytokines that activate cell-mediated immunity pathways. Mucociliary transport is active in the trachea and bronchi; alveolar macrophages do not play a role in that process.

188. The answer is d. (*McKenzie and Klein, pp 375–377, 381–383. Alberts, 3/e, pp 752–753.*) The region shown on the MRI is the olfactory area lined by the olfactory epithelium. The response of rod cells to light causes hyperpolarization, whereas olfactory stimuli result in depolarization. The olfactory epithelium and rod cells are two examples of signal transduction that bypass a protein kinase system. In the case of the olfactory epithelium, an odorant molecule binds to an odor-specific transmembrane receptor found on the modified cilia at the apical surface. The binding activates an odorant-specific G protein (G_{olf}), which binds GTP. The resulting dissociation of the α subunit stimulates adenylate cyclase to produce cyclic AMP. Cyclic AMP directly stimulates the opening of the cation channels on the membrane of the bipolar olfactory receptor cells, leading to Na^+ influx. The resulting change in membrane potential (depolarization) is transmitted from the modified cilia to the olfactory vesicle through the neuron to the basal axon. Axonal processes traverse the lamina propria as the olfactory nerve and pass through the cribriform plate of the ethmoid to terminate in the olfactory bulb. In the case of the rod, the cyclic nucleotide involved is cGMP.

189. The answer is c. (*McKenzie and Klein, p 264, 273, 275. Kumar, 6/e, pp 396–397, 415. Junqueira, 9/e, p 345–346.*) Mucociliary action is critical in protecting the respiratory system, which is exposed to constant assault from the environment. To protect the distal portions of the lung, which under normal conditions are considered a sterile environment, extensive defense mechanisms have evolved. Nasal clearance of material occurs through sneezing, whereas other material located posteriorly may be swept into the nasopharynx. The mucociliary action within the trachea and bronchi is often called the mucociliary, or tracheobronchial, escalator. At the distal end of the system, the alveolar macrophages phagocytose foreign material and secrete and respond to an array of cytokines. The type II pneumocytes resorb as well as secrete surfactant and surfactant associated proteins that have some antiviral and antibacterial function.

In the bronchi, there is extensive associated lymphoid tissue (BALT), which is analogous to the mucosa-associated lymphoid tissue (MALT) of the gut and the skin-associated lymphoid tissue (SALT). There are B and T cell areas throughout the BALT. The B cells are precursors of plasma cells and synthesize immunoglobulins such as IgA associated with the bronchial secretion. Helper T cells recognize foreign antigen in association with class II major histocompatibility complex (MHC) molecules. Cytotoxic T cells recognize fragments of antigen (specifically viral fragments) on the surface of viral-infected cells in association with class I MHC. Antigen-presenting cells (i.e., alveolar macrophages) also function in a similar fashion to those found elsewhere in the body; they present antigen to helper T cells in conjunction with class II MHC. Pores of Kohn are described in feedback for question 190.

190. The answer is a. (*McKenzie and Klein, pp 278–279. Junqueira, 9/e, pp 340–341, 345.*) Oxygen moving from the alveolar air to the capillary blood and carbon dioxide diffusing in the opposite direction pass through a three-component blood-air barrier. This barrier consists of type I pneumocytes, endothelial cells, and their fused basal laminae. Pulmonary capillaries are sometimes in direct contact with the alveolar wall, whereas in other locations, the alveolar wall and capillaries are separated by cells and extracellular fibers. The areas of direct contact are the location of gas exchange, whereas the other areas represent sites of fluid exchange between the interstitium and air spaces. Macrophages are present for the phagocytosis of debris and surfactant. The pores of Kohn are connections from one alveolus to another, and macrophages travel through these passageways. The pores normally equalize air pressure between alveoli and can, in the disease state, provide collateral circulation of air in the event that a bronchiole is blocked. However, they also provide a passageway for the spread of bacteria.

Integumentary System

Questions

DIRECTIONS: Each item below contains a question or incomplete statement followed by suggested responses. Select the **one best** response to each question.

191. The structure indicated by the arrow in the photomicrograph secretes its product by which of the following mechanisms?

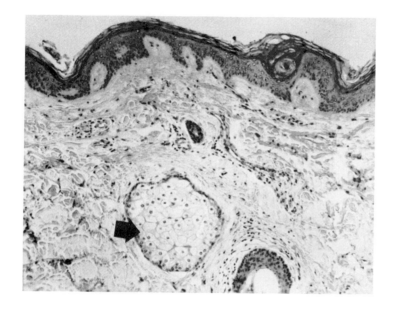

a. Holocrine
b. Merocrine
c. Apocrine
d. Endocrine
e. Autocrine

192. Merkel cells are modified epidermal cells that function primarily in

a. Cytokine secretion
b. Phagocytosis
c. Antigen presentation
d. Cutaneous sensation
e. Expression of Fc, Ia, and C3 receptors

193. The hair is formed by

a. Keratinization
b. Phagocytosis of keratinocytes
c. Fibroblast collagen synthesis
d. Smooth muscle elastin synthesis
e. Continuous, synchronous growth

194. The impermeability of the epidermis is established at the level of the

a. Stratum granulosum
b. Stratum basale
c. Stratum lucidum
d. Stratum corneum
e. Stratum spinosum

195. Which of the following occurs after exposure to ultraviolet (UV) radiation?

a. Reduced protection of the nuclei of dividing keratinocytes by melanin
b. Lightening of melanin
c. Increased melanin synthesis
d. Proliferation of melanocytes
e. Decreased cytocrine secretion of melanin

196. Repair of a deep wound, with removal of the epithelium, involves recruitment of new epidermal cells from

a. Vascular endothelial cells at the site of injury
b. Dermal fibroblasts below the injury site
c. Hair follicles
d. Dedifferentiation of mature keratinocytes
e. Sebaceous glands

197. Perception of fine touch in glabrous skin is performed by which of the following sensory receptors?

a. Ruffini endings
b. Pacinian corpuscle
c. Meissner corpuscle
d. Merkel corpuscle
e. Free nerve endings

Integumentary System

Answers

191. The answer is a. (*McKenzie and Klein, pp 304, 324, 330–331, 351. Young, 4/e, pp 95, 164, 168. Junqueira, 9/e, pp 73, 75, 357–358.*) The structure marked with the arrow is a sebaceous gland, which is located in the dermis and associated with the hair follicles. The sebaceous glands are holocrine (i.e., they shed the cell along with the secretory product). Sebum is a lipid product released into a duct that terminates in a hair follicle. The photomicrograph represents a microscopic section obtained from thin skin. The presence of sebaceous glands identifies the section as thin skin. Sebaceous glands and hair follicles are not found in thick skin. Another difference between thick and thin skin is the virtual absence of the stratum lucidum in thin skin.

The sweat glands are of two different types: merocrine glands and apocrine glands. The merocrine glands release their secretion through exocytosis with conservation of membrane. In the anal, areolar, and axillary regions, the sweat glands are of the apocrine type and empty into the hair follicles. In apocrine glands, the apical part of the cell is released with the secretion. Endocrine secretion occurs into the blood; autocrine secretion is self-stimulation. For example, activated T cells stimulate their own proliferation by secreting IL-2 and synthesizing IL-2 receptors that bind the IL-2.

192. The answer is d. (*McKenzie and Klein, p 329. Junqueira, 9/e, pp 347, 352.*) The Merkel cell is a neuroendocrine cell. It is a modified keratinocyte found in areas in which fine tactile sensation is critical, such as the fingertips. Merkel cells are associated with an ending of an unmyelinated fiber, forming a Merkel's corpuscle. Langerhans cells function in phagocytosis, antigen presentation, cytokine production, and expression of Fc, Ia, and C3 receptors. They phagocytose epidermal antigens and present them in association with class II MHC molecules to a helper T cell. The helper cell assists a B cell in its differentiation into a plasma cell and a memory cell.

193. The answer is a. (*Junqueira, 9/e, pp 355–356. McKenzie and Klein p 330.*) The hair is formed by keratinization, a process similar to epidermal keratinization. Hair formation and growth occur discontinuously and without synchrony. Growth is described as occurring in patches with periods of growth (anagen), followed by a brief hiatus (catagen), and subsequently a lag period in which atrophy of the hair occurs (telogen). The growth process is influenced by a number of hormones: androgens, adrenocortical, and thyroid.

194. The answer is a. (*McKenzie and Klein pp 326–327. Junqueira, 9/e, pp 346–348.*) The cells of the stratum granulosum contain numerous keratohyalin granules. This layer also produces lamellar granules, which form a bidirectional lipid bilayer barrier to penetration of substances. The skin or integument is composed of an epithelial layer (epidermis) and underlying connective tissue (dermis). The epidermis consists of four to five strata (from the basement membrane to the skin surface): stratum basale, stratum spinosum, stratum granulosum, stratum lucidum, and stratum corneum. The basal layer contains most of the mitotic cells and is attached to the basement membrane with hemidesmosomes. The stratum spinosum contains the prickle cells, which have numerous cytoplasmic tonofilaments and intercellular desmosomes. This layer is often classified with the stratum basale as the malpighian layer. The stratum basale and stratum spinosum contain mitotic keratinocytes, and these are the two layers that show a hyperproliferative state in psoriasis. In that disease, increased cell proliferation leads to a thickening of the epidermis with a shortening of the epidermal turnover period. Under normal conditions, there is a gradual replacement process in the epidermis with the production of new cells in the stratum basale and stratum spinosum and their migration toward the surface as they gradually differentiate. The stratum lucidum is a translucent layer typical of thick skin. The stratum corneum contains as many as 20 layers of flattened cells and is filled with keratin.

195. The answer is c. (*Junqueira, 9/e, pp 346, 350–352. McKenzie and Klein, pp 327–328.*) Darkening of the skin in the presence of UV radiation occurs through the darkening of melanin plus an increase in the synthesis and subsequent transfer of melanin (cytocrine secretion). Melanin is responsible for the pigmentation of the skin and protects the nuclei of dividing keratinocytes in the stratum basale and stratum spinosum from UV light. In general, skin color is determined by the number of melanin granules in the skin and not the number of melanocytes per unit area, which is relatively uniform from region to region and between different races.

In melanocytes, melanin is synthesized from tyrosine by the action of tyrosinase forming 3,4-dihydroxyphenylalanine (DOPA). The DOPA is subsequently transformed to melanin. This process occurs in melanosomes (immature granules that contain tyrosinase). Mature granules are transferred to keratinocytes by phagocytosis of part of the melanocyte; this process is called cytocrine secretion and occurs in the stratum basale and stratum spinosum (malpighian layer). Melanin granules remain relatively intact in persons with black skin; in caucasian individuals, there is degradation of the granules by lysosomal systems.

196. The answer is c. (*Kumar, 6/e, pp 55–59.*) In deep wounds, new epithelial cells are obtained from the epithelium of the hair follicles and sweat glands located in the dermis. Reepithelialization is inhibited in wounds that remove all epithelial cells and require skin grafts to enhance the repair process. In those cases there is only minor wound healing by migration from the margins of the wound. Repair of epidermal wounds requires chemoattraction of macrophages to the wound site and removal of damaged tissue by those monocyte-derived infiltrating cells. Repair is mediated by the proliferation of endothelial and smooth muscle cells for the repair of blood vessels and angiogenesis. Proliferation of basal keratinocytes and fibroblasts occurs in small wounds for the repair of the epidermis and dermis, respectively.

197. The answer is c. (*Guyton, 10/e, pp 540–542. Junqueira, 9/e, pp 446–447.*) The Meissner corpuscle is found in glabrous (hairless) skin in areas such as the lips and palms, and responds to low-frequency stimuli (i.e., fine touch). The other listed sensory receptors are all found in the skin and subserve a variety of functions. Free nerve endings are unencapsulated receptors that function in the reception of many different modalities. Pain receptors in the skin are all free nerve endings. The Ruffini endings are the simplest encapsulated receptor and are associated with collagen fibers. Mechanical stress results in displacement of the collagen fibers and stimulation of the receptor. The Pacinian corpuscle is specialized for deep pressure in areas such as the dermis and internal organs (e.g., the pancreas). Its structure resembles an onion with concentric fluid-filled layers surrounding a centrally placed unmyelinated nerve fiber. Displacement of the layers results in the depolarization of the axon. The Merkel corpuscle consists of a Merkel cell, a modified keratinocyte specialized for acute sensory perception, and a neuron terminal that forms a disk apposed to the Merkel cell. Merkel cells are attached to neighboring keratinocytes by desmosomes.

Gastrointestinal Tract and Glands

Questions

DIRECTIONS: Each item below contains a question or incomplete statement followed by suggested responses. Select the **one best** response to each question.

198. The resting parietal cell does not secrete acid because

a. The Na^+/K^+-ATPase is inserted into the apical membrane
b. The chloride channel of the apical plasma membrane is closed
c. The H^+/K^+-ATPase is localized in the apical plasma membrane
d. Carbonic anhydrase is sequestered in tubulovesicles
e. Histamine receptors are uncoupled from their second messengers

199. Enteroendocrine cells differ from goblet cells in

a. The direction of release of secretion
b. The use of exocytosis for release of secretory product from the cell
c. Their presence in the small and large intestine
d. Their origin from a crypt stem cell
e. Secretion by a regulated pathway

200. In regard to the enteroendocrine cells and the cells composing the enteric nervous system of the gut, both types of cells

a. Are derived from neural crest
b. Secrete similar peptides
c. Are essential for the intrinsic rhythmicity of the gut
d. Are turned over rapidly
e. Are found only in the small intestine

201. In the photomicrograph below from the small intestinal epithelium, the area indicated between the arrows is the site of

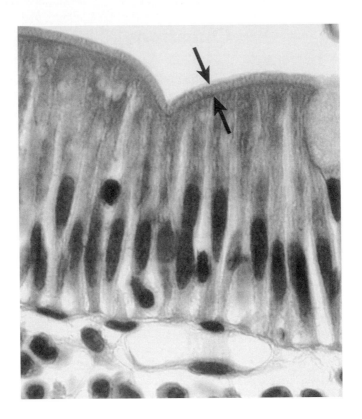

a. Glucose and galactose cotransporters
b. Passive diffusion of monosaccharides
c. Uptake of triglycerides by endocytosis
d. Release of chylomicra by exocytosis
e. Active transport of gycerol into the enterocyte

202. Hirschsprung disease and Chagas disease result in disturbance of intestinal motility. The site of this disruption is most likely which of the layers on the accompanying micrograph?

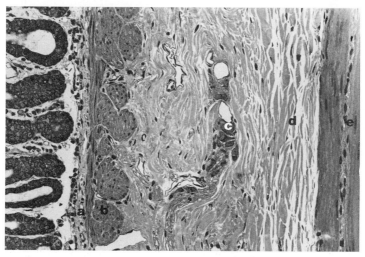

(Courtesy of Dr. John K. Young.)

a. A
b. B
c. C
d. D
e. E

203. As saliva passes through the duct system, which of the following changes occurs?

a. Active secretion of Na^+
b. Secretion of Cl^{2-}
c. Absorption of HCO_3-
d. Secretion of K^+
e. Absorption of Ca^{2+}

204. The primary regulator of salivary secretion is

a. Antidiuretic hormone
b. Autonomic nervous system
c. Aldosterone
d. Cholecystokinin
e. Secretin

205. On the electron micrograph of a hepatocyte below, what are the dark structures indicated by the arrows?

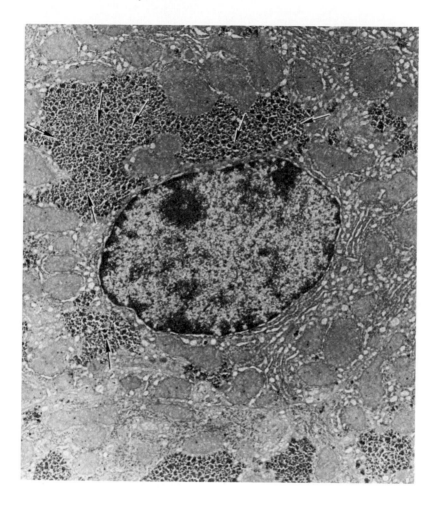

a. Chylomicra
b. Glycogen
c. Mitochondria
d. Peptide-containing secretory granules
e. Ribosomes

Use the figure below to answer the following question. It is a scanning electron micrograph taken from the region between two hepatocytes.

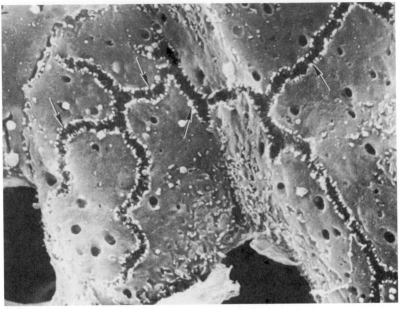

(Courtesy of Dr. Kuen-Shan Hung and Karen Grantham, KUMC Electron Microscopy Center.)

206. The branching structures shown in the photomicrograph are involved in

a. Communication between the hepatocytes
b. Preventing flow between adjacent hepatocytes
c. Bile flow
d. Blood flow
e. Spot welds between hepatocytes

207. In this photomicrograph, the cell labeled with the arrow functions to

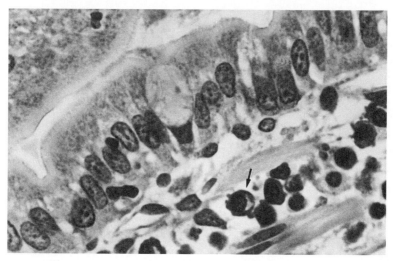

(Courtesy of Dr. John K. Young.)

a. Transport chylomicra from the small intestine
b. Phagocytose antigen-antibody complexes
c. Synthesize IgA
d. Present antigen
e. Inhibit thrombogenic activity

208. The following question refers to the photomicrograph below of a plastic-embedded, thin section. The structure labeled A is

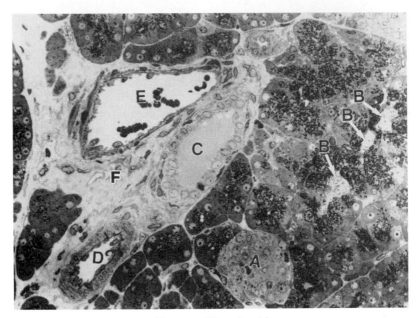

(Courtesy of Eileen Roach.)

a. A parasympathetic ganglion
b. A cluster of hepatocytes
c. A serous acinus
d. An intralobular duct
e. An islet of Langerhans

209. The accompanying photomicrograph illustrates which of the following organs?

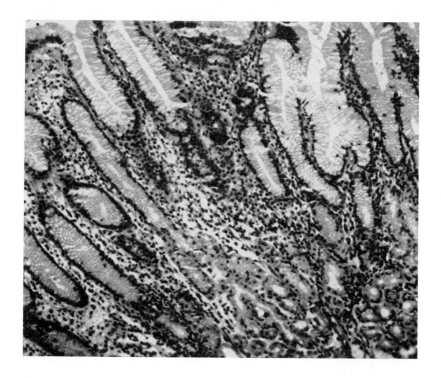

a. Fundus
b. Pylorus
c. Colon
d. Small intestine
e. Esophagus

210. A pathologist views the following tissues (A and B) in a biopsy. She determines that the tissues are normal. The presence of both of these tissues indicates that the sample was taken from the region of the junction between the

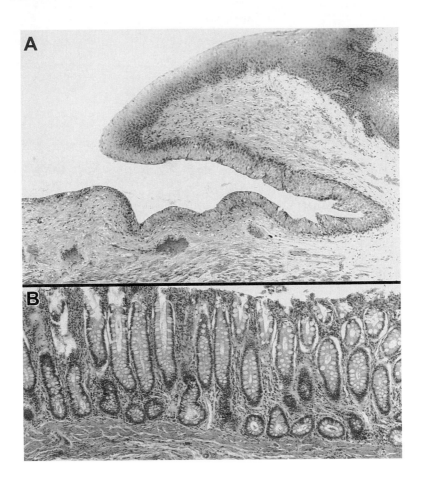

a. Anal canal and rectum
b. Esophagus and stomach
c. Skin of the face and mucous epithelium of the lip
d. Stomach and duodenum
e. Vagina and cervix

211. The structures labeled in the figure with an asterisk produce

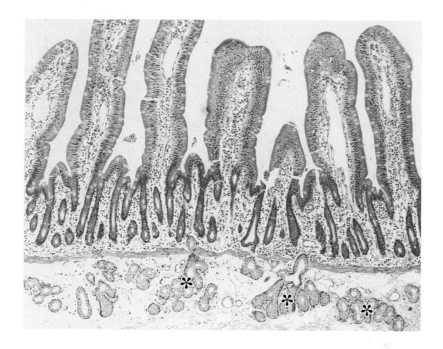

a. Acid
b. Mucus and HCO_3^-
c. Pepsinogen
d. Lysozyme
e. Enterokinase

212. The accompanying photomicrograph is from an organ that primarily

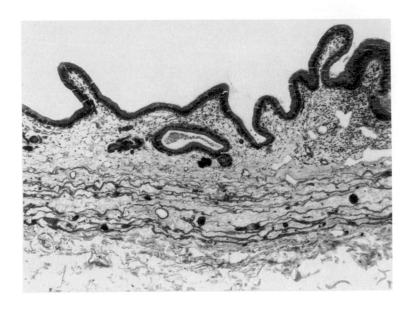

a. Concentrates the bile
b. Synthesizes bile
c. Resorbs water from the colonic lumen
d. Exchanges nutrients and waste products between mother and child
e. Absorbs monosaccharides, amino acids, and glycerol from the lumen

213. The cells labeled with the asterisks in the electron micrograph function in

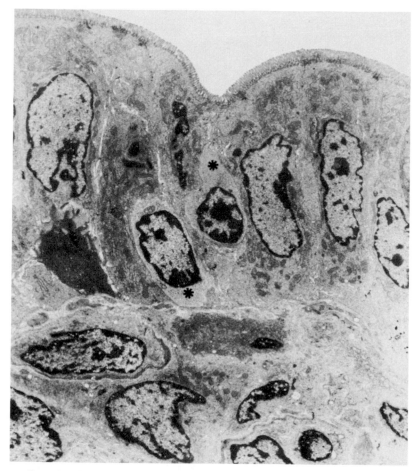

(Reproduced, with permission, from McKenzie, Klein, Am J Anat 164:175–186, 1982.)

   a. Immune defense mechanisms
   b. Mucus secretion
   c. Heparin and histamine secretion and release
   d. Endocrine secretion
   e. Regulation of the flora of the small bowel

214. In hemolytic jaundice, the structure labeled with the arrow in the accompanying photomicrograph will contain

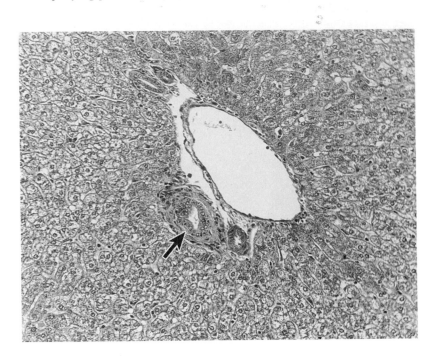

a. Elevated urobilinogen levels
b. Elevated bilirubin levels
c. Decreased urobilinogen levels
d. Decreased bilirubin levels
e. Elevated numbers of lymphocytes undergoing diapedesis

215. A four-day-old male infant weighing 7 lb, 6 oz is brought to the emergency room by his parents. The examining emergency room physician notes that his skin and sclerae are icteric. A blood test indicates elevated unconjugated bilirubin in the serum. The elevated bilirubin levels in this patient are most likely the result of

a. Deficiency of enzymes regulating bilirubin solubility
b. Hepatocellular proliferation
c. Decreased destruction of red blood cells
d. Dilation of the common bile duct
e. Increased hepatocyte uptake of bilirubin

216. A 42-year-old woman (5 ft, 3in., 170 lb) complains of sudden onset of severe pain in the right upper abdomen "under the ribs" accompanied by sweating, nausea, and a feeling of imminent collapse. The pain lasts for about two hours and then persists as a dull ache. When seen several hours later, she has normal bowel sounds, is tender throughout the abdomen, especially in the right upper quadrant, and is faintly icteric. She has noticed her urine is darker than usual but has not passed stool recently. She recalls occasional episodes of "indigestion" referred to the right upper abdomen and radiating to the shoulder. This has occurred especially after eating fried foods or after eating a meal following a long period of fasting. She has no fever but is anxious and tachycardic.

The tests available are a blood count and blood chemistry including liver enzymes, alkaline phosphatase, and bilirubin. She has a WBC of 10,000. Her cellular hepatic enzymes are: AST/SGOT = 52 (2-33) and ALT/SGPT = 70 (4 to 44), alkaline phosphatase = 300 (17 to 91), bilirubin = 6.3 (0.2 to 1.0).

The most probable diagnosis is

a. Hepatitis A
b. Hepatitis B
c. Carcinoma of the head of the pancreas
d. Gallstone obstructing common bile duct
e. Biliary cirrhosis

217. In this diagram of a coronal section of a human tooth, the layer labeled B

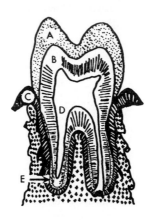

a. Has a composition similar to that of bone and is produced by cells similar in appearance to osteocytes
b. Is formed on a noncollagenous matrix that is resorbed on mineralization by the same cells that secreted it
c. Contains abundant nerves, blood vessels, and loose connective tissue
d. Consists of mineralized collagen secreted by cells derived from neural crest
e. Is the site of inflammation in diabetic patients and is sensitive to deficiency in vitamin C

218. The diagram below shows the relationship between the esophagus, stomach, and duodenum. The area labeled A is the region that contains

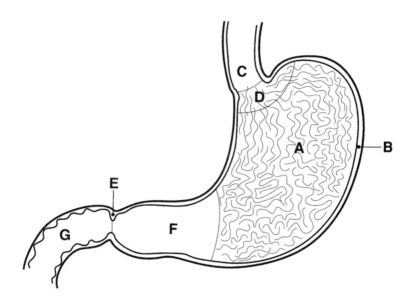

a. Cells that secrete gastric intrinsic factor
b. Most of the Paneth cells
c. Cells that secrete mucus and gastrin
d. Cells that secrete mucus and bicarbonate
e. Cells replaced by renewal from a stem cell in the crypt

219. Cholera toxin exerts its effect through

a. Activation of enterokinase on the brush border of epithelial cells
b. Activation of cholecystokinin effects on pancreatic secretion
c. Closure of chloride channels in the enterocyte cell membrane
d. Inhibition of cyclic AMP in the enterocytes
e. ADP-ribosylation of G_s of the GTP-binding protein in enterocytes

Gastrointestinal Tract and Glands

Answers

198. The answer is d. (*McKenzie and Klein, pp 290–293. Johnson, 3/e, pp 1123–1124. Junqueira, 9/e, pp 283, 285–288.*) In the resting parietal cell, the proton pump (H^+/K^+-ATPase) and carbonic anhydrase are found in the tubulovesicle membranes that are located intracellularly. The sequestration of the proton pump and carbonic anhydrase in intracellular tubulovesicles in the resting state prohibits secretion. On activation of the parietal cell through calcium and diacylglycerol second messengers, the tubulovesicle membranes fuse with the plasma membrane by exocytosis. Histamine, along with gastrin and acetylcholine, activate the parietal cell. In the activated parietal cell, the Na^+/K^+-ATPase and the chloride channel of the apical plasma membrane maintain the appropriate ionic gradients to facilitate acid secretion. Carbonic anhydrase, a cytoplasmic enzyme, catalyzes the formation of carbonic acid (H_2CO_3) from carbon dioxide, which is the source of protons in the parietal cell and other cell types, such as the osteoclast, that also depend on a proton pump. After dissipation of the stimulus (i.e., gastrin, acetylcholine, or histamine) or exposure to an H_2-blocker, the parietal cell returns to the resting state. This involves the recycling (endocytosis) of membrane to reform the tubulovesicular arrangement within the cytoplasm.

199. The answer is a. (*McKenzie and Klein, pp 294, 299. Junqueira, 9/e, pp 75, 292, 294.*) Goblet cells secrete mucus from their apical surface (domain), whereas enteroendocrine cells release peptides from their basal surface (domain). The goblet cells are unicellular mucus-secreting glands analogous to the enteroendocrine cells that are unicellular endocrine glands. Enteroendocrine cells secrete into the bloodstream (endocrine function) or into the local area to affect nearby cells (paracrine function). The enteroendocrine cells may be identified by their staining response to silver or chromium stains; hence the older terms argentaffin and enterochromaffin, respectively. Examination of such preparations indicates that the enteroendocrine cells are rare compared with other mucosal cell types, including the mucous cells. Enteroendocrine and goblet cells are found in both the small and large intestinal mucosa and release granules by a regulated exocytotic secretion. Both cells are formed by stem cells in crypt base of both the small and large intestinal glands (of Lieberkühn).

200. The answer is b. (*McKenzie and Klein, pp 289, 299. Junqueira, 9/e, pp 294, 296–297.*) The enteroendocrine cells and the enteric (intrinsic) nervous system secrete similar peptides and are found throughout the gastrointestinal tract. Enteroendocrine cells are derived from the same stem cell as other epithelial cell types and originate embryonically from the endoderm. These cells turn over at a slower rate than other epithelial cell types. In contrast, the cells that compose the enteric nervous system are neurons, derived from neural crest. There is little cell replacement except in the glial populations. The enteric nervous system, particularly the myenteric (or Auerbach's) plexus, is responsible for the intrinsic rhythmicity of the gut and peristalsis. The enteroendocrine cells function in local paracrine regulation of the mucosa (e.g., acid secretion in the stomach, mucosal growth, small intestinal secretion, and turnover).

201. The answer is a. (*McKenzie and Klein, pp 295–298. Junqueira, 9/e, pp 288, 290, 291–292.*) The structure between the arrows is the brush border containing microvilli. It is the site of monosaccharide cotransport of glucose and galactose, brush border enzymes (e.g., monosaccharidases), and enterokinase, that is important for cleavage of pancreatic zymogens (e.g., trypsinogen) to their active form.

Digestion of lipids occurs through the action of bile (from the liver and bile duct) and lipase (from the pancreas). Bile serves to emulsify the lipid to form micelles, whereas lipase breaks down the lipid from triglycerides to fatty acids, glycerol, and monoglycerides. These three breakdown products diffuse freely across the microvilli to enter the apical portion of the enterocyte by passive diffusion. Triglycerides are resynthesized in the smooth endoplasmic reticulum. Proteins are synthesized in the RER and are combined with sugar and lipid portions in the Golgi to form glycoproteins and lipoproteins. These two types of molecules form the coverings of the triglyceride cores of the chylomicra. The chylomicra are released at the basolateral membranes by exocytosis into the lacteals. From the lacteals, the chylomicra travel into the cisterna chyli and eventually into the venous system by way of the thoracic duct. Digestion of fat occurs to a greater extent in the duodenum and jejunum than in the ileum.

Sugars are broken down by amylase in the oral cavity, with continued digestion by monosaccharidases on the brush border. Proteins are broken down by pepsinogen in the stomach with continued breakdown in the small intestine by the enzymes of the pancreatic jucie (e.g., trypsin, chymotrypsin, and carboxypeptidases). The products of protein digestion are amino acids that are actively transported by transporters also located in the brush border.

202. The answer is e. (*Braunwald, 15/e, pp 1218–1219, 1696, 1897. Junqueira, 9/e, pp 273, 296–297.*) Hirschsprung disease (congenital megacolon) and Chagas disease have different etiologies, but both inhibit intestinal motility by affecting the myenteric (Auerbach's) plexus located between the layers of the muscularis externa (labeled "e") in the figure. The submucosal (Meissner's) plexus is more involved in regulation of lumenal size and, therefore, will affect defecation, but will be less involved in peristalsis. Vascular smooth muscle, the muscularis mucosa, and enteroendocrine cells do not play a major role in the regulation of peristalsis, which is observed even after removal of the gut and placement in a nutrient solution. Hirschsprung disease, also known as aganglionic megacolon, results from failure of normal migration of neural crest cells to the colon, resulting in an aganglionic segment. Although both the myenteric and submucosal plexuses are affected, the primary regulator of intrinsic gut rhythmicity is the myenteric plexus. Chagas disease is caused by the protozoan *Trypanosoma cruzi*. Severe infection results in extensive damage to the myenteric neurons.

The wall of the GI tract contains four layers: mucosa, submucosa, muscularis externa, and serosa. The structure labeled "a" in the photomicrograph is the lamina propria, a loose connective tissue layer immediately beneath the epithelium. Also part of the mucosa is a double layer of smooth muscle cells (b) comprising the muscularis mucosae. In the photomicrograph, an inner circular and outer longitudinal layer of smooth muscle cells is discernible. A thick layer of dense irregular connective tissue, the submucosa (d), separates the muscularis mucosae from the muscularis externa. The structure labeled "c" is a nest of parasympathetic postganglionic neurons forming part of Meissner's plexus. The muscularis externa (labeled "e") generally consists of inner circular and outer longitudinal layers of smooth muscle cells. Slight variations in these components may occur in specific organs of the GI tract. The respiratory, urinary, integumentary, and reproductive systems differ from the gastrointestinal system in their epithelia and arrangement of underlying tissue.

203. The answer is d. (*McKenzie and Klein, pp 285, 305–307. Avery, 2/e, p 366. Guyton, 10/e, pp 740–741.*) The change from isotonic to hypotonic saliva involves the secretion of K^+ from the striated duct cells. The primary secretion produced by the acinar cells consists of amylase, mucus, and ions in the same concentrations as those of the extracellular fluid. In the duct system, Na^+ is actively absorbed from the lumen of the ducts, Cl^- is passively absorbed, K^+ is actively secreted, and HCO_3^- is secreted. The result is a hypotonic sodium and chloride concentration and a hypertonic potassium concentration.

204. The answer is b. (*McKenzie and Klein, pp 305–307. Guyton, 10/e, pp 739–741, 746–749, 855–856.*) The autonomic nervous system is the primary regulator of salivary gland function in contradistinction to the pancreas, which is regulated primarily by hormones (cholecystokinin and secretin). Parasympathetic fibers carry neural signals that originate in the salivatory nuclei of the medulla and pons. The sympathetic nervous system originates from the superior cervical ganglion of the sympathetic chain and stimulates acinar enzyme production. Elevated aldosterone levels affect the amount and ionic concentration of the saliva, resulting in decreased NaCl secretion and increased K^+ concentration. Cholecystokinin (pancreozymin) and secretin are the hormones that regulate acinar and ductal secretions, respectively, in the exocrine pancreas. Antidiuretic hormone can modulate salivary gland production.

205. The answer is b. (*McKenzie and Klein, pp 148, 150, 308. Young, 4/e, p 25. Junqueira, 9/e, pp 48, 319, 322.*) The cytoplasmic inclusions labeled with the arrows in the transmission electron micrograph are glycogen. The hepatocyte, under the regulation of insulin and glucagon, stores glucose in its polymerized form of glycogen. In electron micrographs, glycogen appears as scattered dark particles with an approximate diameter of 15 to 25 nm. Lipid droplets appear as spherical, homogeneous structures of varying density and diameter, although their diameter would be considerably larger than that of the glycogen granules. Ribosomes are found on the rough endoplasmic reticulum or as free structures, in which case they are not found in clusters like glycogen. Mitochondria contain distinctive cristae and are much larger (0.5–1.0 μm in diameter) than glycogen. Chylomicra are located at the basal surface of the hepatocytes and are less dense than glycogen. Secretory granules would also show polarity in their location.

206. The answer is c. (*McKenzie and Klein, p 313. Junqueira, 9/e, pp 315–316, 318, 319, 320.*) The bile canaliculi are labeled with arrows in the scanning electron micrograph. They comprise the space between the lateral surfaces of adjacent hepatocytes. Microvilli line the bile canaliculi and are visible protruding into the lumen. The membranes between the cells are connected by tight (zonula occludentes) and gap junctions, neither of which are visible in the photomicrograph. The zonula occludentes prevent material from passing between the hepatocytes and desmosomes, when they are present between cells, function as spot welds.

207. The answer is c. (*McKenzie and Klein, pp 299, 301–302. Junqueira, 9/e, pp 106–109, 112–113, 295.*) The cell labeled with the arrow is a plasma cell (in the lamina propria) that synthesizes immunoglobulins (antibodies), including secretory immunoglobulin (IgA). IgA is coupled with secretory component synthesized by the enterocyte to protect the IgA from luminal proteolytic contents. The photomicrograph shows a section through a portion of a villus in the small intestine. The core of the villus is occupied by blood and lymphatic capillaries (lacteals). The cell designated by the arrow is within a lymphatic lacteal and is classified as a plasma cell by its characteristic round, eccentric nucleus with heterochromatin arrayed in a clock-face pattern. A distinct, pale-staining perinuclear clear area (region of the Golgi apparatus) is also present. Other plasma cells and smaller lymphocytes are present within the lacteal. The organ is identified as small intestine by the simple columnar epithelium with a brush border (microvilli) and the presence of goblet cells. Macrophages and M cells present antigen in the small intestine. The M cells are found in the follicle-associated epithelium of the Peyer's patches and sample antigens from the lumen. Endocytosis of luminal antigens by M cells is followed by presentation of antigen to intraepithelial lymphocytes. The Peyer's patches form part of the gut-associated lymphoid tissue (GALT). Lacteals transport chylomicra, eosinophils phagocytose antigen-antibody complexes, and vascular endothelial cells possess antithrombogenic properties.

208. The answer is e. (*Young, 4/e, pp 283–284. Junqueira, 9/e, pp 308–309, 395–397.*) The organ in the photomicrograph is the pancreas, and the cells labeled are the islets of Langerhans. The pancreas functions as both an exocrine (secretion of pancreatic juice) and endocrine (secretion of insulin and glucagon) gland. The islets (A) have a heterogeneous distribution within the pancreas (i.e., they decrease from the tail to the head of the gland) and may be used to distinguish the pancreas from the parotid gland. The submandibular and sublingual glands can be ruled out because of the purely serous nature of the acini within the exocrine portion of the gland. The centroacinar cells (B) are modified intralobular duct cells, specifically from the intercalated duct, and are present in the lumen of each acinus. The duct (C) can be distinguished by the presence of a cuboidal epithelium, the absence of blood and blood cells from the lumen, and the absence of a characteristic vascular wall. A pancreatic artery (D) and a vein (E) are shown within the interlobular connective tissue (F).

209. The answer is b. (*McKenzie and Klein, pp 290–291, 394. Young 4/e, pp 256, 259. Junqueira, 9/e, pp 287–288.*) The photomicrograph shows the pylorus of the stomach. The pylorus differs from the fundus of the stomach in the length of the pits of the glands compared with the length of the gland. In the fundus there are short pits and long glands (pit/gland ratio of about 1:4) compared with a pit/gland ratio of 1:2 in the pylorus. There is also an absence of parietal cells in the pylorus. The small intestine contains crypts and villi, the colon has crypts without villi, and the esophagus is lined by a stratified squamous epithelium.

210. The answer is a. (*McKenzie and Klein, pp 290–291, 393, 394. Junqueira, 9/e, pp 279, 287–288, 298, 300, 430, 432, 433.*) Photomicrographs A and B show two distinctly different types of epithelium: stratified squamous epithelium of the anus (top panel) and crypts (without villi) of the rectum (lower panel). The anus has anal valves and an absence of the muscularis mucosa. The esophageal-cardiac junction also represents a junction between stratified squamous and simple columnar epithelium, but the cardiac portion of the stomach forms the mucus-secreting cardiac glands with no goblet cells. The junction of the stomach (pylorus) and duodenum represents the juncture of two simple columnar epithelia, the pylorus containing the short (compared with fundus) pyloric glands and the duodenum with crypts and villi as well as the submucosal Brunner's glands. Skin is keratinized. The cervical mucosa contains extensive cervical glands, and the vaginal epithelium is keratinized. In vagina and cervix, the GI tract pattern [epithelium, connective tissue (CT), muscle, CT, muscle, CT] is not present.

211. The answer is b. (*Young, 4/e, p 261. McKenzie and Klein, pp 290–293, 294, 307. Junqueira, 9/e, pp 285, 288, 290, 292, 296. Kumar, 6/e, pp 479–480, 490, 503.*) The presence of the mucus and bicarbonate (HCO$_3$-) secreting Brunner's glands (labeled with the asterisks) in the submucosal layer of the intestine is an identifying feature of the duodenum. The Brunner's gland secretions function to neutralize the acidic pH of the stomach and establish the appropriate pH for function of the enzymes in the pancreatic juice. Parietal cells are unique to the stomach (with the exception of Meckel's diverticulum and Barrett's esophagus) and synthesize acid and gastric intrinsic factor (required for vitamin B$_{12}$ absorption from the small intestine). Chief cells in the fundic glands produce pepsinogen that is activated by acid to form pepsin. Paneth cells in the base of the crypts make lysozyme and modulate the flora of the small intestine. Enterokinase is made by the duodenal mucosa and is instrumental in the conversion of pancreatic zymogens to their active form (e.g., trypsinogen to trypsin).

212. The answer is a. (*McKenzie and Klein, pp 314–315, 394. Young, 4/e, p 282. Junqueira, 9/e, pp 297–298, 323–324, 325, 438.*) The photomicrograph illustrates the structure of the gallbladder that stores and concentrates the bile. Although the finger-like extensions resemble villi, they represent changes that occur in the mucosa with increasing age. The thinness of the wall is the notable characteristic of the gallbladder. The bile is synthesized by hepatocytes and transported from the liver to the gallbladder. The colon absorbs water from digested material in the colonic lumen. The placenta is responsible for exchange of waste and nutrients between the fetus and the mother. The small intestine absorbs monosaccharides, glycerol, and amino acids.

213. The answer is a. (*McKenzie and Klein, pp 299, 301–302. Junqueira, 9/e, pp 290, 295.*) Intraepithelial lymphocytes (labeled with the asterisks) are lymphocytes that have crossed the basal lamina. These cells may respond to antigen in the lumen of the small intestine or antigen that has been sampled from the lumen and processed by M cells in the Peyer's patches. Enterocytes are the absorptive cells of the gut and possess numerous microvilli on their apical surfaces. Goblet cells synthesize and secrete mucins. Paneth's cells and enteroendocrine cells contain granules but secrete lysozyme (regulation of flora) and endocrine peptides, respectively. Mast cells synthesize and secrete histamine and heparin.

214. The answer is b. (*Braunwald, 15/e, pp 255–259, 1717. Guyton, 10/e, pp 800–801. Young, 4/e, pp 274–279. McKenzie and Klein, pp 313–314. Junqueira, 9/e, pp 323–324.*) The structure labeled with the arrow is a bile duct and would contain elevated levels of bilirubin following hemolytic jaundice. Hemolytic jaundice is associated predominantly with unconjugated hyperbilirubinemia. The overproduction of bilirubin occurs because of accelerated intravascular erythrocyte destruction or resorption of a large hematoma. When the hepatic uptake and/or excretion of urobilinogen is (are) impaired or the production of bilirubin is greatly increased (e.g., with hemolysis) daily urinary urobilinogen excretion may increase significantly. In contrast, cholestasis [arrested flow of bile due to obstruction of the bile ducts (intrahepatic)] or extrahepatic biliary obstruction interferes with the intestinal phase of bilirubin metabolism and leads to significantly decreased production and urinary excretion of urobilinogen. Diapedesis of lymphocytes across the endothelium of the postcapillary high endothelial venules of lymphoid organs (e.g., lymph nodes) increases during inflammation.

Bile is formed by the hepatocytes and is released into bile canaliculi, which are located between the lateral surfaces of adjacent hepatocytes. The direction of flow is from the hepatocytes toward the bile duct, which drains bile from the liver on its path to the gallbladder, where the bile is stored and concentrated. The hepatic artery and hepatic portal vein (shown in the photomicrograph) plus the bile duct comprise the portal triad. Blood flows from the triad (hepatic artery, portal vein, and bile duct) toward the central vein, whereas bile flows in the opposite direction toward the triad.

Bile is synthesized by hepatocytes using the smooth endoplasmic reticulum (SER) and consists of bile acids and bilirubin. Bile acids are 90% reused from the distal small and large intestinal lumen and 10% newly synthesized by conjugation of cholic acid, glycine, and taurine in the SER. Bilirubin is the breakdown product of hemoglobin derived from the action of Kupffer cells in hepatic sinusoids and other macrophages, particularly those lining the sinusoids of the spleen where degradation of RBCs is prominent.

215. The answer is a. (*Junqueira, 9/e, pp 318–319, 323, 324. Braunwald, 15/e, pp 1715–1720.*) Commonly, initial low levels of glucuronyl (glucuronysl) transferase in the underdeveloped smooth endoplasmic reticulum of hepatocytes in the newborn result in jaundice (neonatal unconjugated hyperbilirubinemia); less commonly, this enzyme is genetically lacking. The neonatal small intestinal epithelium also has an increased capacity for absorption of unconjugated bilirubin, which contributes to the elevated serum levels.

Bilirubin, a product of iron-free heme, is liberated during the destruction of old erythrocytes by the mononuclear macrophages of the spleen and, to a lesser extent, of the liver and bone marrow. The hepatic portal system brings splenic bilirubin to the liver, where it is made soluble for excretion by conjugation with glucuronic acid. Increased plasma levels of bilirubin (hyperbilirubinemia) result from increased bilirubin turnover, impaired uptake of bilirubin, or decreased conjugation of bilirubin. Increased bilirubin turnover occurs in Dubin-Johnson and Rotor syndromes, in which there is impairment of the transfer and excretion of bilirubin glucuronide into the bile canaliculi. In Gilbert's syndrome, there is impaired uptake of bilirubin into the hepatocyte and a defect in glucuronyl transferase. In Crigler-Najjar syndrome, a defect in glucuronyl transferase occurs in the neonate.

The ability of mature hepatocytes to take up and conjugate bilirubin may be exceeded by abnormal increases in erythrocyte destruction (hemolytic jaundice, see question 214 and feedback) or by hepatocellular damage (functional jaundice), such as in hepatitis. Finally, obstruction of the duct system between the liver and duodenum (usually of the common bile duct in the adult and rarely from aplasia of the duct system in infants) results in a backup of bilirubin (obstructive jaundice, see question 216 and feedback).

216. The answer is d. (*Braunwald, 15/e, pp 255–259, 1785. Kumar, 6/e, pp 550–552. Junqueira, 9/e, pp 318–319. Guyton, 10/e, pp 800–801.*) The most probable diagnosis is gallstones. The pattern of elevated liver enzymes, alkaline phosphatase, and bilirubin are consistent with obstructive jaundice (see table below). The presence of pain (in the right upper quadrant radiating to the shoulder) after eating a meal consisting of fried foods makes gallstones the most probable diagnosis. Similar pain often occurs in these patients when they have not eaten for long periods of time and then have a large meal. The pain is caused by the obstruction of the cystic duct or common bile duct that produces increased lumenal pressure within the bile vessels, which cannot be compensated for by cholecytokinin-induced contractions. The pain lasts for about one to four hours as a steady, aching feeling.

Enzyme	Obstructive	Parenchymal
Liver enzymes		
(AST and ALT)	↑	↑↑↑
Alkaline phosphatase	↑↑↑	↑
Bilirubin	↑↑↑	↑↑↑

217. The answer is d. (*McKenzie and Klein, pp 285, 286–288. Junqueira, 9/e, pp 276–279.*) The structure labeled B is dentin, which consists of mineralized collagen synthesized by odontoblasts. Odontoblasts are derived from the neural crest. The pulp of a mature tooth (labeled D in the diagram) consists primarily of loose connective tissue rich in vessels and nerves. Odontoblasts lie at the edge of the pulp cavity and secrete collagen and other molecules, which mineralize to become dentin (B). Mineralization of the matrix occurs around the odontoblast processes and forms dentinal tubules. Ameloblasts, which are ectodermal derivatives, lay down an organic matrix and secrete enamel, initially onto the surface of the dentin. As hydroxyapatite crystals form at the apices of ameloblast (Tomes') processes, rods of enamel grow peripherally, and the ameloblasts resorb the organic matrix so that the enamel layer (A) is almost entirely mineral. It contains no collagen, but has unique proteins such as the amelogenins and enamelins.

On eruption of the tooth, enamel deposition is complete and the ameloblasts are shed. Cementum (E) has a composition similar to that of bone, is produced by cells similar in appearance to osteocytes, and covers the dentin of the root. The periodontal ligament (C) consists of coarse collagenous fibers running between the alveolar bone and the cementum of the tooth and separates the tooth from the alveolar socket. Although the periodontal ligament suspends and supports each tooth, the ligament permits physiologic movement within the limits provided by the elasticity of the tissue. It is a site of inflammation in diabetic patients and is affected in scurvy (recall the image of the 18th century British sailor).

218. The answer is a. (*McKenzie and Klein, pp 290–293. Young, 4/e, pp 254–257. Junqueira, 9/e, pp 283–288, 296.*) The cells in the region labeled A synthesize pepsinogen, acid, and gastric intrinsic factor. Region A is the fundus of the stomach. Its mucosa is comprised of gastric glands containing mucous cells, chief cells that synthesize pepsinogen, and parietal cells that synthesize hydrochloric acid and gastric intrinsic factor. Gastric intrinsic factor is required for absorption of vitamin B_{12} from the small intestine. The diagram shows the anatomic relationship between the esophagus, stomach, and duodenum. The esophagus (C) joins the stomach in the cardiac region (D). The pylorus (F) contains shorter glands with deeper pits than those of the fundus and body. These glands contain more mucous cells and many gastrin-secreting enteroendocrine cells. Food entering the pylorus stimulates the release of gastrin, that stimulates HCl production by the parietal cells. The pylorus connects with the duodenum (G), which contains the mucus and bicarbonate-neutralizing secretion of the Brunner's glands. The wall of the stomach consists of the mucosa (epithelium, lamina propria, and muscularis mucosa), submucosa, muscularis externa, and serosa (B) lined by a mesothelium.

219. The answer is e. (*Braunwald, 15/e, pp 834, 983. Junqueira, 9/e, pp 308–309, 323–324.*) Cholera toxin causes secretory diarrhea through the ADP-ribosylation of G_s of the GTP-binding protein, which leads to elevated cyclic AMP and the opening of the chloride channel. The exit of chloride through the open channels is followed by the passage of sodium and water. The result can be dehydration, which can be offset by intravenous feeding or oral rehydration therapy. Pancreatic secretion is regulated by hormones. Secretin regulates ductal secretion, whereas cholecystokinin regulates the release of enzymes (amylase, lipase, DNAse, RNAse, and the other enzymes that compose the pancreatic juice). A number of pancreatic secretions are released into the pancreatic duct system as zymogens (inactive precursors). They are activated only when they arrive in the small intestinal lumen. Enterokinase, a brush border enterocyte enzyme, converts trypsinogen to trypsin. Trypsin and enterokinase are responsible for the activation of chymotrypsinogen, proelastase, and procarboxypeptidase A and B to their active forms: chymotrypsin, elastase, and carboxypeptidase A and B. These hormones are not related to cholera-induced diarrhea.

Endocrine Glands

Questions

DIRECTIONS: Each item below contains a question or incomplete statement followed by suggested responses. Select the **one best** response to each question.

220. The adrenal cortex influences the secretion of the adrenal medulla by

a. Secretion of aldosterone into the intra-adrenal circulation
b. Secretion of glucocorticoids into the intra-adrenal circulation
c. Autonomic neural connections
d. Secretion of monoamine oxidase into the portal circulation
e. Secretion of androgens into the intrarenal circulation

221. A pheochromocytoma is a common tumor of the adrenal medulla. In the presence of this tumor, which of the following symptoms would most likely be observed?

a. Hypotension
b. Hypoglycemia
c. Hirsutism
d. Decreased metabolic rate
e. Paroxysms

222. The anterior lobe of the pituitary is not a good candidate for transplantation compared with other endocrine glands because

a. More severe rejection of neurally related tissue occurs compared with other endocrine organs
b. Its hormonal source is unavailable after its axonal connections to the hypothalamus are disrupted
c. It lacks function when separated from the hypothalamohypophyseal portal system
d. Neogenesis of blood vessels will not occur at the transplant site
e. The vascular wall of the superior hypophyseal arteries is unique

223. The gland shown in the photomicrograph and labeled with the arrow in the MRI

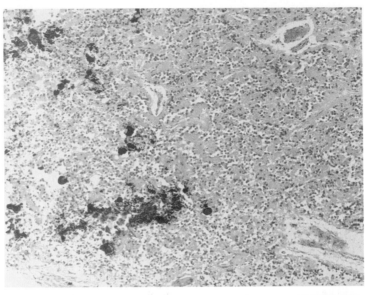

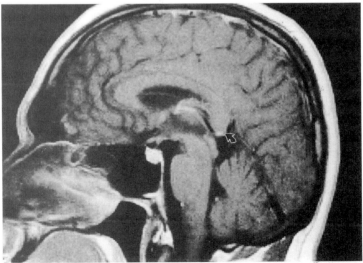

a. Arises as an outgrowth of the midbrain
b. Influences the rhymicity of other endocrine organs
c. Contains many melanocytes
d. Is innervated by preganglionic sympathetic fibers
e. Secretes melanocyte-stimulating hormone (MSH)

224. During the physical examination of a newborn child, it was observed that the genitalia were female, but masculinized. The genotype was determined to be 46,XX. Which of the following would be the most likely cause of this condition?

a. Androgen insensitivity
b. Decreased blood ACTH levels
c. Atrophy of the zona reticularis
d. A defect in the cortisol pathway
e. Hypersecretion of vasopressin

225. Secretion from the gland shown in the photomicrograph

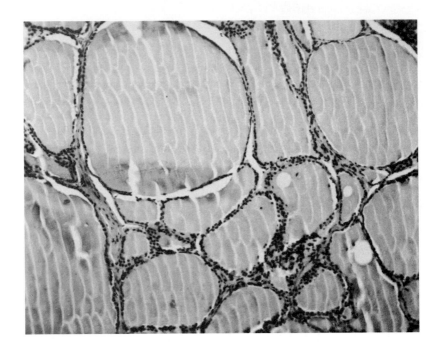

a. Is independent of anterior pituitary regulation
b. Is stored as triiodothyronine (T_3) and thyroxine (T_4) in the follicular colloid
c. Consists of milk and related proteins that are stored and released by exocytosis into the mammary duct system
d. Includes a hormone that transiently increases blood calcium levels
e. Involves phagocytosis of colloid by follicular cells

226. Which of the following cells or parts of the pituitary are derived embryologically from neuroectoderm?

a. Gonadotrophs
b. Pars intermedia
c. Pars tuberalis
d. Herring bodies
e. Lactotrophs

227. A pituitary adenoma is likely to result in

a. Cushing's syndrome
b. Deficiency in T_3 and T_4
c. Diabetes insipidus
d. Osteoporosis
e. Stunted growth or dwarfism

228. A tumor in the specific region denoted by the asterisks will most likely cause

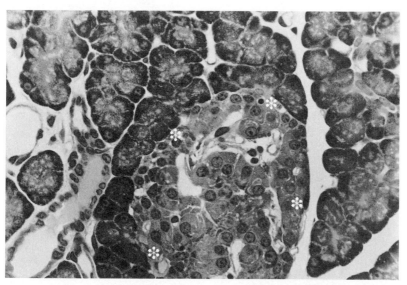

(Courtesy of Dr. John K. Young.)

a. Diabetes
b. Hypoglycemia
c. Elevated blood pressure
d. Decreased blood pressure
e. Increased bone resorption

Questions 229 to 230

Refer to the photomicrographs below in answering these questions. The low-magnification micrograph is on top and is from the same organ as the high-magnification micrograph located below it.

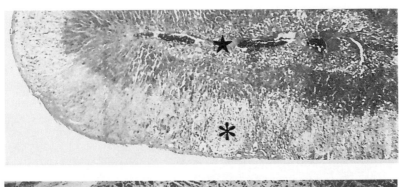

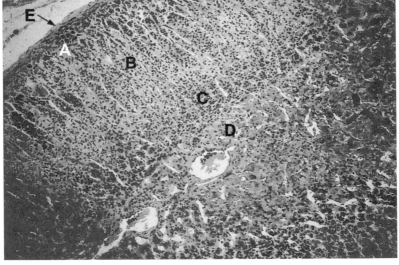

229. In the top panel, the cells located in the region marked with the asterisk and those in the region delineated with the star and dashes have which of the following characteristics in common?

a. Embryologic origin from intermediate mesoderm
b. Storage of appreciable quantities of product
c. Dependence on anterior pituitary regulation
d. Are essential for life
e. Release of stress-related hormones

230. In Addison's disease, which of the following would be a direct effect of the disease?

a. Hypertrophy of zone A only
b. Hypertrophy of zones A, B, and C only
c. Hypotrophy of zones A, B, and C only
d. Hypotrophy of zones A, B, C, and D only
e. Hypertrophy of zones A and B only

Questions 231 to 232

Refer to the drawing below in answering the following questions.

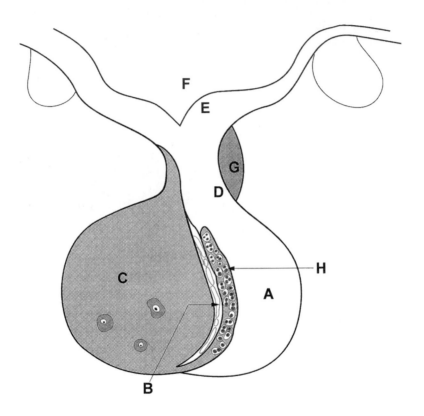

231. The region labeled "C" is the

a. Site of action of corticotropin-releasing hormone (CRH)
b. Storage region for a secretory product that is synthesized in another organ
c. Site of production of TSH-RF
d. Site of storage of the hormone that regulates the milk ejection reflex
e. Origin of a portal system

232. The region labeled "A" is the site where

a. Oxytocin and vasopressin are synthesized for release into the bloodstream
b. Hypothalamic cell bodies are found
c. ACTH-RF acts
d. ACTH is synthesized
e. Hypothalamic axons with dilated terminals are found

Endocrine Glands

Answers

220. The answer is b. (*McKenzie and Klein, pp 321–323. Braunwald, 15/e, pp 439–440, 2088. Junqueira, 9/e, pp 387–389.*) Metabolism in the adrenal medulla is regulated by glucocorticoids because they induce the enzyme phenylethanolamine-N-methyltransferase, which catalyzes the methylation of norepinephrine to epinephrine. Most of the blood supply entering the medulla passes through the cortex. Glucocorticoids synthesized in the zona fasciculata of the adrenal are released into the sinusoids and enter the medulla. The adrenal gland is not usually considered a classic portal system although there are similarities. Monoamine oxidase is a mitochondrial enzyme that regulates the storage of catecholamines in peripheral sympathetic nerve endings.

The adrenal gland functions as two separate glands. The adrenal cortex is derived from mesoderm and the adrenal medulla from neural crest. The blood supply to the adrenal is derived from three adrenal arteries: (1) the superior adrenal (suprarenal) from the inferior phrenic, (2) the middle adrenal from the aorta, and (3) the inferior adrenal from the renal artery.

221. The answer is e. (*Braunwald, 15/e, pp 2105–2109. Junqueira, 9/e, pp 387, 394.*) Patients with a pheochromocytoma often have paroxysms that are the hallmark of this tumor. These are seizure-like catecholamine-induced attacks that include headache, profuse sweating, palpitations, and overall anxiety. Pheochromocytoma is a common tumor of the adrenal medulla that leads to an excess of norepinephrine, which causes hypertension and hyperglycemia. Vasoconstriction of arterioles occurs in conjunction with the increased blood pressure. Epinephrine (e.g., cortisol and growth hormone) have anti-insulin effects, thus causing hyperlycemia.

222. The answer is c. (*McKenzie and Klein, pp 316–318. Junqueira, 9/e, pp 380–383, 393.*) The anterior pituitary is unique in that it depends on the presence of the hypothalamohypophyseal portal system. Releasing and inhibitory factors are transported from the cell bodies in the hypothalamus along axons into the median eminence, where the secretion is released into a primary capillary plexus. The hypothalamohypophyseal portal system carries blood from the primary plexus to the secondary plexus, which comprises the sinusoids of the pars distalis. This system brings the hypothalamic hormones into close proximity with the appropriate cell types in the pars distalis. For example, CTH-RF (corticotropin-releasing factor) is synthesized in the hypothalamus, released into the primary capillary plexus in the median eminence, and subsequently carried in the portal system to the secondary capillary plexus, where it interacts with corticotrophs in the pars distalis. The pars nervosa is the neurally connected portion of the pituitary and contains the dilated axons of hypothalamic cell bodies that produce vasopressin and oxytocin.

223. The answer is b. (*McKenzie and Klein, p 324. Junqueira, 9/e, p 405.*) The photomicrograph and the MRI illustrate the structure of the pineal gland, or epiphysis, which arises as an outgrowth of the diencephalon. The pinealocytes secrete melatonin in response to the light-dark cycle and influence the rhythmicity of other endocrine organs. In a sense, the pineal, therefore, functions as a biologic clock. The pineal contains two main cell types: pinealocytes and neuroglia (the latter appear to be modified astrocytes). The pineal is innervated by postganglionic sympathetic fibers in a fashion similar to other glands in the head and neck region (e.g., salivary glands). The adrenal medulla is innervated by preganglionic sympathetic fibers. Corticotrophs in the pars distalis and possibly cells in the pars intermedia produce MSH. The pineal does not contain melanocytes or secrete MSH. There are age-related changes in the pineal in which the number of concretions and the degree of calcification of the "brain sand" increase. The pineal can be identified and used as a landmark in radiologic procedures by its calcification.

224. The answer is d. (*Junqueira, 9/e, pp 385–386, 393, 395. Moore, Developing Human, 6/e, p 320.*) The newborn described is genotypically female and suffers from adrenogenital or congenital virilizing hyperplasia in which there is a deficiency in the pathway that leads to cortisol synthesis. The inability to synthesize cortisol in turn leads to production of high levels of ACTH and ACTH-releasing factor from the hypothalamus. The result is hypertrophy of the fetal adrenal cortex, which is a critical fetal structure that produces dehydroepiandrosterone. The excessive production of androgens by the fetal adrenal leads to masculinization of the female genitalia. Increased secretion of cortisol cannot occur because of the metabolic defect in this pathway; therefore, negative feedback control is not functional. The fetal cortex is part of maternal-feto-placental unit because the dehydroepiandrosterone is used by the placenta to produce estradiol. The fetal adrenal cortex involutes following birth, causing an overall reduction in the size of the adrenal. The adult cortex (zona glomerulosa, zona fasciculata, and zona reticularis) replaces the fetal adrenal cortex. The zona fasciculata and zona reticularis produce androgens after birth. Vasopressin [AVP; also known as antidiuretic hormone (ADH)] is released by the posterior pituitary and regulates fluid balance. ADH increases the permeability of the collecting duct through an aquaporin-mediated mechanism. Androgen insensitivity is the cause of testicular feminization and is not a factor in the adrenogenital syndrome.

225. The answer is e. (*McKenzie and Klein, pp 319–320. Junqueira, 9/e, pp 83, 146, 397–400, 402, 403. Moore, Before We Are Born, 5/e, pp 206, 213, 214. Moore, Developing Human, 6/e, pp 230–233.*) The thyroid gland, shown in the photomicrograph, contains follicular cells that phagocytose the iodinated thyroglobulin containing colloid, releasing T_3 and T_4 the active thyroid hormones. The thyroid gland is composed of follicles filled with colloidal material and surrounded by follicular cells with a cuboidal-to-columnar epithelium. Connective tissue separates the thyroid follicles. Milk is produced by the lactating mammary gland; the thyroid, unlike the mammary gland, has no ducts.

The activity of the follicular cells is under the influence of the thyrotrophs in the anterior pituitary. The thyroid follicular epithelial cells import iodide and amino acids from the capillary lumen. The follicular cells synthesize thyroglobulin from amino acids. When iodide enters the follicular cells, it undergoes oxidation. Thyroglobulin is iodinated while in the colloid, and iodinated thyroglobulin (not the thyroid hormones) is the storage product in the thyroid colloid. The thyroid follicular cells process iodinated thyroglobulin, and the activity of lysosomes breaks down the colloid to form thyroxine (T_4), triiodothyronine (T_3), diiodotyrosine (DIT), and monoiodotyrosine (MIT). Most of the secretion of the human thyroid gland is composed of thyroxine, although triiodothyronine is more potent.

The thyroid gland also produces calcitonin, synthesized by the interfollicular "C" (parafollicular) cells derived embryologically from the ultimobranchial bodies that form from the fourth pair and possibly fifth pair of branchial pouches. Calcitonin decreases elevated serum calcium levels by transiently inhibiting osteoclastic activity through receptors on osteoclasts.

226. The answer is d. (*McKenzie and Klein, p 319. Junqueira, 9/e, pp 380–383. Moore, Before We Are Born, 5/e, pp 442–445.*) The neurohypophysis containing the Herring bodies is formed from neuroectoderm as an extension of the developing diencephalon. The pars nervosa consists of pituicytes (supportive glia) and the Herring bodies, dilated axons that originate in the supraoptic and paraventicular nuclei. These nuclei produce oxytocin and vasopressin that are stored in the Herring bodies.

Overall, the pituitary gland (hypophysis cerebri) is formed from two types of ectoderm. An outgrowth of the oral ectoderm, Rathke's pouch, forms the structures that compose the adenohypophysis: pars distalis, pars intermedia, and pars tuberalis. The pars distalis includes the classic histologic cell types: chromophils (acidophils and basophils) and chromophobes (acidophils and basophils that are depleted of secretory product). Since the development of immunocytochemistry, the classification scheme for pars distalis cell types has been changed to include acidophils: lactotrophs (prolactin), somatotrophs (growth hormone), and basophils: corticotrophs (ACTH, α-lipotropin, β-MSH and α-endorphin), thyrotrophs (TSH), and gonadotrophs (FSH and LH). The pars intermedia is also formed from the oral ectoderm, is rudimentary in humans, and may produce preproopiomelanocortic peptide. The pars tuberalis forms a collar around the pituitary stalk and is also derived from the oral ectoderm. The pars nervosa (including Herring bodies) and the remainder of the pituitary stalk (infundibular stem and median eminence) are formed from a downgrowth of the diencephalon. The posterior pituitary (pars nervosa and stalk) retains this close relationship with the brain (i.e., hypothalamus) throughout life.

227. The answer is a. (*Junqueira, 9/e, pp 380–383, 394, 402–405.*) Pituitary adenomas are anterior pituitary specific. A corticotroph-adenoma would cause increased levels of ACTH and stimulate excessive production of corticosteroids from the adrenal cortex (Cushing's syndrome). LH and FSH-producing gonadotrophs occur but tend to result in hypogonadism. Somatotropic tumors produce GH and cause giantism. Prolactinomas are the most common form of pituitary adenoma resulting in infertility, galactorrhea (excessive production of milk), and amenorrhea. Diabetes insipidus is caused by absence of vasopressin [arginine vasopressin (AVP)], leading to excretion of a large quantity of dilute fluid (hypotonic polyuria). Overproduction of parathyroid hormone (PTH) leads to osteoporotic changes, but PTH is not regulated by the anterior pituitary.

228. The answer is a. (*Junqueira, 9/e, pp 395–397, 398. Guyton, 10/e, pp 884–893. Braunwald, 15/e, pp 600–601.*) A tumor of the glucagon secreting alpha (α) or A cells delineated with the asterisks results in hyperglycemia and diabetes. This photomicrograph shows both exocrine and endocrine portions of the pancreas. Pancreatic exocrine tissue is found throughout the pancreas with round aggregation of lighter staining cells forming the islets of Langerhans. There are several endocrine cell types within the islets. The more numerous (70% of total) B or β cells are centrally located and secrete insulin that is secreted after a meal and results in a lowering of blood sugar. The smaller population of A or α cells located at the periphery of the islet (*) secrete glucagon. Glucagon is secreted in response to low blood sugar and raises blood sugar levels. A glucagonoma produces excessive amounts of glucagon that results in hyperglycemia and diabetes. The interaction of β and α cells is based on the blood supply. Blood entering the islet initially bypasses the α cells. The result is that blood reaching the α cells already contains insulin, which regulates glucagon production. The absence of normal glucagon regulation by insulin is a further complication in type I diabetes in which insulin is not produced. Other cell types [D (δ) and F)] are variable in location and secrete somatostatin and pancreatic polypeptide, respectively. Somatostatin regulates insulin and glucagon release, whereas pancreatic polypeptide appears to regulate exocrine protein and bicarbonate secretion. The exocrine portion of the pancreas consists of acinar and ductal cells. The acinar cells are pyramidal in shape and possess a very basophilic basal cytoplasm, indicating the presence of abundant rough ER and an acidophilic apical cytoplasm due to the presence of numerous secretory (zymogen) granules.

Other tumors of the islets of Langerhans include insulinomas in which elevated levels of insulin are secreted into the bloodstream. The result is hypoglycemia as blood sugar levels drop. There is decreased storage of glycogen in the liver, inhibition of hepatic phosphorylase (which causes the breakdown of glycogen to form glucose), and increased glucose metabolism in muscle.

229 to 230. The answers are 229-e, 230-c. (*Braunwald, 15/e, pp 2084–2089. Junqueira, 8/e, pp 382, 384, 388–394, 394–395.*) The photomicrograph shows the histology of the adrenal gland showing the cortex (*) and medulla (– – –), which both release stress-related hormones [i.e., glucocorticoids and catecholamines (norepinephrine and epinephrine)]. The adrenal cortex originates from the intermediate mesoderm, whereas the adrenal medulla forms from neural crest. Adrenocortical cells are under the influence of corticotrophs in the anterior pituitary. Adrenocortical cells import cholesterol and acetate and produce the hormones shown in the table below. The zona glomerulosa (A) is found immediately beneath the capsule (E) and is followed by the zona fasciculata (B) and zona reticularis (C) as one moves toward the medulla (D). However, in all zones the cells do not store appreciable quantities of hormones, there is an absence of secretory granules, and the steroid hormones are released by diffusion through the plasma membrane without use of the exocytotic process used by most glands, including the adrenal medulla. The cells of the adrenal medulla (D) may be considered as modified postganglionic sympathetic neurons. Adrenal medullary cells synthesize and secrete norepinephrine, epinephrine, and enkephalins in response to stimulation of preganglionic sympathetic fibers that travel through the abdomen in the splanchnic nerves and innervate the gland. The adrenal cortical hormones are viewed as essential for life because of their regulation of metabolism. In Addison's disease there is a progressive destruction (hypotrophy) of the adrenal cortex (zones A, B, and C). The result in the patient is asthenia (lack of strength, overall weakness, and fatigue), anorexia, nausea, vomiting, weight loss, hypotension, and low blood sugar.

The adrenal hormones are listed in the table below:

Zone	Secretion	Target	Regulatory Factors
Zona glomerulosa	Mineralocorticoids (aldosterone)	Collecting tubules	Angiotensin II
Zona fasciculata	Glucocorticoids (cortisol, hydro-cortisone) and weak androgens	Gluconeogenesis by the liver	ACTH (adrenocortico-tropic hormone)
Zona reticularis	Glucocorticoids and weak androgens	Androgens are precursors of estradiol in the fetus	ACTH
Medulla	Norepinephrine and epinephrine	Preparation for "flight or fight"	Preganglionic sympathetic fibers from the splanchnic nerves

231 to 232. The answers are 231-a, 232-e. (*Young, 4/e, pp 309–314. Moore, Before We Are Born, 5/e, pp 443–445. Moore, Developing Human, 6/e, pp 470–473. Junqueira, 9/e, pp 378–380.*) The region of the pituitary labeled "C" is the pars distalis, which contains corticotrophs that synthesize adrenocorticotropic hormone (ACTH). The region labeled "A" is the posterior pituitary that stores oxytocin and vasopressin in dilated axonal terminals. Overall, the pituitary is derived from the ectoderm of the oral cavity (Rathke's pouch) and the floor of the diencephalon. The anterior (C) and intermediate (H) lobes and pars tuberalis (G) are derived from the oral cavity, whereas the remainder of the pituitary [pars nervosa (A) and the pituitary stalk (D)] is derived from a neuroepithelial origin. The cleft of Rathke's pouch (B) represents the lumen of the structure formed originally from the oral cavity. The pars distalis (C) contains acidophils and basophils regulated by stimulatory and inhibitory hormones produced by the hypothalamus. CRH and TSH-RF are adenohypophyseal regulatory factors synthesized in the hypothalamus, stored in the median eminence, transported to the anterior pituitary through the hypothalamo-hypophyseal portal system and regulating corticotroph and thyrotroph function, respectively. Factors, such as CRH, reach the anterior pituitary through the portal system. In the pars nervosa (A), the major cell type present is the pituicyte, a supportive glial cell. Axons that originate in the supraoptic and paraventricular nuclei of the hypothalamus descend into the pars nervosa. Oxytocin (regulating the milk ejection reflex) and vasopressin [AVP; also known as antidiuretic hormone (ADH); regulates collecting duct permeability] are stored in dilated endings in the pars nervosa called Herring bodies. These secretions are, therefore, synthesized in the another region (hypothalamus) and stored in the pars nervosa of the pituitary. Structure E is the median eminence; F represents the cavity of the third ventricle.

Reproductive Systems

Questions

233. Elevated estrogen levels during the menstrual cycle

a. Decrease LH levels
b. Downregulate FSH receptors on granulosa cells
c. Increase FSH levels
d. Increase the ciliation of the epithelial cells of the oviduct
e. Decrease synthesis and storage of glycogen in the vaginal epithelium

Questions 234 to 235

Refer to the photomicrograph below.

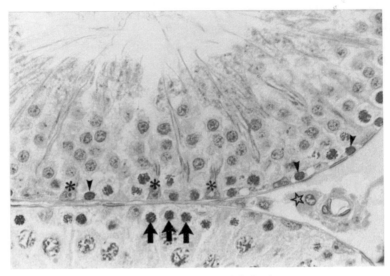

(Courtesy of Dr. George C. Enders.)

234. The activity of the cell labeled with the star is regulated by

a. Follicle-stimulating hormone (FSH)
b. Luteinizing hormone (LH)
c. FSH releasing factor
d. Inhibin
e. Androgen-binding protein

235. Which of the following statements correctly describes the cells marked with asterisks?

a. They divide during each wave of spermatogenic cell division
b. They are found in a 1:1 relationship with spermatogonia, spermatocytes, and spermatids
c. They undergo spermatocytogenesis to form spermatocytes
d. They undergo meiosis and and produce the haploid number associated with the gametes
e. They form tight junctions with each other to establish the blood-testis barrier

236. The structure or structures labeled B in the photomicrograph from the reproductive system below is

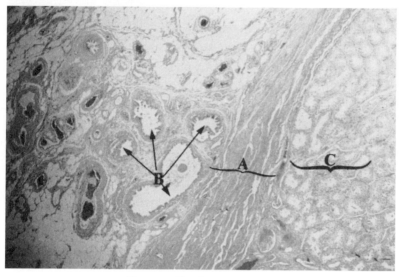

(Courtesy of Dr. George C. Enders.)

a. Rete testis
b. Efferent ductules
c. Seminiferous tubules
c. Vas deferens
e. Oviduct

237. The function of the organ shown in the photomicrograph below is

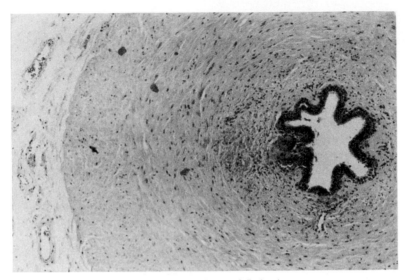

(Courtesy of Dr. George C. Enders.)

a. Passage of urine and sperm in the male
b. Passage of urine in the female
c. Passage of urine from the bladder to the urethrae in males and females
d. Passage of sperm from the epididymis to the urethra
e. Storage of sperm and absorption of fluid

238. Identify the organ below.

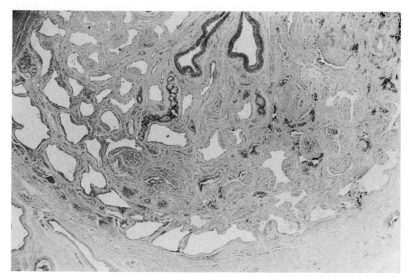

(Courtesy of Dr. George C. Enders.)

a. Female urethra
b. Male urethra
c. Oviduct
d. Ureter
e. Seminal vesicle

239. The portion of this organ in the photomicrograph below that is the primary source of malignancy is

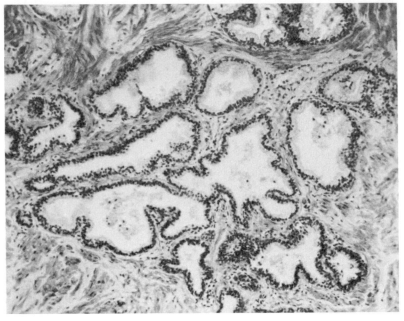

(Courtesy of Dr. George C. Enders.)

a. Mammary duct
b. Periurethral glands
c. Outer peripheral glands
d. Germ cells
e. Mammary alveoli

240. Naturally occurring, nonpathologic cervical eversions ("erosions") are usually naturally corrected by reepithelialization. These eversions are most prevalent in which one of the following reproductive classifications of women?

a. Prepubertal female
b. Postpubertal, premenopausal, nulliparous female
c. Premenopausal, multiparous female
d. Menopausal, nulliparous female
e. Late postmenopausal female

241. The organ shown in this photomicrograph is responsible for production of

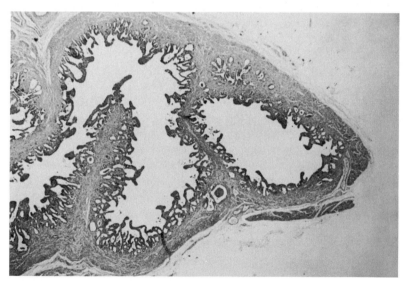

(Courtesy of Dr. George C. Enders.)

a. Spermine and fibrolysin
b. T_3 and T_4
c. Proteins that coagulate semen
d. Acid phosphatase
e. Milk

242. The organ pictured in the photomicrograph performs which of the following functions?

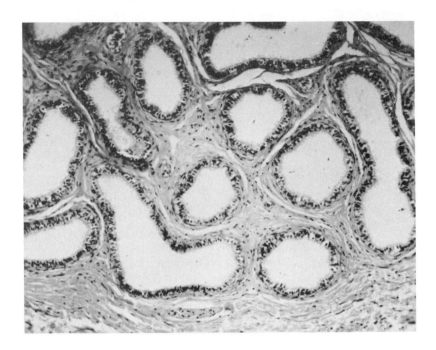

a. The site of spermiogenesis
b. Production of fructose and prostaglandins
c. Phagocytosis of sperm and residual bodies
d. The site of implantation
e. The site of milk production

243. Which of the following is independent of testosterone or other androgens?

a. The structural integrity of the prostatic epithelium
b. The function of the prostatic glands
c. Development of the penis from an indifferent phallus
d. Spermatogenesis
e. Fetal testis development from an indifferent gonad

244. Synthesis of milk by the mammary gland specifically requires

a. Oxytocin
b. Production of prolactin by the corpus luteum
c. The influence of vasopressin
d. Placental lactogen
e. Neurohumoral reflexes

245. The urologist may describe the reattachment of a severed vas deferens (vasovasostomy) as successful, more than 90% of the time. However, it is unsuccessful from the patients' point of view since a much lower percentage of these men can father a child. The difference in success rate is due to the fact that

a. Spermatogonia are exposed to humoral factors
b. Genetic recombination in haploid sperm creates novel antigens
c. Cryptorchid testes are often incapable of producing fertile sperm
d. Vasectomy prevents phagocytosis of sperm by macrophages
e. Sperm coated with autoimmune antibodies are unable to fertilize an egg.

246. Which of the following are characteristic of the secretory phase of the menstrual cycle?

a. It precedes ovulation
b. It depends on progesterone secretion by the corpus luteum
c. It coincides with the development of ovarian follicles
d. It coincides with a rapid drop in estrogen levels
e. It produces ischemia and necrosis of the stratum functionale

247. The low pH in the vagina is maintained by

a. A proton pump similar to that of parietal cells and osteoclasts
b. Acid secretion derived from intracellular carbonic acid
c. Secretion of lactic acid by the stratified squamous epithelium
d. Bacterial metabolism of glycogen to form lactic acid
e. Synthesis and accumulation of acid hydrolases in the epithelium

248. A 33-year-old patient with an average menstrual cycle of 28 days comes in for a routine Pap smear. It has been 35 days since the start of her last menstrual period, and a vaginal smear reveals clumps of basophilic cells. As her physician, you suspect

a. She will begin menstruating in a few days
b. She will ovulate within a few days
c. Her serum progesterone levels are very low
d. There are detectable levels of hCG in her serum and urine
e. She is undergoing menopause

249. If the hormone necessary for maintenance of this structure in the photomicrograph below were absent 12 to 14 days after ovulation in a human female, the result would be

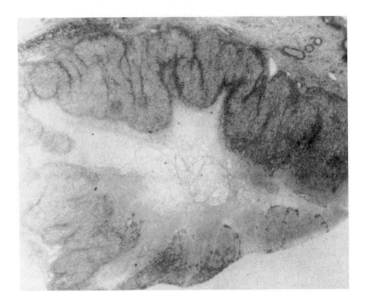

a. The absence of the structure
b. The absence of muscularization
c. Maintenance of the uterine epithelium for implantation beyond 14 days after ovulation
d. Pregnancy
e. The formation of a corpus albicans from the structure

250. The accompanying diagram shows a cross section of a developing human endometrium and myometrium. Hormonal ratios control the development of which of the labeled vessels?

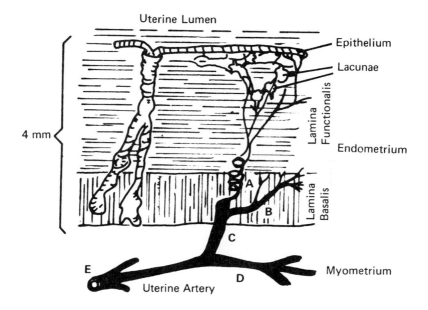

a. A
b. B
c. C
d. D
e. E

251. Which of the following statements is true of the uterus during the menstrual cycle?

a.   Progesterone secretion initiates proliferation in the endometrium
b.   Estrogen secretion stimulates secretory changes in the endometrium
c.   Cessation of estrogen and progesterone secretion results in the degeneration of the endometrium
d.   Incorporation of ^{3}H-thymidine in the uterus of an experimental animal would occur primarily during the secretory phase
e.   Studies with an antibody to the estrogen receptor would demonstrate a peak in immunocytochemically positive endometrial cells after involution of the corpus luteum

252. Cells in the layers labeled A and C in the figure below secrete plasminogen activator and collagenase that is required for

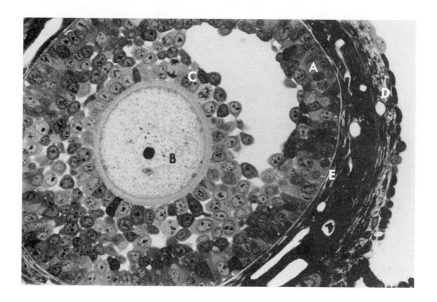

a. Dissolution of the zona pellucida to facilitate sperm penetration
b. pH regulation within the antral cavity
c. Breakdown of the basement membrane between the thecal and granulosa layers, facilitating ovulation
d. Diffusion of androgens between the thecal and granulosa cells
e. Facilitation of follicular atresia through breakdown of the basement membrane between the theca interna and externa

Reproductive Systems

Answers

233. The answer is d. (*Junqueira, 9/e, pp 425–430. McKenzie and Klein, pp 344–347. Guyton, 10/e, pp 930–933.*) Estrogen levels increase during the maturation of ovarian follicles, which results in a concomitant increase in ciliation and height of the oviductal lining cells. Increases in the number of cilia serve to facilitate movement of the ovum. Increased estrogen levels also decrease FSH levels and cause an LH surge. Elevated estrogen levels result in increased secretion of lytic enzymes, prostaglandins, plasminogen activator, and collagenase to facilitate the rupture of the ovarian wall and the release of the ovum and the attached corona radiata. Following ovulation, during the luteal phase of the cycle, the theca and granulosa cells are transformed into the corpus luteum under the influence of LH. Ovulation occurs near the middle of the menstrual cycle and is associated with an increase in basal body temperature that appears to be indirectly regulated by elevated estrogen levels, with IL-1 functioning as the endogenous pyrogen. Estrogen also upregulates FSH receptors on granulosa cell membranes and enhances synthesis and storage of glycogen in the vaginal epithelium.

234 to 235. The answers are 234-b, 235-e. (*Young, 4/e, pp 329–331. McKenzie and Klein, pp 352–356. Junqueira, 9/e, pp 410–417.*) The cell marked with a star is a Leydig cell (i.e., interstitial cell) and is regulated by luteinizing hormone (LH), also known as interstitial cell-stimulating hormone (ICSH), secreted by gonadotrophs in the anterior pituitary. Leydig cells are located between seminiferous tubules and are responsible for the production of testosterone. Sertoli cells function in a nutritive and supportive role somewhat analogous to the glial cells of the CNS. The Sertoli cells produce inhibin, which feeds back on the anterior pituitary and hypothalamus to regulate FSH release. Testosterone is modified by binding to androgen-binding protein (ABP), which is synthesized by the Sertoli cells. The testosterone is necessary for the maintenance of spermatogenesis as well as the male ducts and accessory glands. ABP is regulated by FSH, testosterone, and inhibin. Sertoli cells have extensive tight (occluding) junctions between them that form the blood-testis barrier. Sertoli cells communicate with adjacent cells through gap junctions and extend from outside the blood-testis barrier (basal portion) to luminal to the blood-testis barrier (apical portion). During spermatogenesis, derivatives of spermatocytes cross from the basal to the adluminal compartment across the zonula occludens between adjacent Sertoli cells. Each Sertoli cell is, therefore, associated with multiple spermatogenic cells.

The testis is composed of seminiferous tubules containing a number of spermatogenic cells undergoing spermatogenesis and spermiogenesis. The cells labeled with the arrowheads are spermatogonia, the derivatives of the embryonic primordial germ cells. The spermatogonia are of three types (not distinguishable in the photomicrograph): type A dark cells (Ad), type A pale cells (Ap), and type B cells. Type Ad cells are precursors that divide to form Ad and Ad progeny or Ad and Ap progeny. The Ap cells give rise to B spermatogonia that are capable of differentiating into primary spermatocytes. These cells comprise the basal layer and undergo mitosis (spermatocytogenesis) to form primary spermatocytes, which have distinctive clumped or coarse chromatin (marked by arrows). Secondary spermatocytes are formed during the first meiotic division and exist for only a short period of time because there is no lag period before entry into the second meiotic division that results in the formation of spermatids. The spermatids begin as round structures and elongate with the formation of the flagellum. This last part of seminiferous tubule function is the differentiation of sperm from spermatocytes (spermiogenesis) and is complete with the release of mature sperm into the lumen of the tubule.

236. The answer is b. (*Young, 4/e, pp 329, 335. McKenzie and Klein, pp 356–357.*) The photomicrograph is taken from an area that shows the ductuli efferentes (efferent ductules) (B) with their distinctive wavy epithelium in which adjoining cells are tall (ciliated) and short (nonciliated). Also shown are the seminiferous tubules (C) and the mediastinum testis containing the rete testis (A). Sperm leave the seminiferous tubules through short tubuli recti into the straight tubules of the rete testis, which subsequently drain into the efferent ductules.

237. The answer is d. (*Young, 4/e, p 336. Junqueira 9/e, pp 417–418. McKenzie and Klein, pp 366–367.*) The organ shown in the figure is the vas deferens (ductus deferens). The vas deferens conducts sperm from the epididymis to the urethra. The thick muscular wall is unique in the presence of an inner longitudinal, a middle circular, and an outer longitudinal layer of smooth muscle. The ureter has two thin layers of muscle: inner longitudinal and outer circular. The male and female urethra contain extensive vascular channels. The epididymis consists of a connective tissue stroma and stores sperm, resorbs fluid, and produces sperm maturation factors.

238. The answer is b. (*Young, 4/e, pp 339–340. Junqueira, 9/e, pp 419–420.*) The photomicrograph is the male (penile) urethra. It possesses a primarily pseudostratified columnar type of epithelium. The glands of Littre that produce mucus are also observed in the section. The thick-walled arteries of the penile and cavernous sinuses of penile erectile tissue are also a distinguishing feature of this organ. Helicine arteries supply the sinuses. Action of the parasympathetic nervous system mediates the dilatation of these vessels during erection.

239. The answer is c. (*Young, 4/e, pp 337–339. Junqueira, 9/e, pp 418–419, 444. Kumar 6/e, 1023–1028.*) The photomicrograph is from the prostate. Seventy percent of carcinomas of the prostate arise from the main (external gland), also known as the outer (peripheral) glands. The prostate consists of three parts: (1) a small mucosal (inner periurethral) gland, (2) a transition zone that consists of a submucosal (outer periurethral) gland, and (3) a peripheral portion known as the main, or external, gland. Because of the peripheral location, most prostatic carcinomas (primarily adenocarcinomas) remain undiagnosed until the later symptoms of back pain or blockage of the urethra are detected. They can be detected by rectal digital examination. Benign prostatic hypertrophy, also known as benign nodular hyperplasia, occurs in the mucosal and submucosal glands, which are rarely the sites of inflammation or carcinoma. Benign hyperplasia causes urethral obstruction in its early stages because of its location in the mucosal and submucosal glands. The main gland is sensitive to androgens, whereas the periurethral glands are sensitive to androgens and estrogens. Acid phosphatase levels are valuable in the diagnosis of prostatic carcinoma and its metastasis.

Carcinoma of the breast occurs in about 1 of 10 females in the United States. By definition, a carcinoma is ductal in origin. Carcinoma of the breast metastasizes to the brain, lungs, and bones. The easy access of tumor cells to the extensive axillary blood supply and lymphatic drainage facilitates the spread of the cancer into the blood and lymph supplies. Self-examination and mammography are urged in an attempt to increase early diagnosis, which has reduced mortality of this disease.

Germ cell tumors of the testes (testicular neoplasms) are classified as seminomas (germinomas) of pure germ cells and more heterogeneous cell types (e.g., teratomas and embryonal carcinomas).

240. The answer is c. *(Kumar, 6/e, p 603.)* To a minor extent, the uterine cervical stroma changes during each reproductive cycle; however, during pregnancy (especially parturition) there is a thinning of the uterine stroma. This results in eversions (mistakenly called "erosions"), which are sites of exposed uterine columnar epithelium in the acidic, vaginal milieu. These sites often become reepithelialized as stratified epithelium (squamous metaplasia) and are believed to be the location of cancerous transformation in the cervix. As part of the process of reepithelialization, the openings of cervical mucous glands are obliterated, which results in the formation of nabothian cysts.

241. The answer is c. *(Young, 4/e, pp 337–339. Junqueira, 9/e, pp 418.)* The organ shown in the light microscopic photograph is the seminal vesicle that produces fructose, ascorbic acid, prostaglandins, and proteins responsible for semen coagulation. The seminal vesicle produces about 50% of the seminal fluid on a volume basis and comprises most of the ejaculate. The wall consists of smooth muscle and the mucosa of anastomosing "villus-like" folds. In comparison, the prostate is composed of 15 to 30 tubuloalveolar glands surrounded by fibromuscular tissue. Concretions are often found in the lumina. The prostate secretes a thin, opalescent fluid that contributes primarily to the first part of the ejaculate. Prostatic secretions include acid phosphatase, spermine (a polyamine), fibrolysin, amylase, and zinc. Spermine oxidation results in the musky odor of semen, and fibrolysin is responsible for the liquefaction of semen after ejaculation. Acid phosphatase and prostatic-specific antigen are important for the diagnosis of metastases.

242. The answer is c. *(Young, 4/e, pp 329, 336, 341, 357, 368–371. Junqueira, 9/e, p 417.)* The figure is a light microscopic photograph of the epididymis. The epididymis functions in the storage, maturation, and phagocytosis of sperm and residual bodies. In addition, the epididymis is involved in the absorption of testicular fluid and the secretion of glycoproteins. These glycoproteins may be involved in the inhibition of capacitation. The epithelium of the epididymis is pseudostratified with stereocilia (modified microvilli for absorption), and the wall contains extensive connective tissue. The seminal vesicle produces fructose and prostaglandins and contains a thick smooth muscle layer. Sperm are often found in the lumina. Spermiogenesis occurs in the testes. Milk production occurs in the mammary gland, which contains alveoli and lactiferous ducts. Implantation occurs in the uterus, which is lined by a simple columnar epithelium with endometrial glands that differ in arrangement, depending on the phase of the cycle (long and straight in the proliferative phases and S-shaped in the secretory phase). The myometrium, composed of smooth muscle, is hormone-sensitive and undergoes both hypertrophy and hyperplasia during pregnancy and atrophy after menopause, resulting in a shrinking of the uterus in postmenopausal women.

243. The answer is e. (*Junqueira, 9/e, p 415. Moore, Before We Are Born, 5/e, pp 306–310. Moore, Developing Human, 6/e, pp 325–326.*) The development of the testis from an indifferent gonad depends on the presence of the testis-determining factor, a gene on the short arm of the Y chromosome. During fetal development, the production of androgens by the developing testis results in masculinization of the indifferent gonadal ducts and the indifferent genitalia. In the absence of androgens, female genitalia and female ducts (vagina, oviducts, and uterus) develop. In the mature male, testosterone is required for the initiation and maintenance of spermatogenesis as well as the structural and functional integrity of the accessory glands and ducts of the male reproductive system. Testosterone is bound to androgen-binding protein (ABP), which is synthesized by the Sertoli cells under the influence of follicle-stimulating hormone (FSH). ABP is important for both the storage and delivery of androgens in the male ducts and accessory glands.

244. The answer is d. (*Junqueira, 9/e, pp 443–446. Yen, 4/e, pp 284–288.*) The mammary gland enlarges during pregnancy in response to several hormones, including prolactin synthesized by the anterior pituitary, estrogen and progesterone synthesized by the corpus luteum, and placental lactogen. The alveoli at the end of the duct system respond to these hormones by cell proliferation, which increases the size of the mammary glands. Growth continues throughout pregnancy; however, secretion is most notable late in pregnancy. Milk is synthesized in the alveoli and is stored in their lumina before passage through the lactiferous ducts to the nipples. Secretion of milk lipids occurs by an apocrine mechanism whereby some apical cytoplasm is included with the secretory product. In comparison, milk proteins, such as the caseins, are secreted by exocytosis. Oxytocin is required for the release of milk from the mammary gland through the action of the myoepithelial cells that surround the alveoli and proximal (closer to the alveolus) portions of the duct system. Oxytocin is not required for milk synthesis. Neurohumoral reflexes are involved in the suckling-milk ejection response.

245. The answer is e. (*Braunwald, 15/e, pp 304, 2151.*) Attempts to counteract or repair the effects of a vasectomy (vasovasostomy) are often unsuccessful because of the development of antisperm antibodies. This lack of success occurs despite the fact that 90% of the patients undergoing vasovasostomy have sperm return to the ejaculate. In the case of vasectomy, sperm that have leaked from the severed vas deferens is viewed as foreign by immune surveillance and antibodies develop. The phagocytosis of sperm by macrophages plays a role in the development of antisperm antibodies that occurs following the ligation or removal of a segment of the vas deferens. Attempted reunion of the ligated segments is called vasovasostomy and may return sperm to the ejaculate; however, the presence of antisperm antibodies may prevent normal fertilization. Sperm are immunologically foreign because of a number of factors. Spermatogenesis begins at puberty long after the development of self-recognition in the immune system. The blood-testis barrier protects developing sperm from exposure to systemic factors. The basal compartment containing the spermatogonia and preleptotene spermatocytes is exposed to plasma; however, the adluminal compartment, which contains primary and secondary spermatocytes, spermatids, and testicular sperm, prevents these antigens from entering the blood. The inability of cryptorchid testes to produce fertile sperm is related to the higher temperature in the abdomen than in the normal scrotal location.

246. The answer is b. (*Young, 4/e, pp 341, 351–355. Junqueira, 9/e, pp 432–436.*) The secretory phase of the menstrual cycle depends on progesterone secretion and follows the proliferative (follicular) phase. The menstrual phase occurs after the secretory phase. During the follicular phase (approximately days 4 to 16), estrogen produced by the ovaries drives cell proliferation in the base of endometrial glands and the uterine stroma. The proliferative phase culminates with ovulation. The secretory phase (approximately days 16 to 25) is characterized by high progesterone levels from the corpus luteum, a tortuous appearance of the uterine glands, and apocrine secretion by the gland cells. During this phase, maximum endometrial thickness occurs. The menstrual phase (approximately days 26 to 30) is characterized by decreased glandular secretion and eventual glandular degeneration because of decreased production of both progesterone and estrogen by the theca lutein cells. Contraction of coiled arteries and arterioles leads to ischemia and necrosis of the stratum functionale.

247. The answer is d. (*Young, 4/e, pp 341, 359. Junqueira, 9/e, p 439–440.*) The low pH of the vagina is maintained by bacterial metabolism of glycogen to form lactic acid. The vagina is characterized by a stratified squamous epithelium that contains large accumulations of glycogen. Glycogen is released into the vaginal lumen and is subsequently metabolized to lactic acid by commensal lactobacilli. The low pH inhibits growth of a variety of microorganisms. Treatment for vaginal infections usually includes acidified carriers to reestablish a more acidic pH like that usually seen in midmenstrual cycle.

248. The answer is d. (*Young, 4/e, p 358. Junqueira, 9/e, pp 440–441. Yen, 4/e, pp 714–715.*) The patient described in this question is probably pregnant. The delay in menstruation coupled with the presence of basophilic cells in a vaginal smear are clues. Ovulation is the midpoint of the cycle and should be more than a few days away. She is relatively young for the onset of menopause and there are no other symptoms. The vaginal epithelium varies little with the normal menstrual cycle. Exfoliative cytology can be used to diagnose cancer and to determine if the epithelium is under stimulation of estrogen and progesterone. The presence of basophilic cells in the smear with the Pap-staining method would indicate the presence of both estrogen and progesterone. The data suggest the maintenance of the corpus luteum (i.e., pregnancy).

249. The answer is e. (*Young, 4/e, pp 347, 352. Junqueira, 9/e, pp 428–429.*) The structure in the photomicrograph is a corpus luteum. In the absence of the hormones necessary for maintenance of the corpus luteum [luteinizing hormone (LH) or human chorionic gonadotropin (hCG)], the corpus luteum regresses to form a corpus albicans, which consists primarily of fibrous connective tissue. Without LH or hCG, the uterine epithelium, which has undergone glandular proliferation in preparation for implantation, collapses and degenerates as part of menstruation. The corpus luteum forms from the granulosa and theca layers of the follicle following ovulation. The luteal phase is the second half of the menstrual period and follows the follicular phase during which follicles mature. The corpus luteum synthesizes progesterone in response to high LH levels. In each reproductive cycle, the production of LH stimulates development and maintenance of the corpus luteum, that is well formed by 12 to 14 days following ovulation. In the case of fertilization and subsequent implantation, the corpus luteum of pregnancy is maintained by human chorionic gonadotropin (hCG) produced by the embryo.

250. The answer is a. *(Young, 4/e, pp 349–352. Junqueira, 9/e, pp 432–433. McKenzie and Klein, p 348.)* The spiral arteries of the endometrium (labeled A in the diagram accompanying the question) depend on specific estrogen/progesterone ratios for their development. They pass through the basalis layer of the endometrium into the functional zone, and their distal ends are subject to degeneration with each menses. The straight arteries (B) are not subject to these hormonal changes. In the proliferative phase, the endometrium is only 1- to 3-mm thick, and the glands are straight, with the spiral arteries only slightly coiled. This diagram of the early secretory phase shows an edematous endometrium that is 4-mm thick, with glands that are large, beginning to sacculate in the deeper mucosa, and coiled for their entire length. In the late secretory phase, the endometrium becomes 6- to 7-mm thick.

251. The answer is c. *(Young, 4/e, pp 352–357. Junqueira, 9/e, pp 430–436. McKenzie and Klein, p 348.)* During the uterine cycle, menstruation is initiated by the necrosis of the stratum functionale through the action of the spiral arterioles. After four to five days, proliferation begins in the endometrium in response to estrogen secretion from the granulosa cells. If ^{3}H-thymidine were injected into animals during this period and combined with immunocytochemical staining for antiestrogen receptor, the result would be colocalization of autoradiographic grains and immunocytochemical product over the uterine epithelial and stromal cells as well as vascular endothelial cells. The peak of proliferative activity and estrogen sensitivity would occur after menses and during the proliferative phase. Maintenance of cell proliferation requires continued secretion of estrogen. As progesterone secretion increases, the secretory phase of uterine maturation occurs. The involution of the corpus luteum initiates the degeneration of the endometrial glands, which precedes menses.

252. The answer is c. (*Young, 4/e, pp 342–346, 352. Junqueira, 9/e, pp 421–424.*) The cells labeled A and C in the photomicrograph of the graafian follicle are granulosa cells that produce plasminogen activator and collagenase. These molecules, along with plasmin and prostaglandins, facilitate the rupture of the ovarian follicle, leading to ovulation. The increase in LH in midcycle induces production of collagenase and plasminogen activator. These proteases facilitate ovulation by initiating connective tissue remodeling, including the breakdown of the basement membrane between thecal and granulosa layers. Connective tissue remodeling is involved in the process of follicular atresia. This process occurs throughout life and involves the death of follicular cells as well as oocytes, but there is no basement membrane between the theca interna and externa. In fact, there is an absence of a clear delineation between the theca interna and externa. Development of ovarian follicles begins with a primordial follicle that consists of flattened follicular cells surrounding a primary oocyte. During the follicular phase, these cells undergo mitosis to form multiple granulosa layers (primary follicle) in response to elevated levels of FSH and LH from the anterior pituitary. A glycoproteinaceous coat surrounds the oocyte and is called the zona pellucida. The connective tissue around the follicle differentiates into two layers: theca externa (D) and theca interna (E). The theca externa is closest to the ovarian stroma and consists of a highly vascular connective tissue. The theca interna synthesizes androgens (e.g., androstenedione) in response to LH. Androgens are converted to estradiol by the action of an aromatase enzyme synthesized by the granulosa cells under the influence of FSH. Increased levels of estrogen from the ovary feed back to decrease FSH secretion from gonadotrophs in the anterior pituitary. Liquor folliculi is produced by the granulosa cells and is secreted between the cells. When cavities are first formed by the development of follicular fluid between the cells, the follicle is called secondary. When the antrum is completely formed, the follicle is called a mature (graafian) follicle, and the antrum is completely filled with liquor folliculi. The granulosa cells form two structures. The corona radiata (C) represents those granulosa cells that remain attached to the zona pellucida. The cumulus oophorus (not labeled) represents those granulosa cells that surround the oocyte (B) and connect it to the wall. Structure A is the membrana granulosa.

Urinary System

Questions

DIRECTIONS: Each item below contains a question or incomplete statement followed by suggested responses. Select the **one best** response to each question.

253. In the accompanying transmission electron micrograph of the renal corpuscle, the function of the cell marked with an asterisk is to

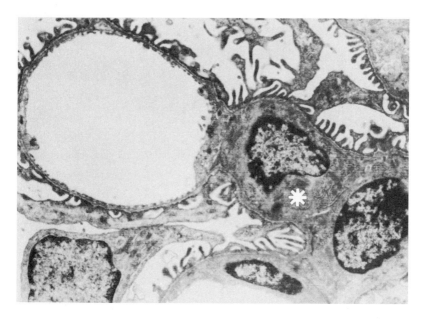

a. Synthesize extracellular matrix for support of the capillary wall
b. Exert an antithrombogenic effect
c. Synthesize vasoactive factors
d. Separate the urinary space and the blood in the capillaries
e. Form the filtration slits through the interdigitations of the pedicels

254. In the accompanying transmission electron micrograph from the renal corpuscle, the structures labeled with arrows are

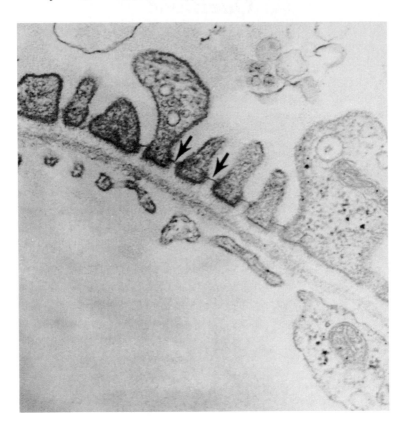

a. Podocyte foot processes
b. Endothelial cell fenestrations
c. Pedicels
d. Filtration slits
e. The lamina rara of the basement membrane

255. The accompanying transmission electron micrograph from the kidney illustrates a cell that is

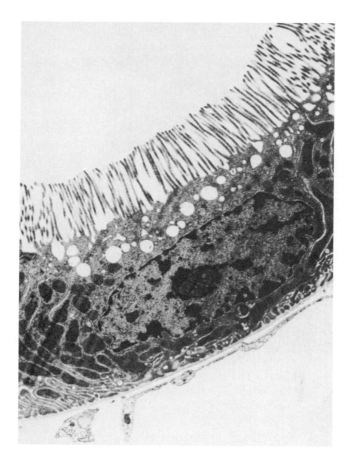

a. Impermeable to water despite the presence of ADH
b. The site of the countercurrent multiplier
c. The site of action of aldosterone
d. The source of renin
e. The primary site for the reduction of the tubular fluid volume

256. The arrows in the accompanying scanning electron micrograph of the renal glomerulus indicate

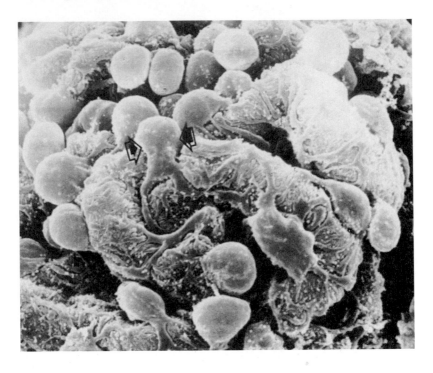

a. A red blood cell
b. A podocyte
c. An endothelial cell
d. A parietal cell
e. The macula densa

257. Renal changes in the kidney in a patient with diabetes mellitus of 30 years duration may result in

a. Decreased permeability to plasma proteins
b. Enhanced selectivity of the filtration barrier
c. Hyperalbuminemia
d. A generalized increase in osmotic pressure
e. Compensatory secretion of aldosterone

258. Which of the following is involved in glomerular filtration?

a. Facilitated diffusion of large anionic proteins
b. Maintenance of a charge barrier
c. A physical barrier consisting of type II collagen
d. Filtration slits between adjacent endothelial cells
e. A positive charge in the basement membrane due to the presence of heparan sulfate

259. Which of the following is found exclusively in the renal medulla?

a. Proximal convoluted tubules
b. Distal convoluted tubules
c. Collecting ducts
d. Afferent arterioles
e. Thin loops of Henle

Urinary System

Answers

253. The answer is a. (*McKenzie and Klein, pp 332–335. Junqueira, 9/e, pp 360–361, 368.*) The cell labeled in the transmission electron micrograph of the renal corpuscle is a mesangial cell that synthesizes extracellular matrix including the basement membrane of the glomerulus for the support of the capillary wall. Mesangial cells are morphologically similar to pericytes found in association with other systemic blood vessels. The mesangial cells surround glomerular capillaries as illustrated in this electron micrograph. Other proposed functions for the mesangial cells include phagocytosis and regulation of glomerular blood flow. A podocyte with its processes in close association with the glomerular capillary is observed below the mesangial cell. The podocytes form the visceral layer of the Bowman's capsule and possess processes that interdigitate to form the pedicels. The outer layer of the Bowman's capsule is formed by parietal cells, one of which is located in the lower left corner of the micrograph. An endothelial cell within a glomerular capillary is also shown below the mesangial cell. Endothelial cells synthesize vasoactive substances (e.g., endothelin) and are antithrombogenic. The urinary space and the blood are separated by the glomerular basement membrane formed from the fusion of the capillary and podocyte-produced basal laminae.

254. The answer is d. (*McKenzie and Klein, pp 334–335. Junqueira, 9/e, pp 360–362, 366.*) The transmission electron micrograph illustrates the filtration barrier of the renal corpuscle. The structures labeled with arrows are the filtration slits, which are located between adjacent pedicels (foot processes of the podocytes). The remainder of the filtration barrier is formed by the glomerular basement membrane, which contains type IV collagen and heparan sulfate. There are three distinct layers within the glomerular basement membrane: (1) an electron-dense lamina densa in the center surrounded by (2) the lamina rara externa on the glomerular side and by (3) the lamina rara interna on the capillary endothelial side.

255. The answer is e. (*McKenzie and Klein, pp 332–340. Junqueira, 9/e, pp 360–375.*) The transmission electron micrograph illustrates a proximal convoluted tubule cell. This cell type is the primary site for reduction of the tubular fluid volume and is, therefore, responsible for reabsorption from the glomerular filtrate. The elaborate microvilli at the apical surface increase the surface area available for absorption. The apical portion of the cell also possesses an extensive endocytic vacuolar arrangement for the reabsorption of proteins. Numerous mitochondria are located basally to provide energy for the reabsorption of water that follows sodium transported actively by a basolateral Na⁺/K⁺-ATPase. In the distal tubule there are very few microvilli.

The afferent arterioles contain the juxtaglomerular cells, modified arterial smooth muscle cells that produce renin, a major factor in blood pressure regulation. The thin loop of Henle is responsible for the production of the countercurrent multiplier, which allows the kidneys to produce a hyperosmotic medulla. The multiplier moves Na⁺ and Cl⁻ out of the ascending limb (which is impermeable to water) and into the medullary interstitial fluid. Subsequently, the descending limb, which is permeable to water, takes up the Na⁺ and Cl⁻ from the interstitium. The vasa recta adjust their osmolarity to that of the medulla.

The distal convoluted tubule has the highest concentration of Na⁺/K⁺-ATPase, pumps Na⁺ ions against a concentration gradient, and is relatively impermeable to water leading to the production of a hypotonic tubular fluid. The distal tubules empty into the connecting and collecting ducts, which are permeable to water under the regulation of ADH. ADH stimulation increases collecting duct permeability to water, allowing the production of hyperosmotic urine. Without ADH, the urine leaving the kidney would be hypoosmotic. The collecting duct principal cells are the ADH responsive cells and contain fewer mitochondria and basal infoldings as occur in the cells of the distal convoluted tubule.

256. The answer is b. (*McKenzie and Klein, pp 333–335. Junqueira, 9/e, pp 362, 364–365.*) The arrows on the scanning electron micrograph illustrate a podocyte. The podocytes surround the glomerular capillaries. The spaces between the foot processes (pedicels) form the filtration slits, an important part of the filtration barrier of the kidney. The macula densa is a portion of the distal tubule that is specialized for determination of distal tubular osmolarity.

257. The answer is e. (*Kumar, 6/e, pp 446, 570. McKenzie and Klein, p 341. Junqueira, 9/e, p 362.*) In patients who have suffered from diabetes mellitus for many years there is compensatory release of aldosterone. The initial change is the thickening of the glomerular basement membrane. The separation of laminae rarae and densa is obliterated, which results in a loss of selectivity of the filtration barrier. This causes the loss of protein from the blood to the urine (proteinuria). The liver adjusts to the proteinuria by producing more proteins (e.g., albumin). After continued proteinuria, the liver is unable to produce sufficient protein, which results in hypoalbuminemia. This leads to an overall decrease in osmotic pressure. The result is edema as fluid leaves the vasculature to enter the tissues. The movement of fluid from the vasculature to the tissues results in reduced plasma volume and decreased glomerular filtration rate (GFR). The overall effect is further edema because of compensatory release of aldosterone coupled with reduced GFR and the already existing edema. These renal changes are known as nephrotic syndrome. The foot processes are affected in many diseases, such as diabetes mellitus, that lead to nephrotic syndrome. Loss of anionic charge and fusion of the foot processes result in the obliteration of the filtration slits.

258. The answer is b. (*McKenzie and Klein, pp 334–335. Junqueira, 9/e, pp 360–364, 372–373.*) The glomerular filtration barrier is a physical and charge barrier that exhibits selectivity based on molecular size and charge. The barrier is formed by three components: (1) glomerular capillary endothelial cells, (2) glomerular basement membrane, and (3) podocyte layer. The presence of collagen type IV in the lamina densa of the basement membrane presents a physical barrier to the passage of large proteins from the blood to the urinary space. Glycosaminoglycans, particularly heparan sulfate, produce a polyanionic charge that binds cationic molecules. Filtration slits are found between adjacent podocyte foot processes and provide a gap of approximately 50 μm. The foot processes are coated with a glycoprotein called podocalyxin, which is rich in sialic acid and provides mutual repulsion to maintain the structure of the filtration slits. It also possesses a large polyanionic charge for repulsion of large anionic proteins.

259. The answer is e. (*McKenzie and Klein, pp 336–340. Junqueira, 9/e, pp 362, 369, 370, 375.*) The collecting ducts are found in both the cortex and medulla of the kidney. Cortical collecting ducts are found in the medullary rays, whereas medullary collecting ducts are found in the medulla and lead into the papillary duct. The convoluted portions of the proximal and distal tubules are found exclusively in the cortex. Afferent arterioles are found adjacent to the vascular pole of the glomeruli within the cortex. Only the thin loops of Henle are found exclusively in the medulla.

Eye and Ear

Questions

DIRECTIONS: Each item below contains a question or incomplete response followed by suggested responses. Select the **one best** response to each question.

260. In the surgical procedure known as radial keratotomy, slits are made in the cornea to flatten it slightly. This will result in

a. Decreased refraction of light by the cornea
b. A decreased amount of light entering through the cornea
c. Conversion of the cornea from a "stationary" to an "adjustable" form of refraction
d. Maintenance of the lens in a more flattened state
e. Focusing of light on the retina at a point other than the fovea

261. Retinal detachment most commonly results from

a. Local swelling in specific retinal layers
b. Leakage of blood from the inner retinal capillaries
c. Fluid accumulation between the retina and the retinal pigment epithelium (RPE)
d. Impaired pumping of water toward the photoreceptors by the retinal pigment epithelium
e. Increased phagocytosis of outer segments by the retinal pigment pithelial cells

262. Visual transduction involves which of the following?

a. Inactivation of phosphodiesterase
b. Increase in cGMP levels
c. Conversion of all-*trans*-retinal to 11-*cis* retinal
d. Closing of a Na^+ channel
e. Depolarization of the rod cell membrane

263. The retinal pigment epithelium (RPE) is characterized by

a. The presence of the photoreceptor (rod and cone) perikarya
b. Phagocytosis of worn-out components of photoreceptor cells
c. Origin from the inner layer of the optic cup during embryonic development
d. Presence of amacrine cells
e. Synthesis of vitreous humor

264. Which of the following occurs in diabetic retinopathy?

a. Reduction in the thickness of the basal lamina of small retinal vessels
b. Microaneurysms
c. Decreased capillary permeability
d. Increased retinal blood flow
e. Loss of phagocytic ability of the pigmented epithelium

265. The structure labeled B in the figure below is

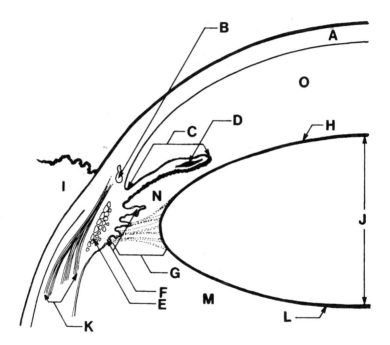

a. Responsible for the production of aqueous humor
b. Site of outflow of vitreous humor from the posterior chamber
c. The site of blockage in glaucoma
d. Involved in the regulation of accommodation
e. The major corneal artery

266. Data from the photoreceptors are integrated in the

a. Outer segment of the rod
b. Inner segment of the rod
c. Ganglion cell layer
d. Inner nuclear layer of the retina
e. Outer plexiform layer of the retina

267. The direction in which vestibular hair cell stereocilia are deflected is important because it

a. Differentiates between type 1 and type 2 hair cells
b. Determines whether cells are depolarized or hyperpolarized
c. Determines whether linear or angular acceleration is detected
d. Determines the direction of blood flow in the stria vascularis
e. Is determined by the frequency of the sound

268. Which of the following is directly involved in sound transduction?

a. Release of neurotransmitter onto the afferent endings of cranial nerve VIII
b. Shearing motion of the basilar membrane against hair cell stereocilia
c. Movement of the tectorial membrane resulting in hair cell depolarization
d. Equalization of the pressure in the middle ear and nasopharynx by the Eustachian tube
e. Vibration at the round window via the stapes

269. Perilymph is located in which of the following structures?

a. Utricle
b. Saccule
c. Semicircular canals
d. Scala media
e. Scala tympani

270. In the structure shown below, the structure labeled D is responsible for

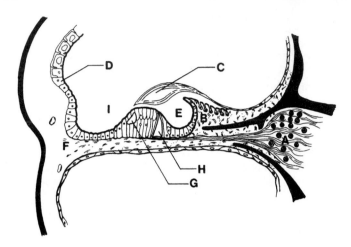

a. Transduction of the sound to a nerve impulse
b. Support of the organ of Corti
c. The characteristic ionic composition of the perilymph
d. Forms the tectorial membrane
e. The characteristic ionic composition of the endolymph

271. The function of the vestibular membrane is to

a. Maintain the gradient between the endolymph and the perilymph
b. Maintain communication between the tympanic and vestibular cavities
c. Transmit sound to the oval window
d. Maintain the concentration gradient necessary for sensory transduction
e. Dampen the action of the auditory ossicles

272. Detection of angular acceleration is accomplished by which of the following structures?

a. Maculae of the utricle and saccule
b. Hair cells of the organ of Corti
c. Cristae ampullaris of the semicircular canals
d. Interdental cells
e. Pillar cells

Eye and Ear

Answers

260. The answer is a. *(Newell, 8/e, pp 230–231, 431–432. Vaughan, 15/e, p 139–140.)* Radial, or refractive, keratotomy decreases the refraction of light by the cornea. It alters corneal (not lens) anatomy to create a new shape that is more flattened in the center and higher at the periphery of the cornea. This occurs because intraocular pressure will cause a reshaping of the cornea due to induced weakness produced by the incisions. The purpose of the procedure is to reduce myopia to eliminate the need for corrective lenses. The reduction in curvature of the central portion of the cornea results in decreased refractive power of the cornea. The slits are made with a laser and the degree of correction required is estimated by computer simulations.

261. The answer is c. *(McKenzie and Klein, pp 374–375. Newell, 8/e, pp 322–324. Vaughan, 15/e, pp 172–173, 187–189.)* Retinal detachment is the result of the accumulation of fluid between the retina and the RPE. In one type of detachment, rhegmatogenous retinal detachment, fluid accumulates after a break occurs in the retina. Detachments without breaks in the retina are called nonrhegmatogenous, or serous, detachments. Vitreous degeneration usually is a prerequisite for retinal detachment that results in the breaking of the retina. The breakdown of the vitreous produces traction on the retina, which may already possess an inherent area of weakness. The site of retinal detachment is the area between the inner and outer layers of the embryonic optic cup and represents a relatively weak area of adherence between the retinal and RPE layers.

262. The answer is d. *(McKenzie and Klein, pp 376–377. Junqueira, 9/e, pp 461–463.)* Visual transduction involves closing of the Na^+ channel in rod cells in response to photons of light. Rhodopsin is the visual pigment of rod cells and is composed of retinal, a vitamin A derivative, bound to opsins. Photons reaching rhodopsin isomerize retinal to the all-*trans* form from 11-*cis* retinal. The result is bleaching, which represents the dissociation of retinal from the opsins. The bleaching process results in a fall in cGMP within the cytosol.

Transducin is a G protein that couples bleaching to cGMP through the action of a phosphodiesterase enzyme that cleaves cGMP to GMP. The closing of the Na⁺ channel results in a reduction in permeability to sodium ions and hyperpolarization of the cell membrane. The signal spreads to the inner segment and through gap junctions to nearby photoreceptor cells. In the presence of cGMP, the Na⁺ channel remains open; in its absence, the channel closes and the cell hyperpolarizes. Therefore, the rods and cones differ from other receptors in that hyperpolarization of the cell membranes occurs rather than the depolarization that occurs in other neural systems. Closing the channel slows down the release of the visual transmitter.

263. The answer is b. *(Junqueira, 9/e, pp 456–459. McKenzie and Klein, pp 374–375.)* The retinal pigment epithelium (RPE) is a single layer of cells that phagocytose old components of photoreceptor cells. It is derived from the outer layer of the optic cup and is continuous from the ora serrata retinae to the optic nerve. Microvilli are prominent on the apical surfaces of the RPE and play an important role in the maintenance of the blood-retinal barrier. In addition, the RPE synthesizes melanin and stores vitamin A for the photoreceptor cells. Rod and cone perikarya and amacrine cells are found in the photosensitive retina derived from the inner layer of the optic cup.

264. The answer is b. *(Junqueira, 9/e, pp 461–463. Newell, 8/e, pp 507–510. Vaughan, 15/e, pp 191–194.)* Retinopathy is one of the major complications of diabetes mellitus. In diabetic retinopathy pathologic changes usually begin with thickening of the basement membrane of small retinal vessels. The abnormal vessels develop microaneurysms, which leak and hemorrhage with resultant ischemia of the retinal tissue. New vessels proliferate in response to ischemia and production of angiogenic factors. Loss of phagocytic capacity of the RPE occurs in retinal dystrophy but is not a characteristic of diabetic retinopathy. Retinopathy also occurs with prematurity when retinal vascularization is disturbed.

265. The answer is c. *(McKenzie and Klein, pp 374–375. Junqueira, 8/e, pp 449–456.)* The structure labeled B is the sinus venosus sclerae (canal of Schlemm), which carries aqueous humor to the scleral veins and the systemic vasculature. Blockage of the canal of Schlemm, the trabecular meshwork, or the scleral veins results in glaucoma. The overall figure shows the region of the iridocorneal angle and other associated structures in the eye.

This region is extremely important in the production and outflow of the aqueous humor and in the distribution of zonule fibers to the lens. The iris (C) contains both sphincter (D) and dilator muscles, which work in opposition to one another and are innervated by parasympathetic and sympathetic fibers, respectively. The center of the iris is a "hole," the pupil.

The ciliary body contains the ciliary muscles (E and K). The ciliary muscles stretch the choroid and relax the lens, which is essential for the process of lens accommodation. The ciliary processes (F) extend from the ciliary body and produce aqueous humor. They are also the origin of the zonule fibers (G), which are similar in structure to elastic fibers and are important for anchorage of the lens. The zonule fibers are involved in accommodation. When the ciliary muscles contract, causing forward displacement of the ciliary body, the tension on the zonule fibers is reduced, which leads to an increase in lens thickness and maintenance of focus. The aqueous humor produced by the ciliary processes (F) is transported into the posterior chamber (N) and flows into the anterior chamber (O) through the pupil. Outflow from the anterior chamber occurs through the trabecular meshwork at the iridocorneal angle and flows through the canal of Schlemm.

The cornea (A) forms the transparent, avascular anterior portion of the eye. The outer anterior surface of the cornea is covered by an epithelium. Beneath the epithelium is Bowman's membrane, the corneal stroma, Descemet's membrane, and the endothelium (at the posterior surface of the cornea), which lines the anterior boundary of the anterior chamber.

The lens (J) is formed embryologically from a thickening of the surface ectoderm called the lens placode, which eventually forms a lens vesicle. Lens fiber production continues throughout life with no turnover. The lens is surrounded by a capsule and an underlying epithelium (H and L). The three compartments of the eye include the posterior and anterior chambers, which are filled with aqueous humor, and the vitreous body (M), which is filled with a gel consisting of hydrated hyaluronic acid and other glycosaminoglycans.

The conjunctiva is the mucosa, or lining, of the eyelid and is labeled I in the figure.

266. The answer is d. (*Klein and McKenzie, pp 374–375. Junqueira, 9/e, pp 449–464.*) The inner nuclear layer is responsible for the integration of data from adjacent photoreceptors. The retina consists of 10 layers:

1. The retinal pigment epithelium (RPE) is derived from the outer wall of the optic cup. The RPE functions in the phagocytosis of rod disks.
2. The photoreceptor layer consisting of the rods and cones is the outer layer of the retina.
3. The outer limiting membrane is formed by the junctional complexes between Muller's cells and the membranes of photoreceptor cells.
4. The outer nuclear layer contains the nuclei of rod and cone cells and the surrounding cytoplasm (perikarya).
5. The outer plexiform layer contains rod and cone synapses as well as the cell processes of bipolar, horizontal, and photoreceptor cells.
6. The inner nuclear (bipolar) layer is composed of the nuclei and perikarya of the bipolar and amacrine cells as well as the nuclei of Muller's cells.
7. The inner plexiform layer consists of amacrine cells dispersed between the processes of bipolar and ganglion cells. This layer is responsible for modulation of signals from the ganglion to the photoreceptor cells.
8. The ganglion cell layer contains the ganglion cells separated by the cytoplasm of astrocyte-like glia (Muller's cells).
9. The nerve fiber layer consists of axons of the ganglion cells that will form the optic nerve.
10. The internal limiting membrane is located between the vitreous body and the retina. The photoreceptors are of two types: rods and cones. The nuclei of the rods and cones are found in the outer nuclear layer and extend across the outer limiting membrane in one direction and toward the outer plexiform layer in the other direction. The outer segment is the photon-sensitive portion of the rod and cone and contains membranous disks. Rhodopsin is composed of opsin and *cis*-retinal. It is responsible for transduction of light (photons) into hyperpolarization of the cell membrane. Rhodopsin is present in the disks of the outer segment of the rod. The inner segment contains numerous mitochondria, glycogen, and protein synthetic apparatus. Rods are responsible for night vision, whereas the cones are responsible for color vision, which is best resolved at the fovea. The fovea, which is the center of the macula, is composed exclusively of cones and is the site of optimal resolution.

The choroid is a highly vascular layer that consists of three parts: stroma, choriocapillaris, and Bruch's membrane. Blood supply to the retina is derived from the choriocapillaris of the choroid. The sclera is a layer of relatively avascular dense connective tissue.

267. The answer is b. (*Kandel, 4/e, pp 597, 614–615, 803. McKenzie and Klein, pp 378–381.*) The vestibular hair cells are the sensory transduction system of the inner ear and are responsible for the conversion of mechanical energy into an electrical signal for cranial nerve VIII. These cells are called hair cells because their surface contains stereocilia. These are modified microvilli that contain a large number of actin filaments and extend from the surface of the cell. The stereocilia are different lengths and are arranged in order by size with a large kinocilium at one end. The arrangement of the stereocilia is very important because bending in one direction (i.e., toward the kinocilium) depolarizes the cell and increases the rate of nervous discharge, whereas bending them in the other direction (i.e., away from the kinocilium) results in hyperpolarization and decreased neural discharge. The classification of type of hair cell (I or II) is based on the pattern of efferent and afferent innervation.

268. The answer is a. (*Junqueira, 9/e, pp 470–472. McKenzie and Klein, pp 378–381.*) Shearing of the hair cell stereocilia against the tectorial membrane results in depolarization, and the release of neurotransmitter onto afferent endings of the auditory cranial nerve leads to initiation of an action potential. Sound waves are directed toward the tympanic membrane by the pinna and the external auditory canal of the external ear. The vibration of the tympanic membrane is transmitted to the oval window by way of the ossicles of the middle ear. Induction of waves in the perilymph results in the movement of the basilar and vestibular membranes toward the scala tympani and causes the round window to bulge outward. The movement of the hair cells is facilitated because the tectorial membrane is rigid and the pillar cells form a pivot. The stabilization of the pressure between the middle ear and the nasopharynx is not directly related to the mechanism of sound transmission.

269. The answer is e. (*Junqueira, 9/e, pp 466. McKenzie and Klein, pp 378–381.*) The scala tympani contains perilymph. Endolymph is similar to intracellular fluid (high K^+, low Na^+). It is found in the utricle, saccule, semicircular canals, and scala media (cochlear duct), which are parts of the membranous labyrinth. Endolymph is synthesized by the highly vascular stria vascularis in the lateral wall of the scala media. The endolymphatic sac and duct are responsible for absorption of endolymph and the endocytosis of molecules from the endolymph.

270. The answer is e. (*Young, 4/e, pp 398–401. Junqueira, 9/e, pp 465–470.*) The stria vascularis (D) is found in the lateral wall of the cochlear duct (scala media, "I") and is responsible for the ionic composition of the endolymph. The organ of Corti is found within the cochlear duct and contains the hair cells that are responsible for transduction of the sound to a nerve impulse. It rests on the basilar membrane, which separates it from the epithelial lining of the tympanic cavity. The inner tunnel (H) of the organ of Corti separates the outer from the inner hair cells. The outer hair cells possess microvilli that are attached to the tectorial membrane (C). In contrast, the inner hair cells are unattached. Supportive cells include the phalangeal and pillar cells, which are not labeled on the figure. The spiral lamina is a bony structure that protrudes from the modiolus. The spiral limbus (B) is a connective tissue structure superior to the unattached edge of the spiral lamina. Along the outer wall of the canal of the organ of Corti is a thickened projection of periosteum known as the spiral ligament (F). The spiral ganglion is labeled A on the figure and contains bipolar cells. Peripheral processes of spiral ganglion cells reach the organ of Corti, whereas central processes terminate in nuclei located in the medulla. The internal spiral tunnel is labeled E in the figure.

271. The answer is a. (*McKenzie and Klein, pp 378–381. Junqueira, 9/e, pp 464–466.*) The vestibular membrane, also known as Reissner's membrane, maintains the gradient between the endolymph of the scala media and the perilymph of the vestibular cavity. The middle ear contains the auditory ossicles, which transmit sound to the oval window and, therefore, serve in the transduction of sound waves to the perilymph. The helicotrema represents the opening that allows communication of the tympanic and vestibular cavities. The epithelium possesses extensive occluding junctions, which serve to maintain the concentration gradient that is essential for sensory transduction. The movement of the middle ear bones is dampened by the stapedius and tensor tympani when an individual is exposed to a loud noise.

272. The answer is c. (*Junqueira, 9/e, pp 466–470. Moore, Before We Are Born, 5/e, pp 471–473. Moore, The Developing Human, 6/e, pp 505–506.*) The semicircular canals, which extend from the utricle, contain the cristae ampullares and detect angular acceleration. The utricle represents the dorsal portion of the otocyst-derived inner ear; the saccule represents the ventral portion. Both the utricle and saccule contain maculae that detect linear acceleration. The maculae of the utricle and saccule are perpendicular to one another. These maculae contain type I and type II hair cells, which differ in their innervation. The hair cells have stereocilia and a kinocilium embedded in a membrane that contains otoconia (statoconia) composed of calcium carbonate. The stereocilia and kinocilia are embedded in the cupola, which does not contain the otoconia found in the maculae. The endolymph turns right when the head turns left and vice versa. Movement stimulates the stereocilia and induces depolarization. The interdental cells produce the tectorial membrane, which is essential for the development of the shearing force in the process of sound transduction in the organ of Corti. It detects sound vibration and is responsive to variation in the frequency of sound waves.

Head and Neck

Questions

DIRECTIONS: Each item below contains a question or incomplete statement followed by suggested responses. Select the **one best** response to each question.

273. Efferent cranial nerves develop from

a. The alar plate
b. The basal plate
c. The floor plate
d. The roof plate
e. Neural crest

274. An elderly gentleman is delivered to the hospital in a febrile and septic condition. The only remarkable recent history was an episode of choking on swallowing a rough object during a meal a few days previously. The choking resolved, but there was some hematemesis the following day that also resolved. The examiner notes edematous pharyngeal tissue and assumes an esophageal laceration with infection within the retrovisceral space. The examining physician suspects that the infection

a. Tracks superiorly and inferiorly within the carotid sheath
b. Extends anteriorly to the trachea
c. Extends into the posterior mediastinum
d. Will not extend below the manubrium

275. A carcinoma in the medial portion of the lower lip is most likely to first metastasize via the

a. Submandibular lynph nodes
b. Parotid lymph nodes
c. Superficial cervical lymph nodes
d. Submental lymph nodes
e. Buccal lymph nodes

276. The arachnoid villi allow cerebrospinal fluid to pass between which of the following two spaces?

a. Choroid plexus and subdural space
b. Subarachnoid space and subdural space
c. Subarachnoid space and superior sagittal sinus
d. Subdural space and cavernous sinus
e. Superior sagittal sinus and jugular vein

277. A tumor in the infratemporal fossa may gain entrance to the orbit through

a. The optic foramen
b. The inferior orbital fissure
c. The pterygoid canal
d. The ethmoidal sinuses
e. The superior orbital fissure

278. A 28-year-old man is treated in an emergency room for a superficial gash on his forehead. The wound is bleeding profusely, but examination reveals no fracture. While the wound is being sutured, he relates that while he was using an electric razor, he remembers becoming dizzy and then waking up on the floor with blood everywhere. The physician suspects a hypersensitive cardiac reflex. The patient's epicranial aponeurosis (galea aponeurotica) is penetrated, which results in severe gaping of the wound. The structure overlying the epicranial aponeurosis is

a. A layer containing blood vessels
b. Bone
c. The dura mater
d. The periosteum (pericranium)
e. The tendon of the epicranial muscles (occipitofrontalis)

279. Which pair of venous structures contributes to the confluence of dural sinuses on the interior surface of the occipital bone?

a. Sigmoid and transverse sinuses
b. Inferior sagittal and cavernous sinuses
c. Occipital and straight sinuses
d. Transverse and inferior petrosal sinuses
e. Superior petrosal and occipital sinuses

280. An elderly man, persuaded to have his eyes examined after a series of minor automobile accidents, was found to have a pituitary adenoma that was producing visual field defects. A pituitary adenoma that expands superiorly and compresses the central portion of the optic chiasm will result in

a. Total blindness
b. Losses of left and right inferior fields of vision
c. Losses of left and right nasal fields of vision
d. Losses of left and right temporal fields of vision

281. Which of the following is the most direct route for spread of infection from the paranasal sinuses to the cavernous sinus of the dura mater?

a. Pterygoid venous plexus
b. Superior ophthalmic vein
c. Frontal emissary vein
d. Basilar venous plexus
e. Parietal emissary vein

282. Most skeletal elements of the face, e.g., bone and cartilages, are derived from

a. Cranial intermediate mesoderm
b. Cervical somites
c. Neural crest cells migrating from the cranial neural tube
d. The somatic layer of cranial lateral plate mesoderm
e. The splanchnic layer of cranial lateral plate mesoderm

Questions 283 to 284

A 53-year-old woman has a paralysis of the right side of her face that produces an expressionless and drooping appearance. She is unable to close her right eye, has difficulty chewing and drinking, perceives sounds as annoyingly intense in her right ear, and experiences some pain in her right external auditory meatus. Physical examination reveals loss of the blink reflex in the right eye on stimulation of either cornea and loss of taste from the anterior two-thirds of the tongue on the right. Lacrimation appears normal in the right eye, the jaw-jerk reflex is normal, and there appears to be no problem with balance.

283. The inability to close the right eye is the result of involvement of the

a. Zygomatic branch of the facial nerve
b. Buccal branch of the trigeminal nerve
c. Levator palpebrae superioris muscle
d. Superior tarsal muscle (of Müller)
e. Orbital portion of the orbicularis oculi muscle

284. The branch of the facial nerve that conveys secretomotor neurons involved in lacrimation is the

a. Chorda tympani
b. Deep petrosal nerve
c. Greater superficial petrosal nerve
d. Lacrimal nerve
e. Lesser superficial petrosal nerve

285. A 55-year-old man was brought into the hospital with a severe burn to his left hand. The man had placed his hand on the hot burner of an electric stove but had not sensed anything wrong until he smelled burning flesh. Neurologic examination revealed loss of pain and temperature sensation over dermatomes C4 through T6 bilaterally. However, pain and temperature were perceived bilaterally both above C4 and below T6. Discriminative touch was present in unburned dermatomes on the left and in the right extremity. Although the left hand was too damaged to accurately assess muscle function, weakness and wasting of small muscles of the right hand was noted. Muscle strength and reflexes were otherwise normal. Pain and temperature sensations from the extremities ascend in the spinal cord in the

a. Intermediolateral cell column
b. Cuneate fasciculus
c. Lateral spinothalamic tract
d. Dorsal columns
e. Fasciculus gracilis

286. Which of the following statements concerning the lacrimal apparatus is correct?

a. The lacrimal gland lies in the medial portion of the orbit
b. Lacrimal fluid is secreted at the puncta in the medial edges of both upper and lower lids
c. The nasolacrimal duct has a blind-ending lacrimal sac at its upper portion
d. The nasolacrimal duct ends in the middle meatus of the nose

Questions 287 and 288

A 70-year-old woman is seen in Outpatient Neurology complaining of strange feelings and numbness in both lower extremities below the knees. She walked with a wide-based gait, slamming her right foot down heavily and dragging her left foot. Subsequent examination revealed diminished two-point discrimination, proprioception, and vibratory senses, especially below the knees. Pain and temperature sensations were intact. Motor examination revealed hyperactive knee and ankle-jerk reflexes with spastic weakness most obvious on the left. The patient tended to tilt to the left when standing with her eyes closed.

287. The afferent fibers involved in this case ascend in the spinal cord in the

a. Lateral spinothalamic tract
b. Cuneate fasciculus
c. Cuneocerebellar tract
d. Anterior spinothalamic tract
e. Fasciculus gracilis

288. Further studies revealed that the patient's symptoms were due to a chronic vitamin B_{12} deficiency (pernicious anemia). This results in decreased activity of B_{12}-dependent enzymes, including methylmalonic CoA mutase, essential for maintenance of myelin sheaths. Demyelinization in which of the following motor pathways would produce the observed symptoms?

a. Lateral corticospinal tract
b. Vestibulospinal tract
c. Lower motor neurons (ventral horn cells)
d. Rubrospinal tract
e. Tectospinal tract

289. The vertebral arteries are correctly described by which of the following statements?

a. They arise from the common carotid artery on the left and the brachiocephalic artery on the right
b. They enter the cranium via the anterior condylar canals
c. They enter the cranium via the posterior condylar canals
d. They pass through the transverse processes of several cervical vertebrae
e. They directly give rise to the posterior cerebral arteries

290. Tic douloureux (trigeminal neuralgia) is characterized by sharp pain over the distribution of the trigeminal nerve. This syndrome involves neurons that have their cell bodies in the

a. Geniculate ganglion
b. Otic ganglion
c. Pterygopalatine ganglion
d. Submandibular ganglion
e. Trigeminal ganglion

291. A cranial fracture through the foramen rotundum that compresses the enclosed nerve results in

a. Inability to clench the jaw firmly
b. Loss of the sneeze reflex
c. Paralysis of the inferior oblique muscle of the orbit
d. Regurgitation of fluids into the nasopharynx during swallowing
e. Uncontrolled drooling from the mouth

292. A 72-year-old male presents in the Emergency Room with dizziness and nystagmus. Examination reveals a loss of pain and temperature sensation over the right side of the face and the left side of the body. The patient exhibits ataxia and intention tremor on the right in both the upper and lower extremities and is unable to perform either the finger-to-nose or heel-to-shin tasks on the right. In addition, he is hoarse and demonstrates pupillary constriction and drooping of the eyelid on the right. Finally, the right side of his face is drier than the left. Following vascular blockage, necrotic damage in which of the following would explain the patient's hoarseness?

a. Nucleus ambiguus
b. Lateral spinothalamic tract
c. Spinal nucleus of CN V
d. Descending sympathetic pathways
e. Inferior cerebellar peduncle

293. In dislocation of the jaw, displacement of the articular disk beyond the articular tubercle of the temporomandibular joint results from spasm or excessive contraction of which of the following muscles?

a. Buccinator
b. Lateral pterygoid
c. Medial pterygoid
d. Masseter
e. Temporalis

294. The pterygomandibular raphe is a useful landmark in the oral cavity. This tendinous tissue marks the juncture of two muscles that are innervated by which of the following cranial nerves?

a. Maxillary (CN V2) and mandibular (CN V3)
b. Mandibular (CN V3) and glossopharyngeal (CN IX)
c. Mandibular (CN V3) and vagus (CN X)
d. Facial (CN VII) and glossopharyngeal (CN IX)
e. Facial (CN VII) and vagus (CN X)

295. A 63-year-old woman was brought into the emergency room by her son, who suspected she had suffered a stroke the previous night. Subsequent examination revealed spastic hemiplegia on the left side with hyperreflexia and a positive Babinski's sign. The left side of the patient's face was paralyzed below the eye, and the right eye was turned out and down. The right pupil made direct and consensual responses to light, but the left pupil was fixed and unresponsive. There were no apparent sensory deficits. Which is the most likely location of the lesion?

a. Left motor cortex
b. Right sensory cortex
c. Right midbrain
d. Left thalamus
e. Right thalamus

296. A 75-year-old man was rushed to the hospital from his retirement community when he suddenly became confused and could not speak but could grunt and moan. The patient could follow simple commands and did recognize his wife and children although he could not name them or speak to them. Additional immediate examination revealed weakness of the right upper extremity. Several days later, a more comprehensive examination revealed weakness and paralysis of the right hand and arm with increased biceps and triceps reflexes. Paralysis and weakness were also present on the lower right side of the face. Pain, temperature, and touch modalities were mildly decreased over the right arm, hand, and face, and proprioception was reduced in the right hand. The patient had regained the ability to articulate with great difficulty a few simple words but could not repeat even simple two or three word phrases. Which artery or major branch of a large artery suffered the occlusion that produced the observed symptoms?

a.   Anterior choroidal artery
b.   Middle cerebral artery
c.   Posterior communicating artery
d.   Ophthalmic artery
e.   Anterior cerebral artery

297. A 53-year-old banker develops paralysis on the right side of the face, which produces an expressionless and drooping appearance. He is unable to close the right eye and also has difficulty chewing and drinking. Examination shows loss of blink reflex in the right eye to stimulation of either right or left conjunctiva. Lacrimation appears normal on the right side, but salivation is diminished and taste is absent on the anterior right side of the tongue. There is no complaint of hyperacusis. Audition and balance appear to be normal. The lesion is located

a.   In the brain and involves the nucleus of the facial nerve and superior salivatory nucleus
b.   Within the internal auditory meatus
c.   At the geniculate ganglion
d.   In the facial canal just distal to the genu of the facial nerve
e.   Just proximal to the stylomastoid foramen

298. The dark structure in the midbrain indicated by the arrow in this midsagittal MRI represents a passage for

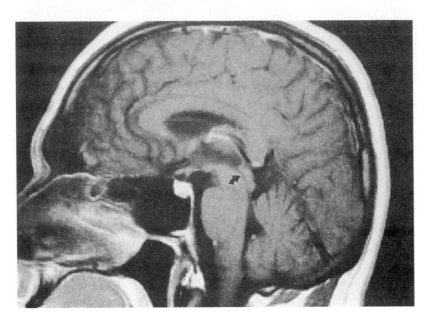

a. Venous blood
b. Arterial blood (in the basilar artery)
c. Neurons of the corticospinal tract
d. Cerebrospinal fluid
e. Spinothalamic (sensory) fibers

299. The palatine tonsils are located between the anterior and posterior faucial folds. The muscles that form these folds are, respectively, the

a. Levator veli palatini and tensor veli palatini
b. Palatoglossus and palatopharyngeus
c. Palatopharyngeus and salpingopharyngeus
d. Styloglossus and stylopharyngeus
e. Superior constrictor and middle constrictor

300. Which of the following is true of neural tube development?

a. Closure of the neural tube proceeds in a craniocaudal sequence
b. The basic organization of the neural tube features peripheral neuronal cell bodies and centrally located myelinated processes
c. The primitive neurectoderm cells of the neural tube give rise to both neurons and all glial components
d. During development, neuronal and glial precursors are born near the central canal and migrate to the periphery
e. Mature neurons migrate out of the spinal cord to form the sensory ganglia

301. Which of the following structures is found in the lateral wall of the tonsillar fossa?

a. Facial nerve
b. Glossopharyngeal nerve
c. Hypoglossal nerve
d. Lingual nerve
e. Vagus nerve

302. A patient is observed to suffer from an alternating hypoglossal hemiplegia. There is atrophy of the tongue on one side and deviation of the tongue toward the right on protrusion. In addition, the patient exhibits upper motor neuron paralysis of the left side of the body. Deviation of the tongue toward the right involves the

a. Left nucleus ambiguus
b. Left pyramidal tract caudal to the decussation
c. Right hypoglossal nerve
d. Right nucleus ambiguus
e. Right pyramidal tract rostral to the decussation

303. A patient is found to have internal (medially directed) strabismus of the left eye, paralysis of the muscles of facial expression on the left side, hyperacusis (louder perception of sounds) of the left ear, and loss of taste from the anterior two-thirds of the tongue on the left. The mouth is somewhat drier than normal. In addition, in the left eye there is a lack of tearing, and a blink reflex cannot be elicited from the stimulation of either the right or the left cornea. There is accompanying upper motor neuron paralysis of the right side of the body. Internal strabismus (deviation of the eye medially) results from paralysis of which of the following cranial nerves?

a. Cranial nerve II
b. Cranial nerve III
c. Cranial nerve IV
d. Cranial nerve V
e. Cranial nerve VI

304. During a neck dissection, the styloid process is used as a landmark. Which of the following statements correctly pertains to one of the four structures that attach to the styloid process?

a. The stylohyoid muscle attaches to the lesser horn of the hyoid bone
b. The styloglossus muscle acts to protrude the tongue
c. The stylohyoid ligament attaches to the lingula of the mandible
d. Distally the stylopharyngeus muscle is split by the digastric muscle

305. An elderly, somewhat obese man is brought to the emergency room complaining of sudden spontaneous flailing movements of his right arm and leg. The arm movements particularly were most severe proximally. No other neurologic deficits were noted. The patient had most likely suffered a hemorrhage in

a. The cerebellum
b. The ventral horn of the spinal cord
c. The hypothalamus
d. Primary sensory cortex
e. The subthalamic nucleus

306. The condition in which the covering of the spinal cord, along with enclosed neural tissue, forms a saclike projection through a dorsal defect in the vertebral column is termed

a. Rachischisis
b. Anencephaly
c. Meningocele
d. Meningomyelocele
e. Hydrocephaly

307. A teenage baseball player was hit in the base of the skull by a loose bat. The patient is hoarse and complains of difficulty swallowing. The cranial x-ray indicates a basal skull fracture that passes through the jugular foramen. The examining physician notes a large hematoma behind the ear on the injured side. If the nerves passing through the jugular foramen were severed as a result of the cranial fracture, one muscle that would remain functional is the

a. Palatoglossus muscle
b. Sternomastoid muscle
c. Styloglossus muscle
d. Stylopharyngeus muscle
e. Trapezius muscle

308. Like all endocrine glands, the thyroid is highly vascular. The thyroid gland receives its blood supply in part from branches of the

a. Internal carotid artery
b. Lingual artery
c. Subclavian artery
d. Transverse cervical artery
e. Vertebral artery

309. Muscle relaxants are used routinely during anesthesia with resultant closure of the vocal folds. Laryngeal intubation by the anesthesiologist is necessary because which of the following muscles is unable to maintain the glottis open?

a. Cricothyroid muscle
b. Lateral cricoarytenoid muscles
c. Posterior cricoarytenoid muscles
d. Thyroarytenoid muscle
e. Transverse arytenoid muscles

310. Your patient is a 30-year-old male who lives in a group home. He was playing with a pencil and, during a fall, accidentally drove the pencil deeply into a nostril. The pencil was angled toward the midline structure indicated by the arrow in this midsagittal MRI. The pencil was driven through the _____ toward the _____ (indicated by the arrow).

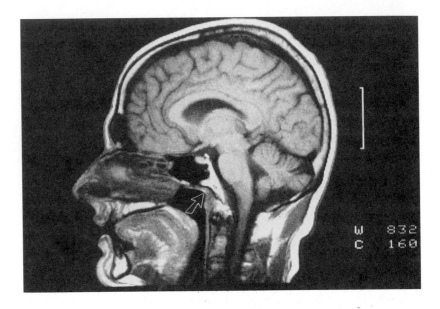

a. Nasal cavity and nasopharynx, toward the pharyngeal tonsil
b. Nasal cavity and sphenoidal sinus, toward the pituitary
c. Nasal cavity and sphenoidal sinus, toward the internal carotid artery
d. Nasal cavity and ethmoidal air cells, toward the circle of Willis
e. Nasal cavity, toward the basilar artery

Questions 311 to 312

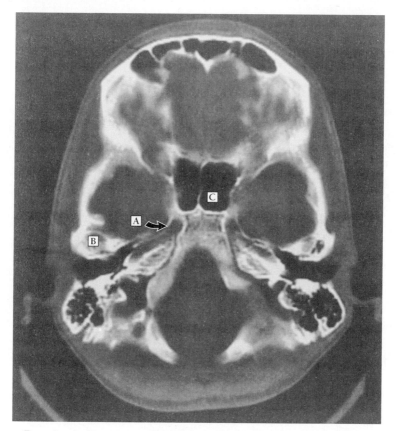

(Reproduced, with permission, from Wicke L: Atlas of Radiological Anatomy, 6/e. Baltimore, MD: Williams & Wilkins, 1998.)

311. A patient has suffered a fracture of the floor of the left middle cranial fossa in a vehicular traffic accident. Bony fragments have crushed a major nerve passing through the opening labeled "A" in the accompanying CT image. Which of the following would you expect?

a. Paralysis of facial muscles
b. Paralysis of masticatory muscles
c. Paralysis of trapezius and sternocleidomastoid
d. Paralysis of the scalene muscles
e. Paralysis of laryngeal muscles

312. In this CT image, the space labeled "C" is the

a. Anterior ethmoid sinus
b. Posterior ethmoid sinus
c. Nasopharynx
d. Sphenoidal sinus
e. Maxillary sinus

DIRECTIONS: Each group of questions below consists of lettered headings followed by a set of numbered items. For each numbered item, select the **one** lettered heading with which it is **most** closely associated. Each lettered heading may be used once, more than once, or not at all.

Questions 313 to 314

For each action, select the muscle that accomplishes it.

a. Buccinator muscle
b. Geniohyoid muscle
c. Lateral pterygoid muscle
d. Medial pterygoid muscle
e. Posterior fibers of temporalis muscle

313. Lateral deviation of the jaw

314. Pure elevation of the jaw

Questions 315 to 316

Certain neurons supplying the head and neck region have their cell bodies located in ganglia. For each of the neurons described, select the ganglion in which the cell bodies are located.

a. Ciliary ganglion
b. Geniculate ganglion
c. Inferior glossopharyngeal (petrosal) ganglion
d. Inferior vagal (nodose) ganglion
e. Otic ganglion
f. Pterygopalatine (sphenopalatine) ganglion
g. Semilunar ganglion
h. Spiral ganglion
i. Submandibular ganglion
j. Superior cervical ganglion
k. Superior glossopharyngeal (jugular) ganglion
l. Superior vagal (jugular) ganglion

315. Cell bodies that bring about accommodation

316. Cell bodies that supply the parotid gland

Questions 317 to 318

Match each of the following questions to the appropriate cranial nerve.

a. Cranial nerve I
b. Cranial nerve II
c. Cranial nerve III
d. Cranial nerve IV
e. Cranial nerve V
f. Cranial nerve VI
g. Cranial nerve VII
h. Cranial nerve VIII
i. Cranial nerve IX
j. Cranial nerve X
k. Cranial nerve XI
l. Cranial nerve XII

317. Provides afferent limb of the gag reflex

318. Innervates the iridic sphincters

Questions 319 to 320

Match each incident of bleeding with the injury that usually produces it.

a. Cerebral vein rupture
b. Hemorrhage within the "danger space"
c. Middle meningeal artery tear
d. Ruptured aneurysm of a branch of the middle cerebral artery

319. Extracranial hematoma

320. Subarachnoid hemorrhage with blood in the cerebrospinal fluid

Questions 321 to 322

For each of the following questions, identify the appropriate labeled structure on the accompanying cross section of the dorsomedian region of the cerebral hemisphere at the sagittal fissure.

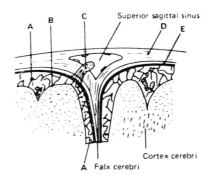

321. Structure through which cerebrospinal fluid filters into the general venous circulation

322. The space that contains the major volume of cerebrospinal fluid

Questions 323 to 327

Match each structure with its embryonic origin labeled in the figure.

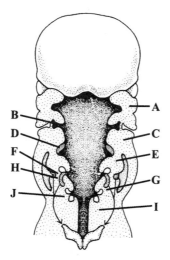

(Modified, with permission, from Sweeney L.: Basic Concepts in Embryology. New York, NY: McGraw-Hill, 2000.)

323. Inferior parathyroid gland

324. Stapes

325. Thymus gland

326. Facial nerve

327. Recurrent laryngeal nerve

Head and Neck

Answers

273. The answer is b. (*Moore, Embryology, 5/e, p 391. Sadler, 7/e, p 376.*) The basal plate of the neural tube gives rise to the motor nuclei of the cranial nerves, which are divided into three groups: general somatic efferent, special visceral efferent, and general visceral efferent. The alar plate contains three similarly divided groups of sensory nuclei and also gives rise to the cerebral hemispheres and the cerebellum. The roof plate consists of a single layer of ependymal cells, which later join with the pia mater to develop into the choroid plexuses of the lateral, third, and fourth ventricles. The floor plate also is devoid of neuroblasts.

274. The answer is c. (*April, 3/e, p 491.*) The retropharyngeal (retrovisceral) space descends into the posterior mediastinum. Infection in the retrovisceral space may track deep into the posterior thorax, a life-threatening condition. Conversely, the pretracheal space, deep to the pretracheal fascia, surrounds the trachea and thyroid gland, but is anterior to the esophagus. It descends into the superior mediastinum to about the level of the manubrium.

275. The answer is d. (*Moore, Anatomy, 4/e, pp 869–870.*) Lymph from the medial portion of the lower lip preferentially drains through the submental nodes in the chin and metastases may first appear here. Lymph from the upper lip and lateral portions of the lower lip drains preferentially through the submandibular nodes on the inferolateral aspect of the mandible. The parotid nodes receive lymph from upper and lateral regions of the face including the forehead, eyelids, and middle ear. Superficial and deep cervical nodes receive lymph from other nodes including the parotid and retroauricular. Buccal lymph nodes drain the cheeks and sides of the nose.

276. The answer is c. (*Carpenter, 4/e, p 7. Noback, 4/e, p 74.*) Cerebrospinal fluid formed in the choroid plexus circulates in the subarachnoid space and is absorbed by the venous sinuses through the arachnoid villi, some of which project into the superior sagittal sinus. Cerebrospinal fluid protects the nervous system from concussions and mechanical injuries and is important for metabolism. It circulates slowly through the ventricles of the brain and through the meshes of the subarachnoid space.

277. The answer is b. (*Moore, Anatomy, 4/e, p 834.*) The infratemporal fossa communicates directly with the orbit via the inferior orbital fissure and the pterygopalatine fossa. The fissure normally transmits branches of the maxillary nerve (V2) and branches of the infraorbital vessels. The optic foramen and superior orbital fissure open into the middle cranial fossa and transmit the optic nerve (CN II) and the oculomotor (CN III), trochlear (CN IV), and abducens (CN VI) nerves, respectively. The pterygoid canal connects the middle cranial fossa with the pterygopalatine fossa and transmits the vidian nerve. The ethmoidal sinuses are mucosa-lined cavities within the ethmoid and adjacent bones. They drain into the nasal cavity.

278. The answer is a. (*Moore, Anatomy, 3/e, p 673.*) A mnemonic device for remembering the order in which the soft tissues overlie the cranium is SCALP: Skin, Connective tissue, Aponeurosis, Loose connective tissue, and Periosteum. The scalp proper is composed of the outer three layers, of which the connective tissue contains one of the richest cutaneous blood supplies of the body. The occipitofrontal muscle complex inserts into the epicranial aponeurosis, which forms the intermediate tendon of this digastric muscle. This structure, along with the underlying layer of loose connective tissue, accounts for the high degree of mobility of the scalp over the pericranium. If the aponeurosis is lacerated transversely, traction from the muscle bellies will cause considerable gaping of the wound. Secondary to trauma or infection, blood or pus may accumulate subjacent to the epicranial aponeurosis.

279. The answer is c. (*Moore, Anatomy, 4/e, pp 879–881.*) The confluence of sinuses is formed by the superior sagittal sinus, both transverse sinuses, the occipital sinus, and the straight sinus. The inferior sagittal sinus and the great cerebral vein join to form the straight sinus. The superior and inferior petrosal sinuses both drain the cavernous sinuses, the former connecting with the ipsilateral transverse sinus and the latter with the origin of the internal jugular vein.

280. The answer is d. (*April, 3/e, p 529.*) A tumor that impinges on and compresses the optic chiasm will produce tunnel vision (bitemporal heteronymous hemianopsia). The reason for this pattern of blindness is that the lens projects reversed and inverted lateral visual fields onto the nasal portions of the retina. The pathways from the nasal retinas cross in the optic chiasm. This decussation collects both right and left visual fields. Thus, nerve fibers from the right nasal retina and left temporal retina, e.g., are collected into the left optic tract for projection to the left lateral geniculate body and then to the left occipital cortex. Injury to a lateral portion of the chiasm produces ipsilateral nasal hemianopsia, the loss of the nasal field from one eye. A lesion of the optic nerve would produce complete blindness of that eye, whereas a lesion to the optic tract produces contralateral homonymous hemianopsia, complete loss of the contralateral visual field.

281. The answer is b. (*Moore, Anatomy, 4/e, pp 880–883.*) The superior ophthalmic vein drains the region of the paranasal sinuses and is directly connected with the cavernous sinus although blood flow is normally away from the brain. The pterygoid venous plexus communicates with the cavernous sinus via the petrosal sinuses. The frontal emissary vein communicates with the superior sagittal sinus via the foramen cecum. The basilar venous plexus communicates with the inferior petrosal sinus. The parietal emissary vein also communicates with the superior sagittal sinus.

282. The answer is c. (*Moore, Embryology, 5/e, p 208.*) Neural crest cells from cranial regions of the neural tube migrate into the presumptive pharyngeal arches and give rise to many structures of both the viscero- and neurocrania. Intermediate mesoderm never forms in the cranial region. Also, somites never develop past the initial stage (somitomere) but do give rise to some mesodermal derivatives of the head including the bones at the base of the skull (visceral chondrocranium). Cervical somites only contribute minimally. In the cranial region, the lateral plate mesoderm forms a solid core. It is not divided into somatic and splanchnic portions separated by a coelom.

283. The answer is a. (*Moore, Anatomy, 3/e, p 660.*) The palpebral portion of the orbicularis oculi muscle (innervated by the zygomatic branch of the facial nerve) produces the blink, whereas the orbital portion is involved

in "scrunching" the eye shut. The buccal branch of the facial nerve innervates muscles of facial expression (including the buccinator muscle)
between the eye and the mouth, whereas the buccal branch of the trigeminal nerve is sensory. The levator palpebrae superioris muscle, which elevates the upper eyelid, is innervated by the oculomotor nerve, whereas the
involuntary superior tarsal muscle is supplied by sympathetic nerves.

284. The answer is c. *(Moore, Anatomy, 4/e, p 951.)* The greater superficial petrosal nerve leaves the facial nerve (CN VII) at the geniculate ganglion. It carries secretomotor neurons from the superior salivatory nucleus
to the pterygopalatine ganglion and joins along the way with the sympathetic deep petrosal nerve to become the nerve of the pterygoid canal.

285. The answer is c. *(Waxman, 24/e, pp 66–67, 203.)* A lesion of the
spinal canal that compresses the ventral commissure (syringomyelia) would
interrupt ascending fibers crossing there but would not interfere with
already crossed fibers ascending in the lateral spinothalamic tracts. Pain and
temperature sensation above and below the level of the cord lesion would be
preserved. The cell bodies of first-order afferent (sensory) neurons are
located in the dorsal root ganglia. Their central processes enter the spinal
cord and ascend one segment before synapsing with a second-order neuron
in the dorsal horn. The central processes of second-order neurons cross in
the ventral white commissure to the opposite side of the cord and ascend in
the lateral spinothalamic tract to the ventral posterior lateral nucleus of the
thalamus where they synapse with third-order neurons, which relay the
message to cortical neurons of the postcentral gyrus of the parietal lobe.
Lesions occurring unilaterally in a peripheral nerve would result in an ipsilateral deficit, whereas lesions in a crossed ascending pathway, in the thalamus, or in the cortex would result in contralateral deficits.

286. The answer is c. *(Moore, Anatomy, 4/e, pp 901–903.)* The lacrimal
gland lies in the upper lateral portion of the orbit. Normally, lacrimal fluid
flows across the cornea to enter puncta in the medial edges of both upper
and lower lids. From the puncta, canaliculi run to enlarged ampullae. The
nasolacrimal duct has a blind–ending lacrimal sac at its upper portion that
is squeezed like a bulb syringe by the opening and closing of the eyelids
and thereby aspirates the lacrimal fluid. The nasolacrimal duct ends in the
inferior meatus of the nose.

287. The answer is e. (*Waxman, 24/e, p 203.*) The fasciculus gracilis consists of afferent fibers carrying information concerning two-point discrimination, vibration, and joint/limb position from the lower extremities and inferior trunk. The cuneate fasciculus (fasciculus cuneatus) carries the same modalities from the superior trunk and upper extremities. Classically, light touch is the modality assigned to afferents in the anterior spinothalamic tract, whereas afferents of the lateral spinothalamic tract convey information regarding pain and temperature. Fibers in the cuneocerebellar tract convey proprioception from the upper extremity.

288. The answer is a. (*Brust, pp 205–207.*) Demyelinization would most profoundly affect the function of well-myelinated large neurons of the lateral corticospinal tract, as well as the lower motor neurons originating in the ventral horn of the spinal cord. However, because reflex pathways were intact and hyperactive, the disease process must be confined to the upper motor neurons of the corticospinal tract. The lateral corticospinal tract carries messages from the contralateral motor cortex to lower motor neurons in the ventral horn of the spinal cord. Loss of this pathway results in spastic, rather than flaccid, paralysis. The other tracts (vestibulo-, rubro-, and tecto-spinal) are composed of fine, sparsely myelinated neurons and would be less affected by the anemia.

289. The answer is d. (*April, 3/e, pp 538–540. Moore, Anatomy, 4/e, p 894.*) The vertebral arteries usually arise from the subclavian arteries and ascend through the transverse foramina of the sixth to the first cervical vertebrae but not the seventh. They enter the cranium through the foramen magnum after which they join to form the basilar artery. The basilar artery terminates by bifurcating into the posterior cerebral arteries. The hypoglossal nerves (CN XII) leave the cranium via the anterior condylar (hypoglossal) canals, whereas the posterior condylar canals transmit emissary veins.

290. The answer is e. (*April, 3/e, pp 529, 535–536. Moore, Anatomy, 4/e, pp 1093–1096.*) The cell bodies of most of the sensory neurons of the trigeminal nerve are located in the trigeminal ganglion. From there they project to the nucleus of the spinal tract and ultimately to the ventral posterior medial nucleus of the thalamus. From this point, they project to the medial portions of the sensory cortex of the postcentral gyrus. The otic, pterygopalatine, and submandibular ganglia are parasympathetic. The geniculate ganglion contains the sensory neurons of the facial nerve.

291. The answer is b. *(Moore, Anatomy, 4/e, p 1096.)* The maxillary division of the trigeminal nerve (CN V2), which passes through the foramen rotundum, is entirely sensory. Damage to this nerve results in sensory deprivation over the maxillary region of the face and loss of the sneeze reflex. The mandibular division of the trigeminal nerve, which passes through the foramen ovale, innervates the masticatory muscles responsible for clenching the jaw as well as the tensor palatini muscle, which assists in the establishment of the velopharyngeal seal. The other muscles of the soft palate are innervated by the pharyngeal branch of the vagus nerve (CN X), which transits the jugular foramen. The orbicularis oris and buccinator muscles are innervated by the facial nerve (CN VII), which transits the stylomastoid foramen. The inferior oblique muscle of the eye is innervated by the inferior branch of the oculomotor nerve, which enters the orbit through the superior orbital fissure.

292. The answer is a. *(Brust, pp 210–213.)* The nucleus ambiguus, along with special visceral efferent (SVE) components of CN IX, X, and XI, is a column of lower motor neurons that innervate muscles of the pharynx, larynx, and palate. Damage to this nucleus results in loss of the gag reflex, difficulty in swallowing, and hoarseness.

The lateral spinothalamic tract passes through the medulla and carries sensory information (pain and temperature) from the contralateral extremities and trunk. Similarly, the spinal tract of CN V carries pain and temperature sensation from the ipsilateral face. Descending sympathetic pathways course through the medulla to reach the intermediolateral cell column of the spinal gray matter. Damage to these fibers would result in loss of ability to dilate the pupil (meiosis), drooping eyelid (ptosis), and loss of sweating ipsilaterally (hemianhydrosis). Damage to nerve fibers passing to and from the cerebellum via the inferior cerebellar peduncle would result in intention tremor and lack of coordination.

293. The answer is b. *(Moore, Anatomy, 4/e, p 921.)* The temporalis, masseter, and medial and lateral pterygoid muscles attach to the mandible and are the major muscles involved in movements of the jaw. The buccinator muscle, which controls the contents of the mouth during mastication, is innervated by the seventh cranial nerve and constitutes the chief muscle of facial expression. The lateral pterygoid muscles, acting bilaterally, protract the jaw and, acting unilaterally, rotate the jaw during chewing. Because the fibers of the superior head of the lateral pterygoid muscle insert onto the anterior aspect of the articular disk of the temporomandibular joint as well as onto the head of the mandible, spasm of this muscle, such as in a yawn, can result in dislocation of the mandible by pulling the disk anterior to the articular tubercle. Reduction is accomplished by pushing the mandible downward and back, so that the head of the mandible reenters the mandibular fossa. The temporalis, medial pterygoid, and masseter muscles primarily elevate the jaw in molar occlusion.

294. The answer is e. *(April, 3/e, pp 626, 633.)* The pterygomandibular raphe extends from the hamulus of the medial pterygoid plate to the mandible and marks the junction of the buccinator and the superior constrictor muscles. The buccinator, a muscle of facial expression, is innervated by the facial nerve (CN VII). The superior constrictor is innervated by the pharyngeal branch of the vagus nerve (CN X).

295. The answer is c. *(Waxman, 24/e, p 94.)* The symptoms indicate that the lesion is at the level of the midbrain. The spastic paralysis, hyperreflexia, and positive Babinski reflect an upper motor neuron lesion. The corticobulbar and corticospinal tracts pass through the cerebral peduncles (basis pedunculi). Those originating in the right cortex will pass through the right peduncle and then cross to the contralateral side in the pyramidal decussation resulting in left-side hemiplegia. It is of interest that the lower motor neurons innervating muscles of facial expression located below the eye receive upper motor neurons (corticobulbar tract) only from the contralateral cortex, whereas lower motor neurons innervating facial muscles above the eye (e.g., frontalis) receive input from both sides of the cortex. This explains why only the lower portion of the left face was paralyzed. The deficit in movement of the right eye indicates damage to the ipsilateral oculomotor nerve (CN III), which passes through the cerebral peduncle en route to the interpeduncular fossa. The "down and out" direction of the right eye is explained by unopposed contraction of the lateral rectus (CN VI) and superior oblique (CN IV) muscles. Because there were no sensory deficits, neither the thalamus nor sensory cortex were involved. The sensory tracts are arranged dorsolaterally in the midbrain and do not pass through the affected area.

296. The answer is b. *(Brust, p 246.)* The middle cerebral artery supplies a large portion of cerebral cortex, including portions of the frontal, parietal, and temporal lobes. These regions include the Broca's and Wernicke's areas and the precentral motor and postcentral sensory regions. Decreased blood flow in these regions explains the observed motor and sensory deficits. The anterior choroidal artery is a branch of the internal carotid artery and is primarily distributed to the basal ganglia, hippocampus, and choroid plexus of the lateral ventricle. The posterior communicating artery connects the internal carotid and vertebral arterial systems. The ophthalmic artery is a direct branch of the internal carotid artery that enters the orbit along with the optic nerve. Although the anterior cerebral artery has a wide distribution and anastomoses with branches of both the middle and posterior cerebral arteries, it primarily supplies medial and superior portions of the cortex.

297. The answer is e. *(April, 3/e, p 613.)* The patient has facial paralysis, which indicates injury to the facial nerve. A problem in the internal auditory meatus usually affects hearing and balance. That the superior salivatory nucleus is normal is indicated by normal lacrimation. Hence, the lesion must be distal to the origin of the greater superficial nerve at the genu of the facial nerve. However, absence of hyperacusis indicates that the branch to the stapedius muscle is functioning normally, and this fact suggests that the lesion is close to the stylomastoid foramen. Loss of taste and diminished salivation locate the lesion proximal to the origin of the chorda tympani nerve. If the lesion were distal to the stylomastoid foramen, taste and salivation would have been normal with facial paralysis as the only sign.

298. The answer is d. *(Moore, Anatomy, 4/e, pp 889–891.)* The arrow indicates the cerebral aqueduct, which is the narrow canal connecting the third and fourth ventricles. The cerebrospinal fluid produced in the lateral and third ventricles must reach the fourth ventricle to escape into the subarachnoid space through the foramina of Luschka and Magendie.

299. The answer is b. *(Moore, Anatomy, 4/e, p 939.)* The tensor veli palatini and levator veli palatini, which arise from opposite sides of the auditory tube and base of the skull, insert into the soft palate. They are innervated, respectively, by the trigeminal nerve and the pharyngeal branch of the vagus nerve.

The anterior faucial pillar, or palatoglossal arch, is formed by the mucosa overlying the palatoglossal muscle. The posterior faucial pillar, or palatopharyngeal arch, likewise is formed by the palatopharyngeus muscle. The palatoglossus and palatopharyngeus muscles insert into the tongue and pharynx, respectively, and both are innervated by the pharyngeal branch of the vagus nerve (CN X).

The salpingopharyngeus muscle, also innervated by the pharyngeal branch of the vagus nerve, arises from the torus tubarius at the opening of the auditory tube and inserts into the pharyngeal musculature. The superior and middle pharyngeal constrictors are also innervated by the pharyngeal branch of the vagus nerve.

The stylopharyngeus and styloglossus muscles originate from the styloid process and insert onto the lesser horn of the hyoid and into the tongue, respectively. They are innervated by the glossopharyngeal and hypoglossal nerves, respectively.

300. The answer is d. (*Moore, Developing Human, 6/e, pp 452–456.*) After closure of the neural tube, cells proliferate and establish three primitive layers: (1) the ventricular zone adjoining the central canal and ventricles; mitoses of neuronal and glial precursors continue in this zone; (2) a mantle zone consisting of cell bodies of neurons and glia that have migrated out of the ventricular zone; and (3) a marginal zone on the periphery containing the myelinated nerve processes characteristic of white matter. Closure of the neural tube begins near the midpoint of its length and proceeds in both directions simultaneously. The neurectoderm of the neural tube will give rise to neurons and some glial cells (astrocytes, oligodendroglia, and ependymal cells), but the precursors of microglia (the monocyte-macrophage lineage) migrate into the nervous system from the blood. The sensory ganglia are formed by neural crest cells that migrated before the development of mature neurons.

301. The answer is b. (*Moore, Anatomy, 4/e, p 1059.*) The location of the glossopharyngeal nerve in the tonsillar bed places it in jeopardy during tonsillectomy. The facial nerve lies superficial on the face, whereas the hypoglossal and lingual nerves pass well inferior to the tonsillar bed.

302. The answer is c. *(Noback, 4/e, pp 214, 245.)* Atrophy of the intrinsic musculature of the tongue on one side is due to a lesion of the ipsilateral hypoglossal nerve. Deviation of the tongue to the right on protrusion results from the unopposed action of the left genioglossus muscle, which is innervated by the left hypoglossal nerve. The hypoglossal nerve also innervates numerous other tongue muscles involved in deglutition.

303. The answer is e. *(Carpenter, 4/e, pp 174–175. Noback, 4/e, p 209.)* The abducens nerve (CN VI) innervates the lateral rectus muscle. Loss of innervation to the lateral rectus results in unopposed tension by the medial rectus, which produces internal strabismus. The oculomotor nerve (CN III) innervates the medial, superior, and inferior recti, the inferior oblique, and the levator palpebrae superioris muscles. Paralysis of this nerve would result in lateral deviation of the eye (external strabismus) accompanied by ptosis (drooping eyelid). In addition, mydriasis (dilated pupil) results from loss of function of the parasympathetic component of the oculomotor nerve. Damage to the trochlear nerve (CN IV) results in paralysis of the superior oblique muscle with impaired ability to direct the eye downward and outward.

304. The answer is a. *(Moore, Anatomy, 4/e, p 1016.)* The stylohyoid muscle inserts onto the lesser horn of the hyoid bone (both derivatives of the second branchial arch) and raises that bone during swallowing. The distal tendon of the stylohyoid muscle is split by the digastric muscle passing through its trochlea attached to the lesser horn. The styloglossus muscle acts to retract the tongue. The sphenomandibular ligament inserts onto the lingula of the mandibular foramen; the stylohyoid ligament inserts onto the lesser horn of the hyoid bone. The stylopharyngeus muscle inserts onto the thyroid cartilage and into the middle pharyngeal constrictor.

305. The answer is e. *(Waxman, 24/e, pp 132, 150.)* An MRI (magnetic resonance imaging) revealed a hemorrhage in the right subthalamic nucleus that is interconnected with the basal ganglia. The basal ganglia participate in feedback regulation of the motor system. The basal ganglia receive information from all regions of the cortex and project back to premotor and association cortex of the frontal lobe via the ventrolateral and ventroanterior thalamic nuclei. A direct pathway facilitates or excites cortical motor activity, whereas an indirect pathway inhibits cortical motor activity. Damage to the subthalamic nucleus decreases the inhibition of excitatory relay neurons in the thalamus, thus increasing the activation of cortical motor neurons, resulting in a characteristic form of jerky movement called ballism. Damage to an appropriate region of the cerebellum would result in loss of fine motor control but not in ballism. Damage to the neurons in the ventral horn of a specific level of the spinal cord would result in a localized flaccid paralysis. The hypothalamus is involved in vegetative functions, not voluntary movement. Damage to a localized portion of primary sensory cortex could not be expected to result in feedback deficits over both upper and lower extremities without other neurologic deficits.

306. The answer is d. (*Moore, Developing Human, 6/e, pp 460–464.*) In the family of conditions known as spina bifida, failure of the dural portions of the developing vertebrae may expose a portion of the spinal cord and its covering. This usually occurs near the caudal end of the neural tube. If there is no projection of the spinal cord or its covering through the bony defect, the condition is generally hidden (spina bifida occulta). However, it is termed *spina bifida cystica* when spinal material traverses the defect. In a meningocele, this is a saclike projection formed only by the meninges. If the projection contains neural material, it is a meningomyelocele. Rachischisis is an extreme example of spina bifida cystica in which the neural folds underlying the vertebral defect fail to fuse, leaving an exposed neural plate. Anencephaly occurs when the cranial neural tube fails to fuse, thus resulting in lack of formation of forebrain structures and a portion of the enclosing cranium. Hydrocephaly results from blockage of the narrow passageways between the ventricles or between the ventricles and the subarachnoid space. Resultant swelling of the ventricles compresses the brain against the cranial vault and may cause serious mental deficits.

307. The answer is c. (*April, 3/e, pp 629–630.*) The styloglossus muscle is innervated by the hypoglossal nerve, which leaves the posterior cranial fossa by way of the anterior condylar canal. In addition to the internal jugular vein, the jugular foramen contains the glossopharyngeal nerve (innervating the stylopharyngeus muscle), the vagus nerve (innervating palatal, pharyngeal, and laryngeal musculature), and the spinal accessory nerve (innervating the sternomastoid and trapezius muscles).

308. The answer is c. (*Moore, Anatomy, 4/e, pp 1030–1033.*) The inferior thyroid artery arises from the thyrocervical trunk, a branch of the subclavian artery. The superior thyroid artery arises from the external carotid artery. An inconsistent thyroid ima artery, when present, may arise from the aortic arch, the innominate artery, or the common carotid artery. There are no branches of the internal carotid artery and infrequent branches of the common carotid artery in the neck. The transverse cervical artery supplies the posterior triangle of the neck. The vertebral arteries give off spinal and muscular branches in the neck.

309. The answer is c. (*April, 3/e, pp 640–641.*) The posterior cricoarytenoid muscles rotate the arytenoids laterally, which swings the vocal process of that cartilage outward to abduct the vocal cords and open the glottis. These are the sole abductors of the vocal folds. The lateral cricoarytenoid muscles and the unpaired transverse arytenoid muscle adduct the vocal folds. The thyroarytenoid muscle and its innermost portion, the vocalis muscle, act to tense the cords. The cricothyroid muscle lengthens the vocal cords.

310. The answer is b. (*Moore, Anatomy, 4/e, pp 843–845.*) The arrow points to the sella turcica, which cradles the pituitary gland. The stalk of the gland can be seen directly above the sella turcica. Surgically, the nasal approach to the pituitary is through the nasal cavity, sphenoidal sinus, and the inferior wall of the sella turcica. The other midline structures are the pharyngeal tonsil (which lies inferior to this region), and portions of the circle of Willis and the basilar artery, which both lie within the cranial cavity.

311. The answer is b. (*Moore, Anatomy, 4/e, pp 843–845, 921–923.*) This CT image was computed close to the floor of the middle cranial fossa as indicated by the mandibular condyle, B. The oval-shaped opening A is the foramen ovale that is traversed by the (1) mandibular nerve (CN V3), (2) the lesser petrosal nerve, (3) an accessory middle meningeal artery, and (4) an emissary vein connecting the pterygoid venous plexus with the cavernous sinus. Because the mandibular nerve is the largest structure passing through the foramen ovale, it is most likely injured if the floor of the middle cranial fossa is fractured. The mandibular nerve supplies the following masticatory muscles: temporalis, masseter, medial and lateral pterygoids, anterior digastric, and mylohyoid. Injury to the nerve causes paralysis of the masticatory muscles. The nerve supply to the other muscles is indicated in parentheses: facial muscles (CN VII); trapezius and sternocleidomastoid (CB XI); scalene muscles (motor branches of the cervical plexus); laryngeal muscles (CN X).

312. The answer is d. (*Moore, Anatomy, 4/e, pp 843–845.*) The space labeled "C" is the sphenoidal sinus. The space is located within the body of the sphenoid bone, which is found in the center of the middle cranial fossa between the nasal cavities anteriorly and the jugum of the sphenoid posteriorly. Its bony roof accommodates the pituitary gland in the hypophyseal fossa, whereas the cavernous venous sinuses are located bilaterally on its lateral walls. The anterior and posterior ethmoidal sinuses are visible anteriorly, and the nasopharynx is located inferiorly. The maxillary sinuses are not found at this level.

313 to 314. The answers are 313-c, 314-d. (*Moore, Anatomy, 4/e, p 921.*) The lateral pterygoid muscles run from the lateral side of the pterygoid plate and from the infratemporal fossa to the head of the mandible and the articular disk of the temporomandibular joint. Contraction of the lateral pterygoid muscles bilaterally protrudes the jaw. Unilateral contraction swings the jaw toward the opposite side.

The medial pterygoid muscle, which originates on the medial side of the lateral pterygoid plate, and the masseter muscle, which originates from the zygomatic arch, pass medially and laterally to the ramus of the mandible to form a sling about the angle of the mandible. These muscles are powerful elevators of the jaw. The muscle bundles of the anterior portion of the temporalis muscle run nearly vertically into the coronoid process of the mandible, acting as a jaw elevator.

The submental muscles, assisted by gravity, are the primary depressors of the jaw. These include the geniohyoid and mylohyoid muscles as well as the anterior belly of the digastric muscle, all of which function in conjunction with the infrahyoid strap muscles.

The posterior muscle bundles of the temporalis originate over the temporal region and pass nearly horizontally into the coronoid process of the mandible and, therefore, function as jaw retractors.

The buccinator muscle fibers are horizontal between the maxilla and mandible so that they cannot act on the mandible. This is a muscle of facial expression and assists mastication by working with the tongue to keep food on the occlusive surfaces of the teeth.

315 to 316. The answers are 315-a, 316-e. *(April, 3/e, pp 534–536.)*

Ganglia Associated with Cranial Nerves		
Nerve (Classification)	**Ganglion**	**Function**
Optic (SSA)	Bipolar cells	Vision
Oculomotor (GVE)	Ciliary	Pupillary constriction, accommodation
Trigeminal (GSA)	Semilunar (trigeminal)	General sensation from the face, nasal and oral cavities, including afferent limbs of blink, sneeze, and jaw-jerk reflexes
Facial (GSA)	Geniculate	General sensation from external ear
(SVA)	Geniculate	Taste from anterior 2/3 of tongue
(GVE)	Pterygopalatine	Secretomotor for lacrimal, nasal, and palatine glands
(GVE)	Submandibular	Secretomotor for sublingual and submandibular glands
Vestibulocochlear (SSA)	Vestibular and Spiral	Balance, audition
Glossopharyngeal (GSA)	Jugular (superior)	General sensation from external auditory meatus
(GVA)	Petrosal (inferior)	Visceral sensation from posterior 1/3 of tongue and pharynx; afferent limb of gag and carotid reflexes
(SVA)	Petrosal (inferior)	Taste from posterior 1/3 of tongue
(GVE)	Otic	Secretomotor for parotid gland
Vagus (GSA)	Jugular (superior)	General sensation from external auditory meatus
(GVA)	Petrosal (inferior)	Visceral sensation from larynx; afferent limb of cough and aortic body reflexes
(SVA)	Nodose (inferior)	Taste from epiglottis
(GVE)	Distal ganglia	Visceral smooth muscle and gland control

*GSA: general somatic afferent; GVA: general visceral afferent; GVE: general visceral efferent; SSA: special somatic afferent; SVA: special visceral afferent; SVA: special visceral afferent.

317 to 318. The answers are 317-i, 318-c. *(April, 3/e, pp 534–536.)*

Course, Distribution & Principal Function of Cranial Nerves			
CN	Foramen	Distribution	Function
I	Cribriform plate	Nasal mucosa	Olfaction
II	Optic canal	Retina	Vision
III	Superior orbital fissure	Levator palpebrae superioris, superior rectus, medial rectus, inferior rectus, inferior oblique muscles	Ocular elevation, depression, adduction, pupillary constriction, accommodation
IV		Superior oblique muscle	Ocular depression and abduction
V_1	Superior orbital fissure	Forehead, conjunctiva	Sensation, afferent limb of blink reflex
V_2	Foramen rotundum, infraorbital foramen	Midface	Sensation, afferent limb of sneeze reflex
V_3	Foramen ovale, mandibular foramen, mental foramen	Jaw, lateral face, anterior tongue	Sensation, afferent limb of jaw-jerk reflex, anterior tongue sensation Motor to muscles of mastication
VI	Superior orbital fissure	Lateral rectus muscle	Ocular abduction
VII	Internal acoustic meatus, facial canal, stylomastoid foramen	Face, lacrimal, nasal, sublingual, and submaxillary glands	Motor to muscles of facial expression and efferent limb of blink reflex; secretomotor for lacrimation, nasal and anterior oral secretion Taste from anterior part of tongue
VIII	Internal acoustic meatus	Cochlear and vestibular apparatus	Audition and balance

Continues

CN	Foramen	Distribution	Function
IX	Jugular foramen	Oropharynx	Sensation to posterior tongue and pharynx, afferent limb of gag reflex; taste from posterior part of tongue, carotid reflex Motor to stylopharyngeus muscle
X	Jugular foramen	Pharynx, larynx	Laryngeal sensation, afferent limb of cough reflex; epiglottic taste Motor to palatine and laryngeal muscles
XI	Foramen magnum, jugular foramen	Sternomastoid and trapezius muscles	Motor to sternomastoid and trapezius muscles
XII	Anterior condylar canal	Tongue	Motor to all intrinsic and most extrinsic tongue muscles

319 to 320. The answers are 319-b, 320-d. *(April, 3/e, pp 502, 517–518, 540–541.)* Bleeding beneath the epicranial aponeurosis (the danger space) produces an extracranial hematoma that is not dangerous unless accompanied by a depressed skull fracture. Hemorrhage from the middle meningeal artery, which is usually the result of a fracture of the temporal bone, produces a life-threatening, high-pressure epidural hematoma. Rupture of an aneurysm of extracerebral branches of the cerebral arteries or of the cerebral arterial circle (of Willis) bleeds into the subarachnoid space. This is confirmed by the presence of blood in a spinal tap. Tearing of a cerebral vein, usually at the point where it enters the superior sagittal sinus, produces a subdural hematoma. Because cerebral venous pressure is low, these hematomas may be chronic, and compensation may occur by decreased production of cerebrospinal fluid.

321 to 322. The answers are 321-c, 322-a. *(Carpenter, 4/e, pp 9–13. Noback, 4/e, pp 67–69.)* The arachnoid villus (labeled C in the diagram accompanying the question) is a projection of the subarachnoid space into the venous blood-filled superior sagittal sinus. It is completely lined by arachnoid membrane, and the dura over the tip of the villus is considerably thinned. The pressure of the cerebrospinal fluid within the subarachnoid space is greater than that of the blood in the dural sinuses, which results in filtration and even bulk flow of cerebrospinal fluid into the superior sagittal sinus.

The subarachnoid space (labeled A on the diagram accompanying the question) is located between the arachnoid membrane externally and the pia mater internally. This space is traversed by numerous trabeculae and varies in size from one region of the cerebral hemisphere to another. Where it is quite large, the space is designated a cistern. The major volume of cerebrospinal fluid is within the subarachnoid space. Because the spinal subarachnoid space is continuous with the cranial subarachnoid space, cerebrospinal fluid is readily obtained by puncture in the lower lumbar region.

The outermost and densest of the meninges, the dura mater (labeled D in the diagram accompanying the question) is primarily composed of fibrous connective tissue with some sensory nerves and blood vessels. A flat sheet of mesenchymal epithelium forms its inner surface. This inner surface is separated from the arachnoid membrane by a fluid-filled, thin space called the subdural space (shown as E on the diagram accompanying the question).

The pia mater (labeled B in the diagram) is a vascular layer of delicate connective tissue that is intimately attached to the brain and spinal cord.

323 to 327. The answers are 323-f, 324-c, 325-h, 326-c, 327-i. *(Moore, Developing Human, 6/e, pp 218–226.)* a, c, e, g, and i denote the first, second, third, fourth, and sixth branchial arches, respectively. b, d, f, h, and j denote the first, second, dorsal third, ventral third, and fourth branchial pouches, respectively. See the following table.

Table of Principal Branchial Derivatives

	Groove	Arch	Pouch
I	Pinna and external auditory meatus	Mandible, malleus, incus, anterior part of tongue, mm. of mastication, tensors tympani and veli palatini mm., mylohyoid m., ant. belly of digastric m., trigeminal nerve	Auditory tube, middle ear cavity
II		Lesser horns of hyoid, styloid process, stapes, mm. of facial expression, stapedius m., stylohyoid m., post. belly of digastric m., facial nerve	Tonsillar fossa
III		Gr. horns of hyoid, post. part of tongue, stylopharyngeus m., glossopharyngeal nerve	Vallecular recess, thymus gland, inf. parathyroids
IV		Thyroid cartilage, cricothyroid m., sup. laryngeal nerve	Superior parathyroid glands
V			Ultimobranchial bodies (parafollicular cells)
VI		Cricoid and arytenoid cartilages, intrinsic laryngeal mm., recurrent laryngeal nerve	Laryngeal ventricle

Thorax

Questions

DIRECTIONS: Each item below contains a question or incomplete statement followed by suggested responses. Select the **one best** response to each question.

328. Specialized cardiac muscle cells that control the rate of the heartbeat are found

a. In the muscular wall of the interventricular septum
b. In the arch of the aorta
c. In the wall of the left atrium between openings of the pulmonary veins
d. In the wall of the right atrium near the opening of the superior vena cava
e. On the surface of the heart

329. Which of the following statements is true of cardiac development?

a. During formation of the heart loop, a single-tube heart remains suspended by a complete dorsal mesocardium (mesentery)
b. The atria are represented by cranial portions of the endocardial tubes
c. The heart bends into an S-shape because the caudal regions of the endocardial tubes grow faster than the cranial regions
d. The left and right sides of the heart result directly from the side-by-side apposition of the left and right endocardial tubes
e. The sinus venosus becomes incorporated into the atrium prior to the formation of the heart loop

Questions 330 to 331

A mammogram of a woman, age 48, reveals macrocalcification within the right breast, indicating the need for biopsy. The surgeon visually and manually examines the breast with negative results. The surgeon closely examines the nipple for indications of ductal carcinoma. At surgery for the biopsy, a locator needle is inserted into the region of macrocalcification and the position confirmed by mammography. The surgeon incised the skin and dissected a block of tissue about the needle. The pathology report indicated ductal carcinoma with microinvasion necessitating surgery. Both patient and surgeon agreed that a modified radical mastectomy offered the best prognosis in her case. At surgery for mastectomy, the surgeon carries the dissection along the major pathway of lymphatic drainage from the mammary gland.

330. The major lymphatic channels parallel the

a. Subcutaneous venous networks to the contralateral breast and abdominal wall
b. Tributaries of the axillary vessels to the axillary nodes
c. Tributaries of the intercostal vessels to the parasternal nodes
d. Tributaries of the internal thoracic (mammary) vessels to the parasternal nodes
e. Tributaries of the thoracoacromial vessels to the apical (subscapular) nodes

331. The surgery appears to have been successful. However, the patient is found to have winging of the scapula when the flexed arm is pressed against a fixed object. This indicates injury to which of the following nerves?

a. Axillary
b. Long thoracic
c. Lower subscapular
d. Supraclavicular
e. Thoracodorsal

Questions 332 to 333

A firefighter, age 34 and a nonsmoker, complains of bouts of dizziness at times of intense exertion. His history reveals having been exposed to intense smoke six months ago when his breathing apparatus malfunctioned during a job. He is scheduled for a pulmonary function test.

332. Regarding the "pump handle" movement during respiration, which statement is correct?

a. There is a decrease in the anterior-posterior diameter of the chest
b. No movement occurs at the costovertebral joints
c. There is an increase in the superior-inferior diameter of the chest
d. Movement occurs at the sternomanubrial joint
e. The primary change in dimension of the chest occurs in the transverse diameter

333. When the patient was asked to exhale forcibly and maximally, the volume of expiration was constant but the rate of flow was diminished, indicating airway constriction likely due to bronchospasm. The smooth muscle of the bronchial airways is innervated by the

a. Intercostal nerves
b. Phrenic nerves
c. Thoracic splanchnic nerves
d. Vagus nerve

334. Special receptors in the walls of the aortic arch and carotid arteries convey information concerning mean arterial blood pressure to reflex pathways in the CNS. The afferent limb of this pathway is carried by

a. CN V
b. CN VII
c. CN IX
d. CN X
e. CN XI

335. Pain referred to the right side of the neck and extending laterally from the right clavicle to the tip of the right shoulder is most likely to involve the

a. Cervical cardiac accelerator nerves
b. Posterior vagal trunk
c. Right intercostal nerves
d. Right phrenic nerve
e. Right recurrent laryngeal nerve

336. An elderly woman visits the hospital emergency room with the recent onset of grotesque swelling of the right arm, neck, and face. Her right jugular vein is visibly engorged and her right brachial pulse is diminished. On the basis of these signs, her chest x-rays might show

a. A left cervical rib
b. A mass in the upper lobe of the right lung
c. Aneurysm of the aortic arch
d. Right pneumothorax
e. Thoracic duct blockage in the posterior mediastinum

Questions 337 to 338

A child suspected of aspirating a small, cloth-covered metal button is seen in the emergency room. Although the child does not complain of pain, there is frequent coughing.

337. Diminished breath sounds should be heard

a. In both lungs
b. In the lingula of the left inferior lobe
c. In the right inferior lobe
d. In the left superior lobe
e. In the right superior lobe

338. Aspiration pneumonia (Mendelson's syndrome) usually is associated with which of the following bronchopulmonary segments?

a. Apical segments of the upper lobes
b. Basal segments of the lower lobes
c. Inferior lingular segment of the left upper lobe
d. Medial and lateral segments of the right middle lobe
e. Superior segments of the lower lobes

339. Lymph from which region of the pleura or lungs may drain into axillary lymph nodes?

a. Visceral pleura and parenchyma of right lung
b. Visceral pleura and superior lobe of left lung
c. Cervical parietal pleura of either lung
d. Visceral pleura and inferior lobe of left lung
e. Costal parietal pleura of either lung

340. Which of the following is a correct characterization of bronchopulmonary segments?

a. They are arranged with their bases directed toward the hilum of the lung
b. They are separated by parietal pleura
c. The arterial supply is located in the periphery of each segment
d. Each segment is supplied by a secondary or lobar bronchus
e. Veins may be used to localize the planes between segments

341. A 28-year-old woman comes into the emergency room exhibiting dyspnea and mild cyanosis, but no signs of trauma. Her chest x-ray is shown below. The most obvious abnormal finding in the inspiratory posteroanterior chest x-ray of this patient (viewed in the anatomic position) is a

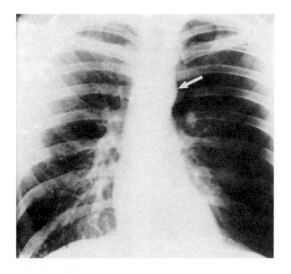

a. Bilateral expansion of the pleural cavities above the first rib
b. Grossly enlarged heart
c. Left pneumothorax (collapsed lung)
d. Paralysis of the left hemidiaphragm
e. Right hemothorax (blood in the pleural cavity)

Questions 342 to 344

A 23-year-old, semiconscious man is brought to the emergency room following an automobile accident. He is tachypneic (breathing rapidly) and cyanotic (blue lips and nail beds). The right lower anterolateral thoracic wall reveals a small laceration and flailing (moving inward as the rest of the thoracic cage expands during inspiration). Air does not appear to move into or out of the wound, and it is assumed that the pleura have not been penetrated. After the patient is placed on immediate positive pressure endotracheal respiration, his cyanosis clears and the abnormal movement of the chest wall disappears. Radiographic examination confirms fractures of the fourth through eighth ribs in the right anterior axillary line and of the fourth through sixth ribs at the right costochondral junction. There is no evidence that bony fragments have penetrated the lungs or of pneumothorax (collapsed lung).

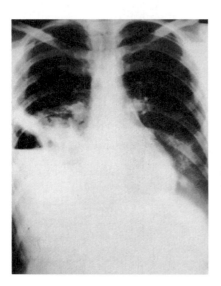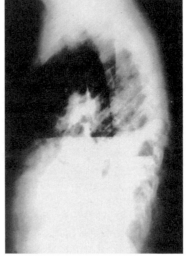

342. The small superficial laceration, once it is ascertained that it has not penetrated the pleura, is sutured and the chest bound in bandages; positive pressure endotracheal respiration is maintained. Several hours later, the cyanosis returns. The right side of the thorax is found to be more expanded than the left, yet moves less during respiration. Chest x-rays are shown above. The most obvious abnormal finding in the inspiratory posteroanterior and lateral chest x-ray of this patient (viewed in the anatomic position) is a

a. Flail chest
b. Right hemothorax
c. Right pneumothorax
d. Paralysis of the right hemidiaphragm

343. A negative pressure drain (chest tube) has to be inserted into the pleural space. Effective locations for the drain include the

a. Apex between the clavicle and first rib
b. Costomediastinal recess on the left, adjacent to the xiphoid process
c. Right fourth intercostal space in the midclavicular line (just below the nipple)
d. Right seventh intercostal space in the midaxillary line
e. Right eighth intercostal space in the midclavicular line (about 4 in. below the nipple)

344. The intercostal neurovascular bundle is particularly vulnerable to injury from fractured ribs because it is located

a. Above the superior border of the ribs, anteriorly
b. Beneath the inferior border of the ribs, posterolaterally
c. Between external and internal intercostal muscle layers
d. Deep to the posterior intercostal membrane
e. Superficial to the ribs, anteriorly

345. Failure of the sixth aortic arch arteries to form would lead to loss of blood supply to the

a. Right side of the heart
b. Face
c. Thyroid gland
d. Lungs
e. Upper digestive tract

346. The sinoatrial node in the heart receives its blood supply principally from

a. The anterior interventricular branch of the left coronary artery
b. The circumflex branch of the left coronary artery
c. The posterior interventricular branch of the right coronary artery
d. The right coronary artery

347. The major venous return system of the heart, the coronary sinus, empties into the

a. Inferior vena cava
b. Left atrium
c. Right atrium
d. Right ventricle
e. Superior vena cava

Questions 348 to 349

A 38-year-old man is seen in the emergency room complaining of severe chest pain. He tends to sit leaning forward. On physical examination he is noted to be tachypneic (breathing rapidly); he has a rapid pulse rate, and on auscultation of the chest, his valve sounds appear distant. A radiograph shows a globular heart shadow. All evidence indicates pericarditis with pericardial effusion.

348. Pericardiocentesis (to drain the exudate) via the costoxiphoid approach passes through which of the following structures?

a. The interchondral portion of an internal oblique muscle
b. The left costodiaphragmatic recess
c. The rectus sheath and rectus abdominis muscle
d. The visceral pericardium
e. The left costomediastinal recess

349. Vessels at high risk during the parasternal approach include the

a. Anterior interventricular artery
b. Left internal thoracic artery
c. Right coronary artery
d. Right marginal artery
e. Nodal artery

350. Your patient reports he spent two weeks on a desert island as part of a television survival show. It rained and was cool the last five days and he developed a cough. He is now in the ER with a productive cough that produces rusty and bloodstained sputum. He also complains of significant pleural pain. You suspect a pneumococcal lobar pneumonia. From this CT scan at the T4 level, which lung lobe (indicated by the *) is involved with the pneumonia?

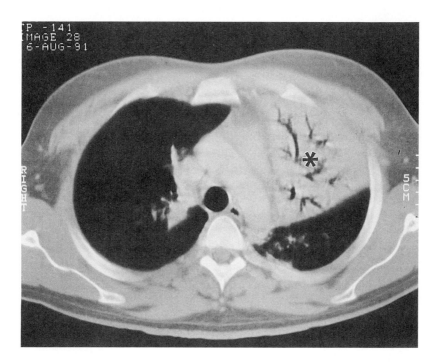

a. Right upper lobe
b. Right middle lobe
c. Right lower lobe
d. Left upper lobe
e. Left lower lobe

Questions 351 to 352

A 36-year-old male office worker comes to the clinic complaining of general weakness and shortness of breath. He also relates a rapid, throbbing pulse after climbing a flight of stairs.

351. Cardiac auscultation reveals a diastolic rumbling murmur attributable to the mitral valve. The mitral valve is best heard on the

a. Left side adjacent to the sternum in the second intercostal space
b. Left side adjacent to the sternum in the fifth intercostal space
c. Left side in the midclavicular line in the fifth intercostal space
d. Right side adjacent to the sternum in the second intercostal space
e. Right side adjacent to the sternum in the fourth intercostal space

352. Which of the following correctly pertains to normal mitral valve function?

a. The papillary muscles are rudimentary and have no major function
b. It prevents regurgitation of blood during ventricular relaxation
c. The chordae tendineae and papillary muscles prevent eversion of the valve cusps
d. The papillary muscles contract to close the valve

Questions 353 to 357

A 64-year-old man is brought into the emergency room after experiencing more than 3 h of increasing chest pain that was unrelieved by rest, antacids, or nitroglycerin. He complains of nausea without vomiting. Further questioning reveals a two-year history of exertional angina pectoris (pressing chest pain that often radiated along the inner aspect of the left arm when the patient climbed one flight of stairs). Propranolol, which reduces the response of the heart to stress, and nitroglycerin, which dilates systemic veins as well as coronary arteries, had been prescribed previously. On physical examination he is found to be acyanotic (normal blood oxygenation), tachypneic (rapid breathing), tachycardiac (rapid pulse rate) with a regular rhythm, and diaphoretic (sweating).

353. This patient's tachycardia probably is mediated by reflex arcs associated with decreased cardiac output and possibly reduced blood pressure. The visceral efferent (motor) pathway of this cardiac response is mediated by the

a. Carotid branches of the glossopharyngeal nerves
b. Greater splanchnic nerves
c. Phrenic nerves
d. Sympathetic cervical and thoracic cardiac fibers
e. Vagus and recurrent laryngeal nerves

354. In angina pectoris, the pain radiating down the left arm is mediated by increased activity in afferent (sensory) fibers contained in the

a. Carotid branch of the glossopharyngeal nerves
b. Greater splanchnic nerves
c. Phrenic nerves
d. Thoracic splanchnic nerves
e. Vagus nerve and recurrent laryngeal nerves

355. The patient is admitted to a coronary care unit for tests and observation. An electrocardiogram reveals a pattern consistent with a small ventricular posteroseptal infarct from ischemic necrosis that resulted from inadequate blood supply. In the diagram of a normal heart shown below, the coronary artery most likely to be involved in a posteroseptal infarct (as in this patient) is indicated by which letter?

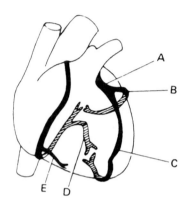

a. A
b. B
c. C
d. D
e. E

356. To improve the blood flow to the interventricular septum, a coronary bypass procedure is elected. During surgery the anterior interventricular artery is located and prepared to receive a graft. The vessel lying adjacent to the anterior interventricular artery is the

a. Anterior cardiac vein
b. Coronary sinus
c. Great cardiac vein
d. Middle cardiac vein
e. Small cardiac vein

357. A section of superficial vein removed from the lower portion of the patient's leg is grafted from the aorta to the coronary artery just distal to the site of occlusion. In coronary bypass surgery, which of the following statements is true?

a. The proximal end of the vein is anastomosed to the aorta
b. The distal end of the vein is anastomosed to the aorta
c. The orientation is unimportant because aortic pressure is always higher than venous pressure
d. The orientation is unimportant because the vein is being used as an artery
e. The orientation would be important only if a coronary vein were being bypassed

358. The first (S$_1$, or "Lub") heart sound and the second (S$_2$, or "Dup") heart sound originate, respectively, from the

a. Closure of the pulmonary valve followed by closure of the aortic valve
b. Closure of the tricuspid valve followed by closure of the mitral valve
c. Closure of the atrioventricular valves followed by closure of the semilunar valves
d. Closure of the atrioventricular valves followed by opening of the semilunar valves
e. Opening of the atrioventricular valves followed by closure of the atrioventricular valves

359. Structures that normally transit the diaphragm by way of the esophageal hiatus include the

a. Aorta
b. Azygos vein
c. Hemiazygos vein
d. Posterior vagal trunk
e. Thoracic duct

360. Which forms the venous coronary sinus?

a. Left horn of the sinus venosus
b. Right horn of the sinus venosus
c. Primitive atrium
d. Bulbus cordis
e. Truncus arteriosus

361. Which of the following correctly pertains to the white rami communicantes?

a. Each contains visceral afferent neurons
b. They consist of unmyelinated nerves
c. They contain postsynaptic neurons
d. Their neurons always synapse in the sympathetic chain
e. They occur at nearly every spinal level

362. What is the identity of the tubular structure indicated by the "P"?

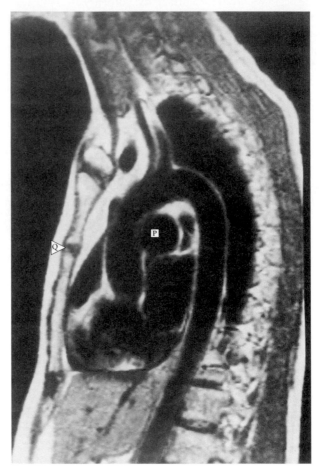

(Reproduced, with permission, from Wicke L: Atlas of Radiological Anatomy, 6/e. Baltimore, MD: Williams & Wilkins, 1998.)

a. Left subclavian artery
b. Pulmonary trunk
c. Left atrium
d. Left brachiocephalic vein
e. Azygos vein

363. In the above image, what is attached to the sternum at the level indicated by "Q"?

a. Clavicle
b. First rib
c. Second rib
d. Third rib
e. Fourth rib

DIRECTIONS: The group of questions below consists of lettered headings followed by a set of numbered items. For each numbered item select the **one** lettered heading with which it is **most** closely associated. Each lettered heading may be used once, more than once, or not at all.

Questions 364 to 365

Movements of the chest wall and diaphragm produce changes in thoracic volume and pulmonary ventilation. For each respiratory muscle action described below, select the factor with which it is most nearly related.

a. A factor in quiet inspiration
b. A factor in quiet expiration
c. An accessory factor in exertional inspiration
d. A factor in exertional expiration
e. Not a factor in respiration

364. Contraction of the interchondral (parasternal) portion of the internal intercostal muscles

365. Contraction of the transverse thoracic muscle

Questions 366 to 367

For each functional event listed below, select the stage of the cardiac cycle during which it is most likely to occur.

a. Atrial diastole
b. Atrial systole
c. Ventricular diastole
d. Ventricular systole

366. Atrioventricular valves close

367. Blood flow through the myocardium is maximal

Thorax

Answers

328. The answer is d. (*Moore, Anatomy, 4/e, pp 137–139.*) Specialized cardiac muscle cells, which form the sinoatrial (SA) node, are the pacemakers of the heartbeat. They have the fastest-paced autorhythmicity of all cardiac muscle cells and are located in the wall of the right atrium near the opening of the superior vena cava. Specialized cardiac muscle cells forming the atrioventricular node are also located in the wall of the right atrium but near the interatrial wall and the opening of the coronary sinus. The left atrium contains no known nodes of pacing cells. Large specialized cardiac muscle cells are the Purkinje's cells, which make up the bundle of His. These cells are found in the subendocardial portion of the interventricular wall and conduct impulses to the ventricular myocytes of both ventricles. The aortic arch contains baroreceptors that control heart rate through a reflex arc connected to parasympathetic ganglia on the surface of the heart.

329. The answer is c. (*Moore, Developing Human, 6/e, pp 350, 356, 358–366. Sadler, 8/e, pp 183–191.*) The heart forms during the third week by the apposition of left and right endocardial tubes as the head fold progresses caudally. The endocardial tubes fuse to form a single-tube heart. This fusion begins cranially in the region of the bulbus cordis (outflow trunks) and proceeds caudally through the ventricles and the atria to the sinus venosus, which is incorporated into the atrium after loop formation. Rapid proliferation of the ventricular region results in the single-tube heart bending into an S-shaped loop. During this process, the dorsal mesocardium partially breaks down, which leaves the heart suspended only at the cranial and caudal ends; the discontinuity in the mesocardium is the transverse sinus. The left and right sides of the heart are established by the subsequent division of the single-tube heart, not by the apposition of left and right endocardial tubes.

330. The answer is b. (*Moore, Anatomy, 4/e, pp 75–77.*) The lymphatic drainage of the mammary gland, which follows the path of its blood supply, generally parallels the tributaries of the axillary, internal thoracic (mammary), thoracoacromial, and intercostal vessels. Because about 75% of the breast lies lateral to the nipple, the more significant lateral and inferior portions of the breast drain toward the axillary nodes. The smaller medial portion drains to the parasternal lymphatic chain paralleling the internal thoracic vessels, whereas the very small superior portion drains toward the nodes associated with the thoracoacromial trunk and the supraclavicular nodes.

331. The answer is b. (*Moore, Anatomy, 4/e, pp 708, 715–716.*) The serratus anterior muscle (protractor and stabilizer of the scapula) is innervated by the long thoracic nerve (of Bell), which arises from roots C5 to C7 of the brachial plexus. During modified radical mastectomy, this nerve is usually spared to maintain shoulder function. However, its location places it in jeopardy during the lymphatic resection. The suprascapular nerves are sensory branches of the cervical plexus. The axillary nerve, deep in the brachial portion of the axilla, innervates the deltoid muscle. The thoracodorsal nerve, which arises from the posterior cord of the brachial plexus, innervates the latissimus dorsi. The lower subscapular nerve innervates the teres major muscle and a portion of the subscapularis muscle.

332. The answer is d. (*Moore, Anatomy, 4/e, p 72.*) Contraction of the intercostal muscles causes rotation of the costovertebral joints and elevation of the sternal ends of the upper (2–6) ribs. Along with slight movement of the sternomanubrial joint, particularly in the young, this "pump-handle movement" increases the anteroposterior (AP) diameter of the chest. The transverse diameter of the thoracic cavity increases when contraction of the intercostal muscles also elevates the midportion of the ribs (bucket-handle movement). Contraction of the diaphragm increases the vertical diameter of the thoracic cavity.

333. The answer is d. (*April, 3/e, pp 268–269.*) Innervation of the bronchial smooth muscle is mediated by parasympathetic neurons carried by the vagus nerve. These nerves also stimulate secretion from the bronchial glands. Excessive vagal activity may initiate bronchospasm or the asthmatic syndrome.

334. The answer is c. (*Waxman, 24/e, p 256.*) Information from baroreceptors in the vascular wall passes via cardiac depressor nerves to the glossopharyngeal nerve (CN IX). The cell bodies of these neurons are located in the petrosal ganglion, and their central processes terminate on second-order interneurons in the nucleus of the solitary tract. These interneurons project to preganglionic parasympathetic cardioinhibitory neurons in the nucleus ambiguus, which reach ganglia on the surface of the heart via CN X (vagus nerve) and branches of the cardiac plexus. CN V (trigeminal) carries general somatic afferents from the face and innervates muscles involved in mastication. CN VII (facial) innervates the muscles of facial expression. CN XI primarily innervates the trapezius and sternocleidomastoid muscles.

335. The answer is d. *(April, 3/e, p 260.)* The phrenic nerve, which arises from cervical nerves C3 through C5, mediates sensation from the diaphragmatic pleura and peritoneum, as well as from the pericardium; in addition, it carries motor fibers to the diaphragm. Therefore, pain from the diaphragmatic pleura or peritoneum, as well as from the parietal pericardium, may be referred to dermatomes between C3 and C5, inclusive. These dermatomes correspond to the clavicular region and the anterior and lateral neck, as well as to the anterior, lateral, and posterior aspects of the shoulder.

336. The answer is b. *(April, 3/e, p 265.)* A Pancoast tumor in the apex of the right lung may compress the right brachiocephalic vein with resultant venous engorgement of the right arm and right side of the face and neck. In addition, there may be compression of the brachial artery, the sympathetic chain, and recurrent laryngeal nerve with attendant deficits. An aneurysm of the aortic arch could reduce pulse pressures as the great vessels are occluded, but it could not explain the venous congestion.

337. The answer is c. *(Moore, Anatomy, 4/e, p 104.)* Large aspirated objects tend to lodge at the carina. Smaller objects usually lodge in the right inferior lobar bronchus because the right mainstem (primary) bronchus is generally more vertical in its course than the left and of greater diameter. In addition, the takeoff angle of the right lower lobe bronchus is less acute than that of the right middle lobe, thereby nearly continuing the direction of both the right mainstem bronchus and trachea. Blockage of the airway will produce absence of breath sounds within the lobe and eventual atelectasis.

338. The answer is e. *(April, Anatomy, 3/e, p 264.)* Because the superior segmental bronchi of the left and right lower lobes are the most posterior and, therefore, most dependent when the patient is supine, they are most frequently involved in aspiration pneumonia. This is easily ascertained by percussive dullness over the superior segment posteriorly, and diminished breath sounds over the same area on auscultation.

339. The answer is c. (*Moore, Anatomy, 4/e, p 110–111.*) The parietal pleura associated with the cupola extends superior to the first rib into the cervical region and may drain directly into axillary lymph nodes. Lymph from the visceral pleura and parenchyma of the right lung drains via superficial and deep plexuses, pulmonary nodes, bronchopulmonary nodes, and tracheobronchial nodes, to the right bronchomediastinal trunk, which may terminate in a short lymphatic duct before reentering the venous system at the juncture of the right subclavian and jugular veins. Lymph from the visceral pleura and superior lobe of the left lung follows a similar pathway on the left, terminating in the thoracic duct. Lymph from the visceral pleura and parenchyma of the inferior lobe of the left lung may enter the right-side pathway at the right tracheobronchial nodes. Lymph from most of the parietal pleura drains via intercostal, parasternal, mediastinal, and phrenic nodes of the thoracic wall.

340. The answer is e. (*Moore, Anatomy, 4/e, pp 104–108.*) Although the segmental bronchus and artery tend to be centrally located, the veins do not accompany the arteries but tend to be located subpleurally and between bronchopulmonary segments. Indeed, at surgery the intersegmental veins are useful in defining intersegmental planes. Bronchopulmonary segments, the anatomic and functional units of the lung, are roughly pyramidal in shape, have apices directed toward the hilum of the lung, and are separated from each other by connective tissue septa. Each bronchopulmonary segment is supplied by one tertiary or segmental bronchus, along with a branch of the pulmonary artery.

341. The answer is c. (*April, 3/e, pp 261–262, 273. Moore, Anatomy, 4/e, p 99.*) The patient has a left pneumothorax. The lucidity of the left pleural cavity with the lack of pulmonary vessels indicates that the left lung has collapsed into a small, dense mass adjacent to the mediastinum. Such a nontraumatic pneumothorax may result from the rupture of a pulmonary bleb, especially in a young person. The right lung is normal. There is no pleural fluid level indicative of hemothorax, and the near symmetry of the domes of the two hemidiaphragms on inspiration indicates normal function of the phrenic nerves. The pleural cavities normally extend superior to the first rib into the base of the neck. The heart, measuring less than one-half of the chest diameter, is of normal size.

342. The answer is b. *(April, Anatomy, 4/e, p 132–135.)* The fluid level in the right pleural cavity is indicative of hemothorax caused by bleeding into the pleural space. As blood collects, lung tissue is displaced and cannot expand fully, thereby impairing ventilation. However, perfusion continues so that the ventilation-perfusion ratio is altered.

343. The answer is d. *(April, 4/e, p 136–137.)* The usual location of choice for a chest tube drain is in the midaxillary or posterior axillary line, i.e., the vertical line commencing at the posterior axillary fold, at the approximate level of the seventh intercostal space. This location is the lowest region of the pleural cavity in the supine position; it is also an appropriate location for a thoracocentesis. The needle is usually inserted just below the level at which percussive dullness occurs.

344. The answer is b. *(Moore, Anatomy, 4/e, pp 87–91.)* The upper two posterior intercostal arteries arise from the costocervical trunk; the remaining arteries arise from the descending thoracic aorta. The posterior intercostal arteries anastomose with the anterior intercostal arteries, which arise from the internal thoracic artery. Laterally, the intercostal neurovascular bundle lies in the costal groove along the internal surface of the inferior border of each rib and between the inner and outer layers of the internal intercostal muscle. Indeed, scalloping of the inferior edge of the rib is a radiographic indication of increased collateral circulation through the intercostal arteries that results from a circulatory deficit elsewhere. Just as a subcostal location offers protection to the intercostal neurovascular bundle, fracture of a rib may involve tearing of these structures. The intercostal neurovascular bundle components give off a smaller accessory bundle, which lies adjacent to the upper border of the ribs. Thoracocentesis usually is performed adjacent to the upper border of the ribs to avoid the main intercostal neurovascular bundle.

345. The answer is d. *(Moore, Developing Human, 6/e, pp 384–389.)* Branches of the arteries of the sixth aortic arches form the pulmonary arteries. In addition, the left sixth arch artery forms the ductus arteriosus. The blood supply to the right side of the heart is primarily derived from the right and left coronary arteries and are derived from the truncus arteriosus. The face and thyroid gland receive blood primarily from the facial and superior thyroid arteries, respectively. These are branches of the common and external carotid arteries which, in turn, are derivatives of the second and third aortic arch arteries. The upper digestive tract is supplied by the celiac and superior mesenteric arteries, derivatives of the vitelline arteries.

346. The answer is d. (*Moore, Anatomy, 4/e, pp 132–135.*) The right coronary artery usually supplies the structures of the right atrium, including the sinoatrial node, right ventricle, and the posterior portion of the interventricular septum. Coronary occlusions involving the right coronary artery are, therefore, often accompanied by rhythm disturbances. The left coronary artery usually supplies the left atrium, the left ventricle, and the anterior portion of the interventricular septum, including the region of the atrioventricular bundle (of His).

347. The answer is c. (*Moore, Anatomy, 4/e, pp 136–137.*) With the exception of the anterior surface of the right ventricle, blood returning from the coronary circulation collects in the coronary sinus, which, in turn, empties directly into the right atrium. During right ventricular systole, venous blood is stored in the right atrium, and during ventricular diastole, blood flows from the right atrium to the right ventricle.

348. The answer is c. (*April, 3/e, pp 272–273.*) In the costoxiphoid approach to the pericardial cavity, a needle angled upward and toward the left passes between the xiphoid process and the costal margin, through the rectus sheath and rectus abdominis muscle, and through the fibrous and serous layers of the parietal pericardium. Because the line of pleural reflection swings away from the midline anteroinferiorly on the left side, the needle should not enter either the left pleural cavity or the left lung. The parasternal approach to the pericardial cavity will pass through the external intercostal membrane and the interchondral portion of an internal intercostal muscle.

349. The answer is b. (*April, 3/e, pp 272–273.*) The parasternal approach is via the left fourth intercostal space adjacent to the sternum so that the internal thoracic artery may be avoided. The low risk of injuring a major blood vessel is the benefit of the costoxiphoid approach. At the level of the costoxiphoid angle, the internal thoracic artery has bifurcated into the musculophrenic and superior epigastric arteries. The former courses later-ally along the costal margin, and the latter enters the rectus sheath some-what lateral to the tract of the needle. Because the heart is tilted on its right side, the right coronary artery lies directly behind and is protected by the sternum. The right marginal branch of the right coronary artery courses anteriorly along the diaphragmatic surface of the heart, anterior and supe-rior to the needle track. The anterior interventricular (descending) artery, which courses to the apex of the heart under the left nipple, is well out of harm's way.

350. The answer is d. (*Moore, Anatomy, 4/e, pp 100–103, 162–163.*) The lobe indicated by the * is the left upper (or superior) lobe. The general ori-entation when viewing CTs is that the observer is looking up from the patient's feet. Therefore, the patient's left is on your right. In addition, on the left, the inferior (lower) lobe begins relatively high in the thoracic cav-ity and is posterior to the upper lobe.

351. The answer is c. (*April, 3/e, pp 288–289.*) The mitral valve is best heard over the apex of the heart, which lies approximately in the fifth inter-costal space along the midclavicular line. The tricuspid valve is heard most distinctly in the fifth intercostal space just to the right of the sternum. The aortic and pulmonary valves are best auscultated in the right and left sec-ond intercostal spaces, respectively, adjacent to the sternum.

352. The answer is c. (*April, 3/e, pp 280–281.*) During the cardiac cycle, differential pressures between the atria and ventricles open and close the atrio-ventricular valves. The papillary muscles attach the chordae tendineae to the heart wall and provide an important dynamic mechanism to ensure the com-petence of the valves. During the ejection phase of ventricular systole, short-ening of the papillary muscle compensates for the decrease in the ventricular chamber size and thereby, prevents eversion of the atrioventricular valve leaflets, thereby preventing regurgitation during ventricular systole.

353. The answer is d. (*Moore, Anatomy 4/e, p 139.*) The afferent limb of the cardiac reflex is mediated by the carotid branch of the glossopharyngeal nerve (CN IX) from the aortic body and sinus as well as by the vagus nerve

(CN X) from the aortic body. The efferent limb, which is carried by the sympathetic division of the autonomic nervous system, mediates increases in heart rate and strength of heart beat through release of norepinephrine at the postganglionic effector site. The sympathetic cardiac accelerator fibers, affecting primarily the ventricles, are derived from the superior, middle, and inferior cervical ganglia (cervical cardiac nerves) as well as from the upper four thoracic ganglia (thoracic cardiac nerves), whence they converge on the cardiac plexus before reaching the heart. Parasympathetic fibers derived from CN X and its recurrent laryngeal branch decrease heart rate and stroke volume through release of acetylcholine, principally in the vicinity of the sinuatrial node.

354. The answer is d. (*April, 3/e, p 286.*) Afferent innervation from the heart and coronary arteries travels to the cardiac plexus along the sympathetic pathways. Once the afferent fibers pass through the cardiac plexus, they run along the cervical and thoracic cardiac nerves to the cervical and upper four thoracic sympathetic ganglia. Having traversed these ganglia, the fibers gain access (via the white rami communicantes) to the upper four thoracic spinal nerves and the corresponding levels of the spinal cord. The visceral afferent fibers associated with the vagus nerve are associated with reflexes and do not carry nociceptive information. The greater, lesser, and least splanchnic nerves convey visceral afferents from the abdominal region.

355. The answer is d. (*April, 3/e, p 275.*) The artery labeled D in the diagram accompanying the question represents the posterior interventricular (descending) artery, which supplies blood to the posterior portions of the interventricular septum as well as to the posterior wall of the right ventricle. This artery usually is a branch of the right coronary artery, and the diagnosis of this patient's disorder is consistent with the results of the ECG, which indicates a posterior septal infarct. The anterior interventricular artery (C) arises from the left coronary artery (A) and supplies the anterior portion of the interventricular septum and the anterior walls of both ventricles. The posterior interventricular artery (D) usually anastomoses with the anterior interventricular artery (C) near the apex of the heart. The circumflex artery (B) circles toward the back of the heart in the coronary sulcus and may occasionally give rise to the posterior interventricular artery (D). The right marginal artery (E) is a branch of the right coronary artery.

356. The answer is c. *(April, 3/e, pp 275–277.)* The great cardiac vein accompanies the anterior interventricular (descending) artery. The anterior cardiac veins pass across the right coronary sulcus to drain directly into the right atrium. The middle cardiac vein lies in the posterior interventricular sulcus with the posterior descending artery. The small cardiac vein accompanies the right marginal vein and the right coronary artery. The coronary sinus, accompanying the circumflex artery in the left coronary sulcus, receives the great, middle, and small cardiac veins before draining into the right atrium.

357. The answer is b. *(Moore, Anatomy, 4/e, p 35.)* In a coronary bypass procedure, the distal end of the vein graft is anastomosed to the aorta so that the presence of a valve or valve leaflets in the graft will not obstruct the flow of coronary blood. In recent years, the reversed saphenous vein graft from the calf has been the choice for this procedure. This vein is closer in size to the coronary arteries than one taken from the thigh.

358. The answer is c. *(April, 3/e, pp 286–289.)* Heart sounds originate from the closure of the atrioventricular and semilunar valves as a result of relative pressure reversals during the cardiac cycle. The first heart sound, heard just after the ventricles begin to contract, occurs when the ventricular pressures exceed atrial pressures and thereby, close the atrioventricular valves. Reverberation within the ventricles causes this S_1 sound ("Lub") to have a low frequency and a relatively long duration. The second heart sound is heard at the beginning of ventricular diastole, when the aortic and pulmonary pressures exceed the respective ventricular pressures and snap shut the aortic and pulmonary semilunar valves. This S_2 ("Dup") is relatively sharp when both aortic and semilunar valves close together. However, deep inspiration, which lowers intrathoracic pressure, results in delayed closing of the pulmonary valve and thus produces a split S_2. Ventricular systole occurs approximately between the S_1 and S_2 heart sounds and diastole between S_2 and S_1. Occasionally, a low, rumbling third heart sound may be heard during diastole and is attributable to ventricular filling. Stenosis or insufficiency of the valves produces turbulence and backflow, respectively, which are heard as murmurs.

359. The answer is d. *(Moore, Anatomy, 4/e, p 294–295.)* The esophageal hiatus, in addition to allowing passage of the esophagus, also passes the anterior and posterior vagal trunks. The aortic hiatus transmits the aorta, the thoracic duct, and occasionally, an azygos or hemiazygos vein. Usually, the azygos and hemiazygos veins either pass lateral to or through a crus of the diaphragm along with the respective left and right sympathetic chains. The phrenic nerves usually penetrate the diaphragm to gain access to the inferior surface; however, the right phrenic may accompany the inferior vena cava through the caval hiatus.

360. The answer is a. (*Moore, Developing Human, 6/e, pp 366, 367.*) The sinus venosus receives the veins (cardinal) from the body. Originally the caudal end of the heart tube, the sinus venosus rotates cranially and dorsally during the looping process. The left horn of the sinus becomes a narrow channel located in the groove between the left atrium and ventricle. The coronary sinus empties into the right atrium. The right horn of the sinus forms the entrance of the two venae cavae into the right atrium and becomes the smooth-walled portion of the right atrium. The primitive atrium becomes the entire left atrium and the trabeculated (rough-walled) portion of the right atrium. The bulbus cordis gives rise to the right ventricle and the muscular portions of the outflow tracts of both ventricles. The truncus arteriosus gives rise to the vascular portions of the outflow tracts, the aorta, and the pulmonary arteries.

361. The answer is a. (*Moore, Anatomy, 4/e, pp 45–52.*) Sympathetic outflow occurs between the first thoracic and second lumbar segments of the spinal cord. The presynaptic sympathetic neurons originate in the lateral cell columns of the spinal cord and pass along the thoracic and upper lumbar spinal nerves. These myelinated neurons leave the respective spinal nerves by white rami communicantes, which convey the sympathetic neurons to the chain of sympathetic ganglia. Some of the sympathetic neurons pass through the chain as splanchnic nerves to reach prevertebral ganglia associated with the viscera. Others may ascend in the cervical portion of the chain or descend to the lower lumbar or sacral portions before synapse occurs. Visceral afferent neurons conveying sensation from the viscera reach the sympathetic chain via the splanchnic nerves and then continue along the white rami communicantes to reach the spinal nerves.

362. The answer is c. (*Moore, Anatomy, 4/e, p. 153.*) This sagittally angled MR image shows the heart and some of the great vessels and associated structures. These include the contents of the superior mediastinum (aortic and pulmonary arches) and the inferior mediastinum (the heart and descending thoracic aorta). The level indicated by Q is the manubriosternal joint (the sternal angle), an important clinical landmark that, when projected dorsally, passes through T4/T5 level. This plane separates the superior and inferior mediastina. Thus, structure P is the pulmonary trunk that is located inferior to the aortic arch. Located between it and the posterior part of the aortic arch is the left bronchus. At this location we find the second esophageal constriction caused by the pressure of the aortic arch.

363. The answer is c. (*Moore, Anatomy, 4/e, p. 93.*) The level indicated by Q is the manubriosternal joint (angle of Louis); it is a symphyseal joint (fibrocartilaginous) that locates the junction of the cartilaginous portions of the second ribs and the sternum. This is an important clinical level that marks the division of the mediastinum into its superior and inferior parts. A transverse line passing through the sternal angle meets the vertebral column at T4/T5 level. This level defines (1) the aortic arch, (2) bifurcation of the trachea into primary bronchi, and (3) the approximate location of the second constriction of the esophagus.

364 to 365. The answers are 364-a, 365-d. (*April, 3/e, pp 254–255, 257.*) In quiet inspiration, the external intercostals and the interchondral (parasternal) portion of the internal intercostals function to elevate the ribs and thereby, increase the transverse diameter of the thoracic cage. Concomitantly, contraction of the diaphragm increases the vertical diameter of the thoracic cage. The relative contribution of each group of muscles depends on the sex and age of the person. Generally, children and older men use the diaphragm and abdominal musculature; women, especially if pregnant, tend to breathe thoracically.

Exertional expiration is accomplished by contraction of the internal intercostal and transverse thoracic muscles, thereby decreasing the transverse diameter of the thoracic cage, as well as by contraction of the abdominal musculature, including the rectus abdominis, external and internal oblique muscles, transversus abdominis muscle, and quadratus lumborum. In addition, the perineal muscles may tense. Contraction of the abdominal muscles moves the viscera under the diaphragm, which forces the diaphragm upward into the thorax and thereby, decreases thoracic volume.

366 to 367. The answers are 366-d, 367-c. *(April, 3/e, pp 277, 286–289.)* The atrioventricular valves open during ventricular diastole so that the ventricles fill during late atrial diastole, ventricular diastole, and atrial systole. The atrioventricular valves close early in ventricular systole as ventricular pressure exceeds atrial pressure. The aortic and pulmonary valves open in midventricular systole when the pressures in the great vessels are exceeded and then close as ventricular diastole begins. Blood flow through the coronary circulation occurs only during diastole (relaxation), or approximately half the cardiac cycle. During ventricular systole, there is no pressure gradient between the aorta and ventricular walls; therefore, no flow. This intermittent nature of coronary blood supply means that, compared with other vital organs, the heart has a correspondingly reduced margin of safety.

Abdomen

Questions

DIRECTIONS: Each item below contains a question or incomplete statement followed by suggested responses. Select the **one best** response to each question.

368. The last segment of the gastrointestinal tract to become fully closed into a tube and separated from the yolk sac is the

a. Anal canal
b. Appendix
c. Cecum
d. Ileum

Questions 369 to 375

A 46-year-old bakery worker is admitted to a hospital in acute distress. She has experienced severe abdominal pain, nausea, and vomiting for two days. The pain, which is sharp and constant, began in the epigastric region and radiated bilaterally around the chest to just below the scapulas. Subsequently, the pain became localized in the right hypochondrium. The patient, who has a history of similar attacks after hearty meals over the past five years, is moderately overweight and the mother of four. Palpation reveals marked tenderness in the right hypochondriac region and some rigidity of the abdominal musculature. An x-ray without contrast medium shows numerous calcified stones in the region of the gallbladder. The patient shows no sign of icterus (jaundice).

369. Diffuse pain referred to the epigastric region and radiating circumferentially around the chest is the result of afferent fibers that travel via which of the following nerves?

a. Greater splanchnic
b. Intercostal
c. Phrenic
d. Vagus

370. The patient receives a general anesthetic in preparation for a chole-cystectomy. A right subcostal incision is made, which begins near the xiphoid process, runs along and immediately beneath the costal margin to the anterior axillary line, and transects the rectus abdominis muscle and rectus sheath. At the level of the transpyloric plane, the anterior wall of the sheath of the rectus abdominis muscle receives contributions from the

a. Aponeuroses of the internal and external oblique muscles
b. Aponeuroses of the transversus abdominis and internal oblique muscles
c. Aponeuroses of the transversus abdominis and internal and external oblique muscles
d. Transversalis fascia
e. Transversalis fascia and aponeurosis of the transversus abdominis muscle

371. Exploration of the peritoneal cavity disclosed a distended gallblad-der. It is located

a. Between the left and caudate lobes of the liver
b. Between the right and quadrate lobes of the liver
c. In the falciform ligament
d. In the lesser omentum
e. In the right anterior leaf of the coronary ligament

372. The lesser omentum is incised close to its free edge, and the biliary tree is identified and freed by blunt dissection. The liquid contents of the gallbladder are aspirated with a syringe, the fundus incised, and the stones removed. The entire duct system is carefully probed for stones, one of which is found to be obstructing a duct. In view of the observation that the patient is not jaundiced, the most probable location of the obstruction is

a. The bile duct
b. The common hepatic duct
c. The cystic duct
d. Within the duodenal papilla proximal to the juncture with the pancreatic duct
e. Within the duodenal papilla distal to the juncture with the pancreatic duct

373. The biliary duct system is carefully dissected. The cystic artery and cystic duct both are identified, ligated, and divided, the duct at a point about an eighth of an inch from its juncture with the common hepatic duct. The gallbladder is then freed from the inferior surface of the liver by blunt dissection and removed. However, the operative field suddenly fills with arterial blood. To locate and ligate the bleeder, hemorrhage should be controlled by

a. Ligating the common hepatic artery
b. Ligating the proper hepatic artery distal to the origin of the right gastric and gastroduodenal arteries
c. Ligating the left hepatic artery, especially if there are additional (aberrant) left hepatic arteries present
d. Ligating the hepatic portal vein
e. Temporarily compressing the hepatic pedicle

374. It is ascertained that an accessory right hepatic artery inadvertently had been torn. There is no choice but to ligate the accessory artery. The effect of this ligation most probably will be

a. Ischemic necrosis of the quadrate lobe of the liver
b. Ischemic necrosis of a discrete portion of the right lobe of the liver
c. No necrosis in any lobe because of the integrity of the hepatic portal vein
d. No necrosis in any lobe because of extrahepatic collateral blood supply
e. No necrosis in any lobe because of intrahepatic collateral blood supply

375. The subcostal incision, which parallels the costal margin anteriorly, is closed in layers. The patient is allowed up on her first postoperative day; on the third day the drain (which shows no bile leakage) is withdrawn, and on the tenth day the patient is discharged. As a result of the location and direction of the incision, one might expect healing to result in

a. Loss of blood supply and necrosis of a portion of the rectus abdominis muscle
b. Significant paralysis of a portion of the rectus abdominis muscle
c. Minimal scarring
d. Negligible possibility of subsequent abdominal herniation

376. A full-term male infant displays projectile vomiting 1 h after suckling. There is failure to gain weight during the first two weeks. The vomitus is not bile-stained and no respiratory difficulty is evident. Examination reveals an abdomen neither tense nor bloated. The most probable explanation is

a. Congenital hypertrophic pyloric stenosis
b. Duodenal atresia
c. Patent ileal diverticulum
d. Imperforate anus
e. Tracheoesophageal fistula

377. In Hirschsprung's disease, neural crest cells fail to migrate to, or invade, the wall of the lower colon, resulting in a loss of peristalsis in that region and often fatal obstruction. Preganglionic neurons, which would innervate the absent intramural ganglia, originate in

a. The nucleus ambiguus
b. Cervical intermediolateral cell column
c. Sacral levels two to four of the spinal cord
d. The motor nucleus of the vagus nerve (CN X)
e. The ventral horn at spinal levels L1–L2

Questions 378 to 380

A 37-year-old man with a history of alcohol abuse was seen in the emergency room complaining of stomach cramps in the region of the umbilicus. He reported several recent incidents of vomiting that contained no noticeable blood, although he had in the past vomited bright red blood. He insisted that he had been on the wagon for the past several months. Physical examination revealed a mass about the umbilicus with indications of periumbilical peritoneal inflammation. His white blood cell count was high and he had a temperature of 39.4°C (103°F). He was admitted to the surgical service for emergency reduction of an umbilical hernia with suspected strangulation.

378. The crampy abdominal pain referred to the umbilical region and knowledge of peritoneal structure would lead the examining physician to suspect that the strangulated section of gut was most likely the

a. Ascending colon
b. Descending colon
c. Small intestine
d. Sigmoid colon
e. Stomach

379. After the herniated segment of gut was placed into the abdominal cavity, its color changed from purple to pink, which indicated that the vasculature was functional. The small intestine normally receives significant collateral circulation from the

a. Descending branch of the left colic artery
b. Renal arteries
c. Splenic artery
d. Superior pancreaticoduodenal artery

380. On manual exploration of the abdominal cavity, the liver was felt to be hard and nodular. This, in addition to the history of hematemesis, indicated that control of the portal hypertension was necessary. In a patient with cirrhosis of the liver, venous hypertension would be expected in the

a. Hepatic vein
b. Renal vein
c. Short gastric veins
d. Suprarenal vein

381. The lateral umbilical fold on each side is created by the underlying

a. Falx inguinalis
b. Inferior epigastric artery
c. Lateral border of the rectus sheath
d. Obliterated umbilical artery
e. Urachus

382. A 24-year-old male visited the community clinic complaining of a draining abscess on his anterior thigh. Subsequent testing revealed an active tuberculosis infection localized in the lumbar vertebrae. The spread of infection most likely occurred via

a. The ischiorectal fossa
b. The sheath of the psoas muscle
c. The inguinal ligament
d. A paracolic gutter

383. A posteriorly perforating ulcer in the pyloric antrum of the stomach is most likely to produce initial localized peritonitis or abscess formation in the

a. Greater sac
b. Left subhepatic and hepatorenal spaces (pouch of Morison)
c. Omental bursa
d. Right subphrenic space
e. Right subhepatic space

384. Which of the following is most likely to lead to intestinal volvulus in a newborn?

a. Failure of fixation of the ascending or descending colon
b. Long mesenteric support of the transverse colon
c. Mesenteric support for the sigmoid colon
d. Retrocecal appendix
e. Situs inversus

385. The lesser sac (omental bursa) is directly continuous with which of the following recesses or spaces?

a. Infracolic compartment
b. Left colic gutter
c. Left subphrenic recess
d. Right subphrenic space
e. Hepatorenal recess

386. Mucosal necrosis of the rectum usually will not result from occlusion of the inferior mesenteric artery because

a. Arterial supply to the rectum is from anastomotic connections from the superior mesenteric artery
b. Arterial supply to the rectum is from the left colic artery with anastomoses to branches of the internal iliac artery
c. The inferior mesenteric artery does not supply the rectum
d. A principal branch of the external iliac artery is a major supplier to the rectum
e. The middle rectal artery, a branch of the internal iliac artery, supplies the rectum

387. Sympathectomy may occasionally relieve intractable pain of visceral origin, inasmuch as visceral afferent pain fibers run along the sympathetic pathways in the abdomen. Autonomic control of peristalsis in the descending colon should not be affected by bilateral lumbar sympathectomy because

a. The descending colon is controlled chiefly by parasympathetic innervation from the pelvic splanchnic nerves
b. The descending colon receives its parasympathetic innervation from the vagus nerve
c. The descending colon receives its sympathetic innervation from thoracic splanchnic nerves
d. Lumbar splanchnics from L1, L2, and L3 only innervate the pelvic viscera via the hypogastric nerve
e. Only presynaptic sympathetic fibers have been severed

388. A man, the victim of several knife wounds to the abdomen during a barroom brawl, subsequently developed a direct inguinal hernia. Damage to which of the following nerves is most likely responsible for the predisposing weakness of the abdominal wall?

a. Genitofemoral nerve
b. Ilioinguinal nerve
c. The subcostal nerve
d. Pelvic splanchnic nerves
e. The nerve of the tenth intercostal space (T10)

389. Molecules secreted into the circulation by the renal cortex include

a. Aldosterone and antidiuretic hormone
b. Angiotensinogen and angiotensin II
c. Erythropoietin and renin
d. Glucocorticoids and mineralocorticoids

390. Which of the following gives rise to all structures of the kidney?

a. Somitic mesoderm
b. Intermediate mesoderm
c. Splanchnic lateral plate mesoderm
d. Somatic lateral plate mesoderm

Questions 391 to 392

A middle-aged woman describes flushing, severe headaches, and a feeling that her heart is "going to explode" when she gets excited. At the beginning of a physical examination her blood pressure (130/85) is not significantly above normal. However, on palpation of her upper left quadrant, the examining physician notices the onset of sympathetic signs. Her blood pressure (200/135) is abnormally high. A subsequent CT scan confirms the suspected tumor of the left adrenal gland. The patient is scheduled for surgery.

391. The symptoms that the patient correlated with the onset of excitement were due to nervous stimulation of the adrenal glands. The adrenal medulla receives its innervation from

a. Preganglionic sympathetic nerves
b. Postsynaptic sympathetic nerves
c. Preganglionic parasympathetic nerves
d. Postganglionic parasympathetic nerves
e. Somatic nerves

392. The adrenal gland is located, and the venous drainage is ligated to prevent life-threatening quantities of adrenalin from entering the bloodstream on manipulation of the gland. Normally, the left adrenal venous drainage is into the

a. Inferior vena cava
b. Left azygos vein
c. Left inferior phrenic vein
d. Left renal vein
e. Superior mesenteric vein

393. Which of the following statements concerning a direct inguinal hernia is correct?

a. It protrudes through Hesselbach's triangle
b. It is the most common type of abdominal hernia
c. It traverses the entire length of the inguinal canal
d. It contains all three fascial layers of the spermatic cord
e. It exits the inguinal canal via the superficial inguinal ring

Questions 394 to 397

While moving furniture, an 18-year-old man experiences excruciating pain in his right groin. A few hours later he also develops pain in the umbilical region with accompanying nausea. At this point he seeks medical attention. Examination reveals a bulge midway between the midline and the anterior superior iliac spine, but superior to the inguinal ligament. On coughing or straining, the bulge increases and the inguinal pain intensifies. The bulge courses medially and inferiorly into the upper portion of the scrotum and cannot be reduced with the finger pressure of the examiner. It is decided that a medical emergency exists, and the patient is scheduled for immediate surgery.

394. Nausea and diffuse pain referred to the umbilical region in this patient most probably are due to

a. Compression of the genitofemoral nerve
b. Compression of the ilioinguinal nerve
c. Dilation of the inguinal canal
d. Incarceration of a loop of small bowel
e. Ischemic necrosis of the cremaster muscle

395. During surgery, one would expect to find which of the following arteries in the inguinal region?

a. Aberrant obturator (if present)
b. Deep circumflex iliac
c. External iliac
d. External pudendal
e. Inferior epigastric

396. The external oblique aponeurosis is incised and the superficial ring is opened. The inguinal canal is then opened by blunt dissection. Abdominal wall structures that usually contribute directly to the spermatic cord include which of the following?

a. External oblique muscle
b. Falx inguinalis
c. Internal oblique muscle
d. Rectus sheath
e. Transversus abdominis muscle

397. At this point in the surgical procedure, it is noticed that a nerve has been inadvertently sectioned. This nerve exited through the superficial inguinal ring and was applied to the anterior aspect of the spermatic cord. As a result of this operative error, it is probable that the patient will

a. Be unable to produce spermatozoa in the right testis
b. Become impotent
c. Lose the cremasteric reflex on the right side
d. Lose the dartos response to cold
e. Lose sensation over portions of the base of the penis and anterior scrotum

398. The femoral ring usually contains the

a. Femoral artery
b. Femoral nerve
c. Femoral vein
d. Iliopsoas muscle
e. Lymphatics

399. Allen is a 30-year-old bachelor who frequents singles bars. He is cautious and always uses a condom in his sexual encounters. Recently, he has felt "off," experiencing a sore throat, malaise, and a slight fever. When you see him in your office, he has a few swollen lymph nodes and has a large palpable structure in the left upper abdomen indicated by the * in the accompanying radiograph. He had a positive monospot test and an elevated sedimentary rate. Your diagnosis is infectious mononucleosis. The structure you palpated was

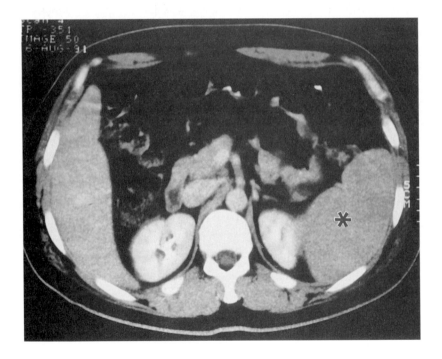

   a. An enlarged liver (hepatomegaly)
   b. An enlarged spleen (splenomegaly)
   c. The stomach
   d. A tumor of the liver
   e. Liver cirrhosis

400. A patient complained of severe abdominal pain on several occasions, but no cause could be identified. She was recently diagnosed with polyarteritis nodosa, so you ordered this abdominal arteriogram to determine whether there were abdominal vascular changes that would explain her abdominal pain. On this arteriogram there is a tortuous vessel indicated by the arrow. What is this vessel?

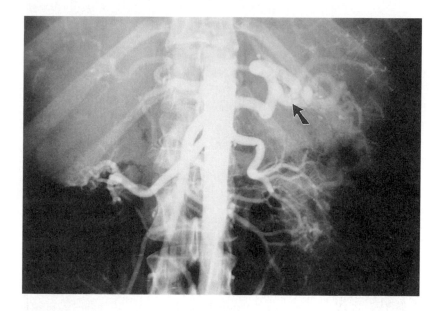

a. Left gastric artery
b. Superior mesenteric artery
c. Splenic artery
d. Right gastric artery
e. Right gastro-omental artery

Questions 401 to 402

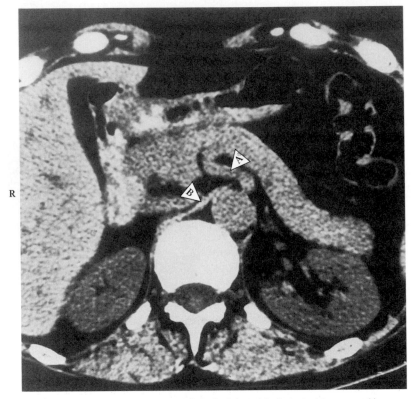

(Reproduced, with permission, from Wicke L: Atlas of Radiological Anatomy. 6/e. Baltimore, MD: Williams & Wilkins. 1998.)

401. What is the identity of the structure indicated by "A" in the above magnetic resonance image (MRI)?

a. Common hepatic artery
b. Left gastric artery
c. Gastroduodenal artery
d. Splenic artery
e. Left renal artery

402. Which structure is indicated by "B" in the above image?

a. Right renal artery
b. Right renal vein
c. Right crus of the diaphragm
d. Common hepatic artery
e. Short gastric artery

DIRECTIONS: Each group of questions below consists of lettered headings followed by a set of numbered items. For each numbered item select the **one** lettered heading with which it is **most** closely associated. Each lettered heading may be used once, more than once, or not at all.

Questions 403 to 404

For each question, select the appropriate innervation.

a. Lumbar sympathetic chain
b. Pelvic splanchnic nerves (nervi erigentes)
c. Pudendal nerve
d. Sacral sympathetic chain
e. Vagus nerve

403. Sensation of fullness in the rectum

404. Control of the external anal sphincter

Questions 405 to 406

Match each description with the appropriate artery.

a. Common hepatic artery
b. Inferior phrenic artery
c. Left gastric artery
d. Splenic artery
e. Superior mesenteric artery

405. Principal supply to the body and tail of the pancreas

406. Principal supply to the left side of the gastric fundus

Questions 407 to 408

Several major anatomic structures pass through hiatal openings in the diaphragm. Abdominal contents may herniate into the thorax, either through one of these hiatuses or through developmental defects in the diaphragm. For each of the following questions, select from the diagram below the lettered opening that is most appropriate.

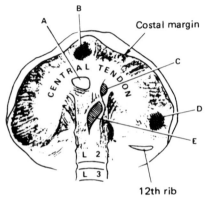

Diaphragm — Inferior Surface

407. Frequently transmits the right phrenic nerve

408. Transmits the left vagus nerve

Questions 409 to 410

Match each question to a hernia from the list below.

a. Diaphragmatic hernia
b. Epigastric hernia
c. Lumbar hernia
d. Spigelian hernia in the lower abdomen
e. Umbilical hernia

409. Usually iatrogenic in the linea alba

410. Frequently a congenital, midline herniation

Questions 411 to 412

Match each structure with the referral area of its afferent innervation.

a. Upper thoracic region and postaxial arm
b. Lower thorax and epigastric region
c. Umbilical region
d. Subcostal and hypogastric regions
e. Lumbar and inguinal regions; anterior thigh

411. Appendix

412. Pancreatic papilla

Abdomen

Answers

368. The answer is d. (*Moore, Developing Human, 6/e, pp 154, 292–294. Sadler, 8/e, pp 258–261.*) During the first month of development, the midgut communicates over its entirety with the yolk sac. This connection narrows during the next month to form the vitelline duct (yolk stalk, omphalomesenteric duct) as the midgut closes and usually disappears during the ninth week. Because the vitelline duct joins the ileum, this section of the gastrointestinal tract is the last to close. Failure of closure results in a persistent vitelline fistula, whereas partial obliteration results in an ileal diverticulum (of Meckel).

369. The answer is a. (*April, 3/e, pp 359–360.*) Visceral afferent pain fibers from the gallbladder travel through the celiac plexus, thence along the greater splanchnic nerves to levels T5–T9 of the spinal cord. Thus, pain originating from the gallbladder will be referred to (appear as if coming from) the dermatomes served by T5–T9, which include a band from the infrascapular region to the epigastrium.

370. The answer is a. (*Moore, Anatomy, 4/e, pp 182–186.*) The rectus sheath is formed by the aponeuroses of the abdominal wall musculature. Between the costal margin and the umbilicus, the aponeurosis of the internal oblique muscle splits; one portion passes anterior and the other posterior to the rectus abdominis muscle. The aponeurosis of the external oblique muscle fuses with the anterior leaflet of the aponeurosis of the internal oblique muscle to form the anterior wall of the rectus sheath. The aponeurosis of the transversus abdominis muscle fuses with the posterior leaflet of the aponeurosis of the internal oblique muscle to form the posterior wall of the rectus sheath. Approximately midway between the umbilicus and symphysis pubis, the aponeuroses of the internal oblique and transversus abdominis muscles pass anterior to the rectus abdominis muscle to contribute to the anterior leaf of the rectus sheath. This abrupt transition results in a free edge to the posterior rectus sheath, known as the arcuate line (of Douglas). Between this line and the pubis, only the transversalis fascia separates the rectus abdominis muscle from the peritoneum. It is here, where the inferior epigastric artery gains access to the rectus sheath, that ventral lateral (spigelian) herniation may occur.

371. The answer is b. *(Moore, Anatomy, 4/e, p 274–276.)* The gallbladder lies on the inferior surface of the liver between the right and quadrate lobes. The caudate lobe lies posteriorly between the right and left lobes. The falciform ligament, a portion of the lesser omentum, attaches to the liver at the incisura between the quadrate and left lobes as well as along the fissure for the round ligament. Toward the superior surface of the liver, the falciform ligament splits to form the left and right coronary ligaments, which define the bare area of the liver. The coronary ligaments come together again to form the gastrohepatic ligament of the lesser omentum.

372. The answer is c. *(Moore, Anatomy, 4/e, p 276–277.)* Obstruction of any portion of the biliary tree will produce symptoms of gallbladder attack. If the common hepatic duct or bile duct is occluded by stone or tumor, biliary stasis with accompanying jaundice occurs. In addition, blockage of the duodenal papilla (of Vater), distal to the juncture of the bile duct with the pancreatic duct, can lead to complicating pancreatitis. If only the cystic duct is obstructed, jaundice will not occur because bile may flow freely from the liver to the duodenum. Bile duct obstruction also may arise as a result of pressure exerted on the duct by an external mass, such as a tumor in the head of the pancreas.

373. The answer is e. *(April, 3/e, pp 339, 354–355.)* Compressing the hepatic pedicle and its contained vascular structures between the forefinger placed in the omental foramen (of Winslow) and the thumb placed anteriorly is a convenient way to stem extrahepatic hemorrhage until the source of bleeding can be located and ligated. The blood supply to the liver is variable; several potential anastomotic loops exist between branches of the extrahepatic arterial system. Thus, ligation of the common hepatic artery proximal to the gastroduodenal artery will enable arterial blood to reach the liver from branches of the splenic artery (via anastomotic left and right gastroepiploic arteries) and the superior mesenteric artery (via the anastomotic inferior and superior pancreaticoduodenal arteries). Ligation of the proper hepatic artery proximal to the origin of the right gastric artery will enable arterial blood to reach the liver from branches of the celiac artery (via anastomotic left and right gastric arteries). However, ligation distal to the juncture of the right gastric artery will terminate most of, if not all, the blood supply to the liver and incur a danger of ischemia, if not necrosis, of hepatic tissue. Because accessory or aberrant hepatic arteries usually are not sources of collateral blood supply to the liver, they cannot be relied on to provide intrahepatic anastomotic connections.

374. The answer is b. (*April, 3/e, pp 355–356.*) Because few intrahepatic arterial anastomoses exist, ligation of a left or right hepatic artery or of an aberrant (accessory) hepatic artery will result in ischemic necrosis of the region of the liver supplied by that vessel. The left hepatic artery supplies the left lobe and the quadrate lobe, as well as half the caudate lobe. The right hepatic artery supplies the right lobe and the other half of the caudate lobe; it also usually supplies the gallbladder through the cystic artery. No major extrahepatic anastomotic connections distal to the right gastric artery exist, and the hepatic portal vein has far too low a partial pressure of oxygen to supply the metabolic requirements of liver parenchyma.

375. The answer is b. (*Moore, Anatomy, 4/e, p 186–187.*) The rectus abdominis muscle receives an abundant collateral blood supply. The nerve supply to the rectus abdominis muscle is derived from abdominal extensions of the lower seven intercostal nerves and from the iliohypogastric nerve. These nerves run between the internal oblique and transversus abdominis muscles to reach the lateral border of the rectus sheath, which they pierce to reach the rectus abdominis muscle. Consequently, a subcostal incision from the xiphisternal angle to the anterior axillary line is apt to sever one or two of these nerves and thus paralyze a significant portion of the ipsilateral rectus abdominis muscle. An affected patient may be predisposed to subsequent abdominal herniation. Although the direction of an incision along the costal margin is perforce perpendicular to the dermal cleavage lines (of Langer) and thus may produce discomfort and healing with significant scarring, such an incision is justified by the required operative exposure that it provides.

376. The answer is a. (*Moore, Developing Human, 6/e, p 276.*) Blockage of the foregut in the newborn produces projectile vomiting. Congenital hypertrophic pyloric stenosis, occurring in 0.5 to 1.0% of males and rarely in females, involves hypertrophy of the circular layer of muscle at the pylorus. This usually does not regress and must be treated surgically. During the fifth and sixth weeks of development, the lumen of the duodenum is occluded by muscle proliferation but normally recanalizes during the eighth week. Failure of recanalization results in duodenal atresia. Because this occurs distal to the hepatopancreatic ampulla, the vomitus will occasionally be stained with bile. Annular pancreas, rare in itself, seldom completely blocks the duodenum. Imperforate anus results in intestinal distention with bloating.

377. The answer is c. *(Moore, Anatomy, 4/e, p 253.)* Preganglionic parasympathetic neurons to the lower colon arise from the spinal cord at sacral levels two to four and reach the wall of the colon via pelvic splanchnic nerves. The nucleus ambiguus is the source of preganglionic parasympathetic neurons that innervate the heart via the vagus nerve and cardiac plexus. Neurons arising in the cervical intermediolateral cell column are sympathetic preganglionics. Preganglionic parasympathetic neurons arising from the motor nucleus of the vagus innervate the upper GI tract. Neurons arising from the ventral horn are primary somatic motor neurons to skeletal muscle.

378. The answer is c. *(April, 3/e, pp 383–384.)* The umbilical region is innervated by the tenth intercostal nerve. The afferent nerve fibers from the jejunum and ileum as well as from the ascending colon and transverse colon travel through the superior mesenteric plexus and along the lesser splanchnic nerve to spinal nerves T10 and T11. Thus, pain originating from these portions of the gastrointestinal tract will refer pain to the umbilical region. The ascending colon and descending colon, which are secondarily retroperitoneal, are unlikely to be involved in the umbilical herniation. The mobile transverse colon could be involved, but the referred pain would tend to be subumbilical, not periumbilical.

379. The answer is d. *(Moore, Anatomy, 4/e, pp 235, 241.)* The jejunum and ileum receive their principal blood supply from the superior mesenteric artery. A strong collateral circulation is derived from the superior pancreatic artery, a branch of the pancreaticoduodenal artery that arises from the hepatic branch of the celiac artery. The superior pancreatic artery anastomoses with the inferior pancreatic artery, the first branch of the superior mesenteric artery. The collateral circulation is weak between the right colic artery and the ileal branches. There are no possibilities for superior mesenteric anastomoses from the splenic, the descending branch of the left colic, or renal arteries.

380. The answer is c. (*Moore, Anatomy, 4/e, p 229.*) The short gastric veins are branches of the splenic vein and, therefore, would experience the portal pressure. The short gastric veins also anastomose with the esophageal veins and produce esophageal varices. The hepatic vein, between the liver and inferior vena cava, drains the liver and is not part of the portal system. There are no communications between the portal system and the renal or suprarenal veins.

381. The answer is b. (*Moore, Anatomy, 4/e, p 191.*) The lateral umbilical folds are produced by the underlying inferior epigastric arteries as they course from the external iliac artery in the inguinal region toward the rectus sheath. The medial umbilical folds are peritoneal elevations produced by the obliterated umbilical arteries. In the midline, the median umbilical ligament is formed by the underlying urachus, a remnant of the embryonic allantois.

382. The answer is b. (*Moore, Anatomy, 4/e, p 299.*) Tuberculous infections of the lumbar vertebrae are frequently communicated to the sheath of the adjacent psoas muscles. Subsequently, pus may travel inferiorly over the pelvic brim and erupt on the anterior thigh near the insertion of the psoas on the lesser trochanter of the femur. Abscesses in the ischiorectal fossae may drain into the pelvis or the anal canal. The inguinal ligament passes laterally to medially superficial to the psoas muscle to transmit contents to the scrotum or labia. Its origin in the anterolateral abdominal wall is not in close approximation to the lumbar vertebrae. The paracolic gutters can spread infection or metastases into the pelvis or the subphrenic region, depending on whether the patient is erect or supine.

383. The answer is c. (*Moore, Anatomy, 4/e, p 217.*) The omental bursa (lesser sac) is the remnant of the right coelomic cavity, which, owing to rotation of the gut and differential growth of the liver, lies behind the stomach. A posterior gastric perforation or an inflamed pancreas could lead to abscess formation in the lesser sac. The right subhepatic space might become secondarily involved via communication through the omental foramen (of Winslow). The pouch of Morison, which is the combined right subhepatic and the hepatorenal spaces, may be the seat of abscess formation related to gallbladder disease or perforation of a duodenal ulcer. The right subphrenic space is between the liver and the diaphragm and communicates with the pouch of Morison. All these spaces are in communication with the greater sac of the peritoneal cavity.

384. The answer is a. (*Moore, Developing Human, 6/e, pp 290, 292*) Malrotation by failure of either the ascending or descending portions of the abdominal wall to fixate to the posterior peritoneal wall and become secondarily retroperitoneal increases the probability of the bowel twisting about itself (volvulus). This not only produces intestinal obstruction but also may strangulate the vascular supply with intestinal ischemia and life-threatening intestinal infarct. Situs inversus (normal, but reversed) does not predispose to volvulus. The transverse and sigmoid colons are both supported by mesenteries of variable length. A retrocecal appendix is very common.

385. The answer is e. (*Moore, Anatomy, 4/e, p 217.*) The omental (epiploic) foramen connects the lesser sac with the hepatorenal (subhepatic) recess of the greater sac. The hepatorenal recess then communicates with the right subphrenic recess and right paracolic gutter. The subhepatic recess is perhaps the most frequently infected intra-abdominal space as a result of appendicitis, liver abscess, perforated duodenal and gastric ulcers, or perforation of the biliary tree.

386. The answer is e. (*Moore, Anatomy, 4/e, p 386.*) The rectum receives blood from the superior rectal (hemorrhoidal) artery and from the paired middle and inferior rectal arteries. The superior rectal artery is a direct continuation of the inferior mesenteric artery, but the middle and inferior rectal arteries are branches of the internal iliac artery and continue to supply the distal rectum despite occlusion of the inferior mesenteric artery. It should be noted that Sudeck's point, between the last sigmoidal artery and the rectosigmoid artery, is an area of potentially weak arterial anastomoses.

387. The answer is a. *(Moore, Anatomy, 4/e, p 255.)* Control of peristalsis is principally a function of the parasympathetic division of the autonomic nervous system. Although removal of the lumbar sympathetic chain (lumbar sympathectomy) does sever the sympathetic fibers innervating the descending colon as well as the pelvic viscera, the action of sympathetic fibers to the descending colon is apparently confined to vasoconstriction. Because the parasympathetic innervation to the descending colon is derived from the sacral outflow (S2–S4) through the pelvic splanchnic nerves (nervi erigentes), peristalsis will occur normally after lumbar sympathectomy.

388. The answer is b. *(Moore, Anatomy, 4/e, pp 187, 191, 205–207.)* The ilioinguinal nerve innervates the portion of the internal oblique muscle inserting in the lateral border of the conjoint tendon. Paralysis of these fibers would create weakness in the conjoint tendon, allowing herniation to occur medial to the inferior epigastric vessels. The genitofemoral nerve supplies sensory innervation to the skin of the femoral triangle and scrotum/labia majora. The subcostal nerve (T12) supplies lower portions of the external abdominal oblique muscle. The pelvic splanchnic nerves supply autonomic (parasympathetic) innervation to the pelvic viscera. The tenth thoracic spinal nerve (T10) supplies abdominal muscles superior to the inguinal region.

389. The answer is c. *(April, 3/e, p 388.)* In response to the decreased blood pressure in the afferent glomerular arteriole, increased chloride concentration in the distal convoluted tubule, or sympathetic nerve stimulation, the juxtaglomerular cells secrete renin into the circulation. Renin reacts with a plasma α-globulin (angiotensinogen) to produce angiotensin I, which is converted in the lung to vasoactive angiotensin II. Angiotensin II also stimulates the adrenal zona glomerulosa to produce aldosterone, which promotes sodium, chloride, and water uptake by the distal tubule and thereby, raises blood volume and pressure. The renal cortex is the principal source of erythropoietin. The stimuli for production appear to be decreased partial pressure of oxygen (indicative of insufficient erythrocytes) and high-chloride concentration in the distal tubule (indicative of decreased blood volume). Although the cellular source is unknown, the most likely candidates are the juxtaglomerular cells and the lacis cells, both of which contain granules. Glucocorticoids and mineralocorticoids, as well as sex hormones, are products of the adrenal cortex.

390. The answer is b. *(Moore, Developing Human, 6/e, pp 304–309.)* The kidney forms in three stages. The pronephric, metanephric, and mesonephric kidneys all form from the urogenital ridge, an extension of intermediate mesoderm into the coelomic cavity. Mesoderm derived from the somites (somitic) gives rise to components of the axial skeleton and associated muscle and connective tissues. Splanchnic lateral plate mesoderm gives rise to the smooth muscle and connective tissue tunics of the abdominal viscera. Somatic lateral plate mesoderm contributes substantially to the skeleton, connective tissue, and muscle mass of the appendages.

391. The answer is a. *(Moore, Anatomy, 4/e, pp 47–49, 287.)* The adrenal medulla is innervated from thoracic levels of the spinal cord mediated by preganglionic sympathetic nerve fibers traveling in the lesser and least splanchnic nerves, with some contribution from the greater splanchnic and lumbar splanchnic nerves. Because both the adrenal medulla and postganglionic sympathetic neurons are adrenergic and derived from neural crest tissue, the homology of the chromaffin cells and postganglionic sympathetic neurons is apparent. There appears to be no parasympathetic innervation to the adrenal medulla and no innervation whatever to the adrenal cortex.

392. The answer is d. *(Moore, Anatomy, 4/e, pp 286–287.)* The venous drainage from each adrenal gland tends to be through a single vein. The left adrenal gland usually drains into the left renal vein superior to the point where the gonadal vein enters the left renal vein. The left adrenal vein usually anastomoses with the hemiazygos vein and may provide an important route of collateral venous return. The right adrenal gland usually drains directly into the inferior vena cava.

393. The answer is a. *(Moore, Anatomy, 4/e, pp 205–207.)* A direct inguinal hernia protrudes through a space bounded superolaterally by the inferior epigastric vessels and medially by the rectus abdominus muscle. It is found superior to the inguinal ligament in Hesselbach's triangle. The other statements are true only of an indirect inguinal hernia, which is the most common. A direct hernia traverses only the most medial part of the inguinal canal and is not covered by the most internal layers of spermatic cord fascia.

394. The answer is d. (*April, 3/e, pp 383–384.*) The diffuse central abdominal pain in the patient presented is probably referred pain from the loop of small bowel incarcerated within the herniated peritoneal sac. Compression of the bowel results in compromise of the blood supply and subsequent ischemic necrosis. The visceral afferent fibers from the distal small bowel travel along the blood vessels to reach the superior mesenteric plexus and lesser splanchnic nerves, which they follow to the T10–T11 levels of the spinal cord. The pain, therefore, is referred to (appears as if originating from) the T10–T11 dermatomes, which supply the umbilical region. Because the gut develops as a midline structure, visceral pain tends to be centrally located regardless of the adult location of any particular region of the gut. As a result of dilation of the inguinal canal by the hernial sac, however, the patient also experiences localized somatic pain mediated by the iliohypogastric, ilioinguinal, and genitofemoral nerves.

395. The answer is b. (*Moore, Anatomy, 4/e, pp 188–189.*) The deep circumflex iliac artery, which arises from the internal iliac artery opposite the inferior epigastric artery, parallels the inguinal ligament as it courses toward the anterosuperior iliac spine. The external pudendal and superficial epigastric arteries are branches of the femoral artery that supply, respectively, the superficial pubic (hypogastric) region, the inguinal regions, and the anterior surfaces of the scrotum or labia majora. The inferior epigastric artery, a branch of the external iliac artery, courses superomedially beneath the aponeuroses of the abdominal wall to gain access to the rectus sheath by passing anterior to the arcuate line (of Douglas). An aberrant obturator artery (present in about 30% of the population) usually arises from the inferior epigastric artery and courses inferiorly deep to the pubic ramus to the obturator foramen.

396. The answer is c. (*Moore, Anatomy, 4/e, p 200.*) Several abdominal structures are involved in the formation of the spermatic cord. The deep fascia contributes the external spermatic fascia. Although some references include the external oblique muscle or aponeurosis, no contribution is derived from that layer owing to a hiatus in the aponeurosis. The cremaster muscle, a contribution of the internal oblique muscle, joins the spermatic cord as the inguinal canal passes through that layer. The transversus abdominis muscle, which usually terminates as the falx inguinalis just superior to the deep ring, contributes to the cremaster muscle in less than 5% of all males. The transversalis fascia contributes the internal spermatic fascia.

397. The answer is e. *(April, 3/e, pp 325–326.)* The ilioinguinal nerve exits the abdominal wall through the superficial inguinal ring, where it is applied to the anterior surface of the spermatic cord. Section of this nerve will result in paresthesia over the base of the penis and scrotum. The femoral branch of the genitofemoral nerve innervates the upper medial surface of the thigh, where it mediates the afferent limb of the cremasteric reflex. The efferent limb of this reflex is carried by the genital branch of the genitofemoral nerve, which lies within the cremaster layer. The dartos response, which is sympathetic, arises from the sacral sympathetic chain and reaches the pudendal nerve via gray rami communicantes.

398. The answer is e. *(April, 3/e, p 327.)* The femoral canal provides a lymphatic pathway from the lower extremity, as well as from the lower abdominal region, to the external iliac nodes. An invariable occupant of the femoral ring is a large lymph node known as Cloquet's gland that becomes swollen as a result of foot or leg infections. The femoral nerve is located in the muscular compartment with the psoas muscle lateral to the femoral artery and vein.

399. The answer is b. *(Moore, Anatomy, 4/e, pp 256–257.)* Infectious mononucleosis is a virus-induced illness leading to swollen lymph nodes and spleen. The splenomegaly is evidenced by the very rounded contours of the organ. Infectious mononucleosis can exhibit liver involvement; however, the organ indicated is not the liver but the spleen in the upper left hypochondrium. The bright organ between it and the vertebra is the left kidney. The liver is on the opposite side of the abdominal cavity.

400. The answer is c. *(Moore, Anatomy, 4/e, p 231.)* The splenic artery originates from the celiac trunk and courses tortuously along the posterior aspect of the pancreas. The left gastric artery is a separate branch of the celiac trunk and courses along the lesser curvature of the stomach where it anastomoses with the right gastric artery, a branch of hepatic artery. The right gastro-omental (gastroepiploic) artery is a branch of the gastroduodenal artery and courses along the greater curvature of the stomach.

401. The answer is d. (*Moore, Anatomy, 4/e, p. 315.*) This MR image is taken at the L1 level (upper abdomen). It shows the abdominal aorta lying against the lumbar vertebra (to the left of it). It is flanked by the two crura of the respiratory diaphragm (the one on the right is labeled "B"). The vessel that originates from the abdominal aorta at this level is the celiac trunk. Therefore, the vessel labeled "A" is the splenic artery that winds to the right to supply the pancreas, which stretches from the duodenum (R) to the anterior end of the left kidney. Although the common hepatic and left gastric arteries originate from the celiac trunk at about the same level as the splenic artery, they are not recorded at this precise level. These vessels branched off the aorta at a slightly higher level. The gastroduodenal artery does occur at this level, but it is located further to the right.

402. The answer is c. (*Moore, Anatomy, 4/e, p. 315.*) Structure "B" is the right crus of the diaphragm. The right and left crura of the diaphragm form the aortic hiatus (T12 level), which is traversed by the descending aorta, thoracic duct, and the azygos vein (variably).

403 to 404. The answers are 403-b, 404-c. (*Moore, Anatomy, 4/e, pp 285, 386–387, 395.*) Sensation produced by distention of the rectum travels along the pelvic splanchnic nerves to sacral levels S2–S4. Fecal continence is effected by nerves from the S2–S4 segments of the spinal cord. The principal effector, the puborectalis portion of the levator ani muscle, is innervated by somatic twigs from the sacral plexus. Control of the external anal sphincter is by the pudendal nerve, which also carries pain sensation associated with external hemorrhoids.

405 to 406. The answers are 405-d, 406-d. (*April, 3/e, pp 375–377.*) The body and tail of the pancreas receive most of their blood supply from the splenic artery via the great pancreatic, dorsal pancreatic, and caudal pancreatic arteries. The head of the pancreas is supplied by the superior pancreaticoduodenal artery that arises from the gastroduodenal branch of the common hepatic artery. In addition, the pancreatic head is supplied by the inferior pancreaticoduodenal arteries that arise from the superior mesenteric artery.

The chief supply to the left side of the gastric fundus is from the splenic artery via the short gastric branches. The splenic artery also gives rise to the left gastro-omental artery that runs along the greater curvature to anastomose with the right gastro-omental branch that arises indirectly from the common hepatic artery.

407 to 408. The answers are 407-a, 408-c. *(Moore, Anatomy, 4/e, pp 294–295.)* The diaphragm possesses three principal hiatuses shown in the diagram accompanying the question: the hiatus for the inferior vena cava (A), the esophageal hiatus (C), and the aortic hiatus (E). Potential diaphragmatic developmental defects include the foramen of Morgagni (B), just lateral to the xiphoid attachment of the diaphragm, and the pleuroperitoneal canal of Bochdalek (D), which is the most common site for congenital hernias.

The inferior vena cava and frequently small branches of the right phrenic nerve pass through a hiatus (A) slightly to the right of the midline at the T8 level. The left phrenic nerve usually passes through the central tendon of the diaphragm on the left side to innervate the left hemidiaphragm from below. The esophageal hiatus (C) just to the left of the midline at the T10 level transmits the esophagus, the left and right vagus nerves, and the esophageal branches of the left gastric artery and vein. An acquired hiatal hernia usually is the consequence of a short esophagus or of a weakened esophageal hiatus.

The two diaphragmatic crura are joined superiorly by the median arcuate ligament to form an opening (E) at the T12 level. The aortic hiatus transmits the aorta, thoracic duct, and a continuation of the azygos vein into the abdomen. The splanchnic nerves penetrate the crura on each side of the aortic hiatus to reach the abdomen.

409 to 410. The answers are 409-b, 410-e. *(April, 3/e, pp 32, 394.)* Epigastric herniation is a frequent postoperative complication to a midline incision through the linea alba, but rare otherwise. Congenital umbilical hernia, which has an embryologic basis, occurs in about 1 in 50 births. It may be apparent at birth (omphalocele), or it may occur spontaneously in infants and children. Spigelian hernia may also occur along the linea semilunaris inferior to the arcuate line. In addition, a spigelian hernia may enter the rectus sheath at the arcuate line.

411 to 412. The answers are 411-c, 412-b. *(April, 3/e, pp 345, 362, 370, 374.)*

Abdominal Visceral Afferent Pathways			
Organ	**Afferent Pathway**	**Level**	**Referral Area**
Heart	Thoracic splanchnic nn.	T1–T4	Upper thorax, postaxial arm
Foregut (region supplied by celiac artery)	Greater splanchnic n.	T5–T9	Lower thorax; Epigastric region
Midgut (region supplied by superior mesenteric artery)	Lesser splanchnic n.	T10–T11	Umbilical region
Kidneys, upper ureter	Least splanchnic n.	T12	Subcostal and hypogastric regions
Hindgut (region supplied by inferior mesenteric artery)	Lumbar splanchnic nn.	L1–L2	Lumbar, and inguinal regions; Lateral and anterior thigh

Pelvis

Questions

DIRECTIONS: Each item below contains a question or incomplete statement followed by suggested responses. Select the **one best** response to each question.

413. Which of the following is a characteristic of the male (compared with the female) pelvis?

a. An oval-shaped (as opposed to a heart-shaped) pelvic inlet
b. A relatively shallow (as opposed to deep) false pelvis with ilia that are flared
c. A pelvic outlet of larger diameter
d. A narrow subpubic angle between the pubic rami

414. Which of the following is unchanged during childbirth?

a. The diameter between the sacral promontory and the pubic symphysis
b. The separation between the pubic rami
c. The distance between the pubic symphysis and the tip of the coccyx
d. The width of the pelvic outlet

415. The gubernaculum is a continuous mesenchymal condensation extending from the caudal pole of each testis through the inguinal canal to the scrotal swelling, inferiorly. In the female it becomes the

a. Canal of Nuck
b. Ligament of the ovary
c. Round ligament of the uterus
d. Round ligament of the uterus and the ligament of the ovary

416. An extension of the abdominal cavity is present in the scrotum. It is represented in the adult male by the

a. Cremaster muscle
b. Gubernaculum
c. Spermatic cord
d. Tunica vaginalis

417. Following childbirth, a woman experienced urinary incontinence, particularly when coughing. This was most likely caused by tearing of the

a. Puborectalis muscle
b. Obturator internus muscle
c. Pubococcygeus muscle
d. Superficial transverse perineus muscle
e. Piriformis muscle

418. The efferent limb of the cremaster reflex is provided by the

a. Femoral branch of the genitofemoral nerve
b. Genital branch of the genitofemoral nerve
c. Ilioinguinal nerve
d. Pudendal nerve
e. Temperature differential between core body temperature and scrotal temperature

Questions 419 to 420

A 36-year-old man complained to his physician of occasional dull throbbing pain associated with the right testis and scrotum. Examination indicated varicocele of the pampiniform plexus. The physician remarked that in all probability the patient had this condition since adolescence and should not be bothered by it. The patient was emphatic that the condition had arisen within the last few months. Surgery was considered.

419. Factors that should be considered by the physician at this point include the fact that varicocele of the pampiniform plexus on the right side

a. Is very uncommon
b. Occurs about as often as that on the left side
c. May be the result of testicular torsion
d. May be associated with a long, redundant mesorchium

420. On gaining access to the peritoneal cavity and locating the testicular vein, it was noted that the vein was inexplicably dilated. Further exploration revealed a large retroperitoneal mass in the vicinity of the lower pole of the kidney that encroached on the vein so that it did not drain freely into the

a. Hepatic portal vein
b. Inferior vena cava
c. Internal iliac vein
d. Right renal vein
e. Right suprarenal vein

421. Following surgery involving the lateral wall of the pelvis, a patient reported anesthesia over the medial thigh. Subsequent examination revealed weakened adduction of the thigh. Which nerve was most likely injured during the pelvic surgery?

a. Pudendal nerve
b. Genitofemoral nerve
c. Superior gluteal nerve
d. Femoral nerve
e. Obturator nerve

422. Which of the following statements correctly pertains to the dartos tunic of the scrotum?

a. It is formed by the fusion of the two layers of superficial fascia of the perineum
b. It is invested with adipose tissue
c. It participates in the cremaster reflex
d. It receives innervation from the genital branch of the genitofemoral nerve
e. It responds to cold temperatures by lowering the testes away from the body

423. Fructose, a source of energy for spermatozoa, is found primarily in secretions from the

a. Bulbourethral glands
b. Epididymis
c. Prostate
d. Seminal vesicles
e. Testis

424. In this CT of the pelvis, the muscle indicated by the arrow is the

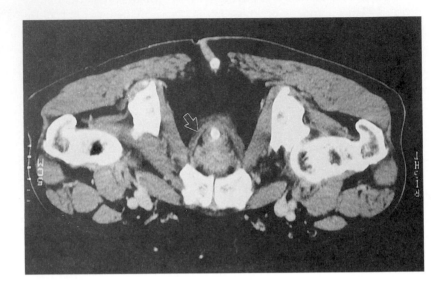

a. Sphincter urethrae/urogenital diaphragm
b. Levator ani/pelvic diaphragm
c. Obturator internus
d. Obturator externus

425. Benign prostatic hypertrophy results in obstruction of the urinary tract. This specific condition is associated with enlargement of the

a. Entire prostate gland
b. Lateral lobes
c. Median lobe
d. Posterior lobes

426. The external urethral sphincter in the female is

a. A modified portion of the pelvic diaphragm
b. Continuous completely around the urethra
c. Innervated by the pudendal nerve
d. Subject to involuntary control

427. In the male, the homologue of the vaginal artery is the

a. Obturator artery
b. Internal pudendal artery
c. Middle rectal artery
d. Umbilical artery
e. Inferior vesical artery

Questions 428 to 431

A 24-year-old woman seeking assistance for apparent infertility has been unable to conceive despite repeated attempts in five years of marriage. She revealed that her husband had fathered a child in a prior marriage. Although her menstrual periods are fairly regular, they are accompanied by extreme lower back pain.

428. The lower back pain during menstruation experienced by this woman probably is referred from the pelvic region. The pathways that convey this pain sensation to the central nervous system involve the

a. Hypogastric nerve to L1–L2
b. Lumbosacral trunk to L4–L5
c. Pelvic splanchnic nerves to S2–S4
d. Pudendal nerve to S2–S4

429. Which of the following would be found immediately inferior to the left cardinal (lateral cervical) ligament?

a. Ovarian neurovascular bundle
b. Uterine tube
c. Round ligament of the uterus
d. Ureter
e. Uterine artery and vein

430. The patient is scheduled for a hysterosalpingogram, in which radiopaque material is injected into the uterus and uterine tubes. Examination of subsequent radiographs discloses bilateral spillage of the contrast medium into the peritoneal cavity, an indication that

a. The uterine tubes are normal
b. The mesonephric ducts failed to form properly
c. The paramesonephric ducts failed to form properly
d. There is a rectouterine fistula
e. There is a vesicovaginal fistula

431. The most important measurement of the pelvic outlet, indicating the LEAST dimension, is the transverse midplane diameter. It is measured between the

a. Ischial spines
b. Ischial tuberosities
c. Lower margin of the pubic symphysis to the sacroiliac joint
d. Sacral promontory to the inferior margin of the pubic symphysis

432. At delivery, caudal analgesia is induced by administration of anesthetic into the epidural space in the sacral region. The needle is introduced via the

a. Anterior sacral foramina
b. Dural sac
c. Intervertebral foramina
d. Posterior sacral foramina
e. Sacral hiatus

433. Which of the following structures is most susceptible to unintentional damage during a hysterectomy?

a. Uterine artery
b. Ureter
c. Urinary bladder
d. Urethra
e. Kidney

434. The patient is a 45-year-old male with a history of colonic diverticulosis. He complains of fever with pain and swelling in the rectal area. You are concerned that the colonic diverticulum may have become infected (diverticulitis) and ruptured into the space indicated by the * in this CT scan. Which of the following is correct regarding the indicated space?

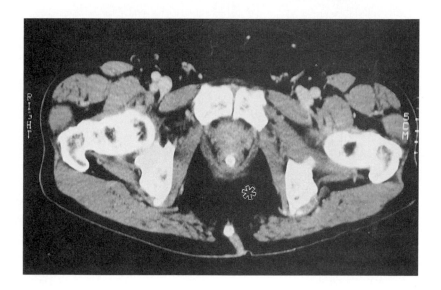

a. It is called the paracolic gutter
b. The space is largely filled with muscle
c. The space is located superior to the pelvic diaphragm
d. Pus from the abscessed diverticuli in that space can extend anteriorly to the perineal body, inferior to the urogenital diaphragm
e. Pus from the abscessed diverticuli in that space can extend superiorly anterior to the sacrum

435. Which of the following arteries may occasionally arise as a branch of the external iliac artery or inferior epigastric artery instead of as a branch of the internal iliac artery?

a. Internal pudendal artery
b. Obturator artery
c. Superior gluteal artery
d. Umbilical artery
e. Uterine artery

436. Sympathetic and parasympathetic nerves reach the pelvic plexus by different pathways. If, during surgical resection of the rectum, the sympathetic nerves were excised bilaterally, which of the following complications would ensue?

a. A dilated and neurogenic bladder
b. Loss of control of the external urethral sphincter
c. Impotence (inability to obtain erection)
d. Inability to ejaculate

437. The role of the sympathetic chain in the pelvis is primarily

a. Bladder contraction
b. Cutaneous function (sudomotor, vasomotor, pilomotor)
c. Ejaculation in males
d. Erection in both male and female
e. Urinary continence

438. Which of the following statements concerning erection, emission, and ejaculation in the male is correct?

a. Contraction of the urethra is under control of the sympathetic nervous system
b. The parasympathetic nerves stimulate closure of the sphincter of the urinary bladder
c. Sympathetic neurons stimulate the helicine arteries to dilate and increase blood flow to the corpora cavernosum
d. Parasympathetic innervation stimulates emission of seminal fluid
e. Contraction of the bulbospongiosus and ischiocavernosus muscles impedes the drainage of blood from the corpora cavernosa

439. A 45-year-old man was riding a snowmobile and hit a snow-covered rocky outcropping. While recovering from the accident, he slipped and fell on the outcropping and now is experiencing pain in the gluteal region. In this CT scan, the dark linear structure indicated by the arrow is

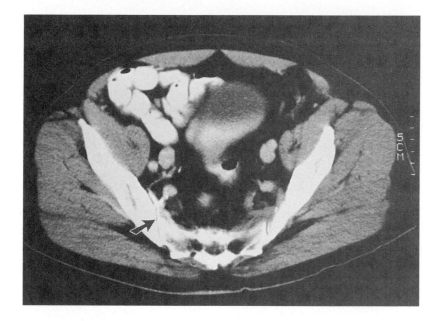

a. A fracture of the ilium
b. The sacroiliac joint
c. A spinal nerve
d. The superior gluteal artery
e. The inferior gluteal artery

Questions 440 to 441

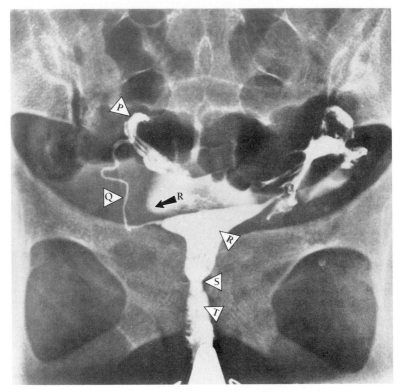

(Reproduced, with permission, from Wicke L: Atlas of Radiological Anatomy, 6/e. Baltimore, MD: Williams & Wilkins, 1998.)

440. The area labeled "P" in the above hysterosalpingogram is the most likely site for which of the following events?

a. Ovulation
b. Fertilization
c. Morula formation
d. Blastocyst formation
e. Implantation

441. Which of the following enters the area marked "R" on the fourth/fifth day following fertilization?

a. A 2-cell preembryo
b. A 16-cell preembryo
c. A morula
d. A secondary oocyte
e. A blastocyst

442. Which of the following contains the ovarian neurovascular bundle?

a. Broad ligament
b. Mesosalpinx
c. Mesovarium
d. Suspensory ligament
e. Transverse cervical ligament

443. Which of the following empties into the penile urethra?

a. Ampulla of the vas deferens
b. Bulbourethral gland
c. Ejaculatory duct
d. Prostate gland
e. Seminal vesicle

444. Match the uterine cervix with the referral area of its afferent innervation.

a. Epigastric region
b. Lateral thigh and buttock
c. Inguinal and pubic regions, anterior scrotum or labia majora, medial thigh
d. Lateral leg and foot, perineum
e. Subcostal and umbilical regions

445. The diagram below represents a frontal section through the bladder and prostate gland. Select the lettered structure that forms the external urethral sphincter.

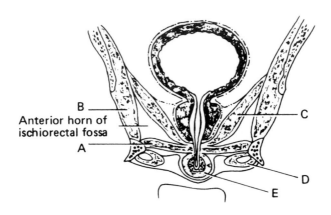

Questions 446 to 447

For each female pelvic structure, select the appropriate male homologue.

a. Corpus cavernosum
b. Corpus spongiosum
c. Penile (cavernous) urethra
d. Scrotal raphe
e. Scrotum

446. Vestibular bulbs

447. Glans clitoridis

Questions 448 to 449

Match each region to the lymph nodes to which it principally drains.

a. Deep inguinal nodes
b. Internal iliac nodes
c. Para-aortic nodes
d. Superficial inguinal nodes

448. Subcutaneous tissues of the penis

449. Vulva and inferior vagina

Pelvis

Answers

413. The answer is d. (*April, 3/e, p 410. Moore, Anatomy, 4/e, p 337.*) The male pelvis is generally heavier than the female pelvis, with stronger bone structure and more definitive muscle markings, which reflect the larger male musculature and generally heavier male build. The generally wider and shallower female pelvis is more suited to childbearing. In the female the false pelvis tends to be shallower with flared ilia, the pelvic inlet more oval, and the pelvic outlet larger than in the male. Also, the subpubic angle between inferior pubic rami is significantly greater in the female than in the male and is perhaps the best identifying feature of the female pelvis.

414. The answer is a. (*Moore, Anatomy, 4/e, pp 340–341.*) During childbirth, sex hormones and the release of relaxin allow loosening of several joints including the sacroiliac joints and the pubic symphysis. This, however, does not change the position of the sacral promontory relative to the pubic symphysis. Loosening of the pubic symphysis does allow the pubic rami to separate slightly, increasing the lateral diameter of the pelvis. Posterior rotation of the coccyx increases the anteroposterior dimension of the pelvic outlet.

415. The answer is d. (*Moore, Anatomy, 4/e, p 197.*) The gubernaculum, which runs from the gonadal anlage to the sexually undifferentiated labioscrotal fold, guides the descent of the testes into the scrotum in the male and the descent of the ovary into the deep pelvis in the female. In the female, the developing uterus grows into the gubernacular tract and divides it into the proper ligament of the ovary and the round ligament of the uterus. Thus, the proper ligament of the ovary runs within the broad ligament from the medial pole of each ovary to the uterus. It then continues within the broad ligament as the round ligament of the uterus into the deep inguinal ring and thereby gains access to the canal of Nuck (the female homologue of the inguinal canal) to insert into the major labial folds.

416. The answer is d. (*April, 3/e, p 429.*) The peritoneal sac extends through the spermatic cord as the processus vaginalis, which continues into the scrotum as the tunica vaginalis testis. After the neonatal period, the processus vaginalis loses its patency, and thereby separates the tunica vaginalis from the peritoneal cavity. The gubernaculum is a band of connective tissue that extends between the inferior pole of the testis to the scrotal fold and directs the descent of the testis into the scrotum. The cremaster muscle is derived from the internal oblique muscle of the abdominal wall.

417. The answer is c. *(Moore, Anatomy, 4/e, p 345.)* The puborectalis, pubococcygeus, and iliococcygeus comprise the levator ani, the main muscular component of the pelvic floor. The pubococcygeus is the part of the levator ani most frequently damaged during parturition. Because the pubococcygeus surrounds and supports the neck of the bladder and the proximal urethra, urinary leakage is a common result, particularly during increased abdominopelvic pressure, e.g., during coughing. Damage to the puborectalis would result in fecal incontinence under similar situations. Both the obturator internus muscle and the piriformis are parts of the lateral wall of the pelvis and assist in lateral rotation of the thigh.

418. The answer is b. *(April, 3/e, p 429.)* The cremaster reflex is mediated by the genitofemoral nerve. The femoral branch supplies the afferent limb, and the genital branch supplies the efferent limb. The ilioinguinal nerve provides sensory innervation to the medial aspects of the thigh and the anterior aspects of the mons or the base of the penis. The pudendal nerve provides sensation to most of the skin of the perineum as well as the motor supply to the perineal muscles. The involuntary scrotal reflex is based on temperature: warmth causes relaxation of the dartos muscle, whereas cold causes contraction.

419. The answer is a. *(April, 3/e, pp 456–457.)* Varicocele usually occurs on the left side and is rare on the right. Left varicocele results from local venous congestion caused by compression of the testicular vein as it passes beneath the usually full sigmoid colon. Testicular torsion, wherein a long mesorchium is a contributing factor, strangulates the testicular artery and produces testicular ischemia.

420. The answer is b. *(April, 3/e, p 457.)* The right testicular vein normally empties into the inferior vena cava. The left testicular vein usually drains into the left renal vein. Although variations are not uncommon, the testicular veins never drain into the hepatic portal system.

421. The answer is e. (*Moore, Anatomy, 4/e, pp 300, 347–348.*) The obturator nerve runs on the lateral surface of the pelvic wall and exits the pelvis through a canal in the obturator membrane. It innervates the adductor muscles of the medial thigh (a. magnus, a. longus, a. brevis, pectineus, and gracilis). The pudendal nerve exits the pelvic cavity via the greater sciatic foramen and enters the perineum via the lesser sciatic foramen. It innervates the perineal muscles and the skin of the genitalia. The genitofemoral nerve supplies skin over the femoral triangle and scrotum/labia majora. The superior gluteal nerve innervates the gluteus medius and gluteus minimus, which are powerful abductors of the thigh. The femoral nerve innervates the quadriceps muscles, which extend the leg at the knee joint.

422. The answer is a. (*April, 3/e, pp 428, 429–430.*) The two layers of superficial perineal fascia, i.e., the superficial layer of subcutaneous fascia (Cruveilhier's) and the deep layer of subcutaneous fascia (Colles'), fuse to form the dartos tunic of the scrotum. However, the superficial layer loses its fat and picks up smooth muscle. The smooth muscle of the dartos is responsive to temperature. The dartos muscle relaxes when too warm, which drops the testes away from the body, and contracts when too cool, which brings the testes closer to the body. This provides a thermoregulatory mechanism that helps maintain the optimum temperature for spermatogenesis. The cremaster reflex is associated with the spermatic cord and raises the testes within the scrotum as a protective measure. The afferent limb and efferent limbs of the cremaster reflex are provided, respectively, by the femoral and genital branches of the genitofemoral nerve.

423. The answer is d. (*April, 3/e, p 459.*) The thick secretion from the seminal vesicles contributes substantially to the ejaculate volume that conveys the spermatozoa. The high fructose content of secretions of the seminal vesicles provides the primary metabolic energy source for sperm motility. The flavins that are contributed to the ejaculate by the seminal vesicles fluoresce strongly in ultraviolet light, a phenomenon that supplies a useful forensic test for the presence of semen.

424. The answer is b. (*Moore, Anatomy, 4/e, pp 395–399, 555–556.*) The muscle indicated is attached to the pubic bone and extends around the rectum. It is the puborectalis portion of the levator ani (pelvic diaphragm).

The puborectalis is responsible for fecal continence. The urogenital diaphragm is positioned inferior to the pelvic diaphragm and includes the deep transverse perineus muscle. The obturator internus covers the lateral wall of the lesser pelvis. The obturator externus is found in the deep thigh.

425. The answer is c. (*April, 3/e, pp 460–461.*) Benign prostatic hypertrophy is the result of enlargement of the median lobe, which may compress the prostatic urethra to the point of obstruction. This hypertrophic tissue may also protrude into the urinary bladder to prevent complete emptying. The posterior lobes are commonly associated with malignant transformation. The lateral (anterior) lobes tend to be asymptomatic.

426. The answer is c. (*Moore, Anatomy, 4/e, pp 396–398.*) The external urethral sphincter, which partially surrounds the membranous portion of the urethra in the female, is a modified portion of the deep transverse perineal muscle of the urogenital diaphragm. Somatically innervated by the deep perineal branches of the pudendal nerve, the sphincter, in addition to contracting with the musculature of the pelvic and urogenital diaphragms on coughing or sneezing, can be voluntarily contracted to maintain urinary continence once the desire to micturate is experienced. However, the effectiveness of this muscle is greater in the male, where it completely surrounds the membranous urethra.

427. The answer is e. (*Moore, Anatomy, 4/e, 350–351.*) All of the listed choices are branches of the internal iliac artery. The inferior vesical artery in the male supplies the seminal vesicle, prostate, fundus of the bladder, distal ureter, and the vas deferens. In the female, the vaginal artery supplies the vagina, urinary bladder, and pelvic portion of the urethra. The obturator artery gives off muscular and nutrient branches within the pelvis and then leaves the pelvis via the obturator canal to supply the thigh. The internal pudendal artery crosses the piriformis muscle, exits the pelvic cavity via the greater sciatic foramen, and enters the ischiorectal fossa via the lesser sciatic foramen. It supplies the external genitalia (penis and clitoris). The middle rectal artery supplies the inferior rectum and forms important anastomoses with other rectal arteries. The umbilical artery gives off the superior vesical artery in both sexes. Its distal portion degenerates to form the medial umbilical ligament.

428. The answer is a. *(April, 3/e, p 470.)* The visceral afferent fibers that mediate sensation from the fundus and body of the uterus, as well as from the oviducts, tend to travel along the sympathetic nerve pathways (via the hypogastric nerve and lumbar splanchnics) to reach the upper lumbar levels (L1–L2) of the spinal cord. Thus, uterine pain will be referred to (appear as if originating from) the upper lumbar dermatomes and produce apparent backache. The visceral afferent fibers that mediate sensation from the cervical neck of the uterus travel along the parasympathetic pathways (via the pelvic splanchnic nerves [nervi erigentes]) to the midsacral levels (S2–S4) of the spinal cord. In this instance, pain originating from the cervix will be referred to the midsacral dermatomes and produce pain that appears to arise from the perineum, gluteal region, and legs.

429. The answer is d. *(Moore, Anatomy, 4/e, p 378.)* The ureter, lying just medial to the internal iliac artery in the deep pelvis, passes from posterior to anterior immediately inferior to the lateral cervical ligament. This ligament contains the uterine artery and vein to which the ureters pass inferior approximately midway along their course between internal iliac artery and uterus. The ureter continues inferior to the anterior portion of the lateral cervical ligament (where it can sometimes be palpated through the walls of the vagina at the lateral fornices) to gain access to the base of the urinary bladder. The close association between uterine vessels and ureter is of major importance during surgical procedures in the female pelvis.

430. The answer is a. *(Moore, Anatomy, 4/e, p 382.)* The uterus is formed by fusion of the paired paramesonephric ducts. The uterine tubes are the unfused portions of these ducts. Patency of the uterine tubes may be ascertained by hysterosalpingography, wherein radiopaque material is injected into the uterine cavity and uterine tubes through a catheter inserted into the external cervical os. Radiographs delineate the cavity of the body of the uterus and the uterine tubes. Spillage of the contrast material through the abdominal ostia into the peritoneal cavity demonstrates normal patency of the uterine tubes. The abdominal ostia of the uterine tubes permit passage of infection, air, and spermatozoa into the female peritoneal cavity. The rare rectouterine fistula would result in the appearance of contrast media in the rectum. A vesicovaginal fistula between the vagina and urethra or bladder would not be evident on a hysterosalpingogram.

431. The answer is a. *(April, 3/e, p 410.)* The transverse midplane diameter is measured between the ischial spines. It can be approximated by the somewhat greater transverse diameter measured between the ischial tuberosities. The distance from the lower margin of the pubic symphysis to the sacroiliac joint defines the sagittal diameter, which is usually the greatest dimension and, therefore, unimportant.

432. The answer is e. *(Moore, Anatomy, 3/e, pp 334–337.)* Caudal analgesia can be induced by injection of anesthetic through the sacral hiatus into the sacral epidural space of the vertebral canal well caudal to the termination of the dural sac. The sacral hiatus represents the absence of a complete neural arch of the fifth sacral vertebra. The four anterior and posterior sacral foramina on either side of the midline join the intervertebral foramen and provide egress for the anterior and posterior primary rami of the sacral spinal nerves. The level to which the anesthesia blocks the spinal nerves is a function of the amount delivered.

433. The answer is b. *(Moore, Anatomy, 4/e, p 382.)* The uterine artery crosses anterior and superior to the ureter near the lateral fornix of the vagina. Some clinicians and anatomists used to refer to the uterine artery as "the bridge over troubled waters." Because of its close proximity to the artery, the ureter may be accidentally ligated or severed during tying off of the artery. Of course, the bladder and the kidney are large structures and should not be mistaken or unnoticed. The urethra should be far out of the operating field.

434. The answer is d. *(Moore, Anatomy, 4/e, p 395.)* The ischioanal fossa is a fat-filled space that extends from below the levator ani muscle (puborectalis, pubococcygeus, and iliococcygeus muscles). It also extends anteriorly in the area between the pelvic diaphragm (superiorly) and the urogenital diaphragm (inferiorly). It cannot extend superiorly above the pelvic diaphragm and, therefore, cannot extend superiorly anterior to the sacrum.

435. The answer is b. *(Moore, Anatomy, 4/e, pp 546–547.)* The obturator usually arises from the anterior trunk of the internal iliac artery. However, in 25 to 30% of the population, it arises from the inferior epigastric or the external iliac artery. There is considerable variation as to the origins of the branches of the posterior and anterior trunks of the internal iliac artery. The internal pudendal artery, umbilical artery, and uterine artery almost always arise from the anterior trunk. The superior gluteal usually arises from the posterior trunk.

436. The answer is d. *(Moore, Anatomy, 4/e, p 411.)* Loss of sympathetic innervation to the pelvic plexus results in an inability to ejaculate. Parasympathetic innervation in this region mediates penile erection, without which ejaculation probably cannot occur. The afferent and efferent limbs of the detrusor reflex, which controls reflex emptying of the bladder, also travel in the nervi erigentes with the parasympathetics. Thus, injury to this pathway would result in a dilated bladder. Voluntary control of the external anal sphincter and levator ani muscles is mediated through branches of the pudendal nerve.

437. The answer is b. *(April, 3/e, pp 32–33.)* Postsynaptic sympathetic neurons destined for the skin lie in the ganglia of the sympathetic chain. Although the preganglionic fibers arise between T1 and L2, each of the sacral ganglia has a gray ramus that brings postganglionic fibers to the associated spinal nerve. These sympathetic neurons mediate sweating, vasodilation, and piloerection in dermatomes S1–S5. The preganglionic sympathetic fibers regulating male ejaculation travel via the lumbar splanchnic nerves, thereby bypassing the sympathetic chain ganglia.

438. The answer is e. *(Moore, Anatomy, 4/e, p 411.)* The bulbospongiosus and ischiocavernosus muscles are innervated by the pudendal nerve (S2–S4). Concomitant with dilation of the helicine arteries under parasympathetic innervation, which allows blood to flow into the cavernous spaces, contraction of the bulbospongiosus and ischiocavernosus muscles at the base of the cavernous bodies prevents blood from leaving, resulting in engorgement and penile erection. Contraction of the smooth muscle of the urethra (ejaculation) is a parasympathetic function, whereas closure of the sphincter of the urinary bladder is under sympathetic control. Emission of seminal fluid and prostatic secretions is due to contraction of smooth muscle under sympathetic control.

439. The answer is b. *(Moore, Anatomy, 4/e, pp 339–341, 418–423.)* The indicated line represents the sacroiliac joint. These structures are seen bilaterally between the alae of the sacrum and the ilia. The sacroiliac ligaments might have been sprained by the trauma of the fall. The pathway for spinal nerves is through foramina of the sacrum, not through long bony canals. Similarly, the pathway for the gluteal arteries is through the greater sciatic foramen between the ilium and the sacrum. However, the bones are not contiguous at that level.

440. The answer is b. *(Sadler, 8/e, pp 37, 45; Moore, Anatomy, 4/e, pp 418–423.)* Ovulation occurs at the midpoint of the ovarian cycle (± day 14). The secondary oocyte at metaphase 1 stage is expelled from the graafian follicle and passes through the peritoneal cavity before being "captured" by the fimbriae of fallopian tube and wafted into this tube. Fertilization normally occurs in the dilated ampullary region of the fallopian tube. Site "P" locates this area. Ovulation occurs at the surface of the ovary; the morula and the blastocyst form in the more distal parts of the fallopian tube; implantation occurs in the uterine cavity (R).

441. The answer is e. *(Sadler, 8/e, pp 42–45; Moore, Anatomy, 4/e, pp 418–423.)* On the fourth or fifth day following fertilization, the developing preembryo becomes the blastocyst, which contains the embryoblast. It enters the uterine cavity at the site indicated by R. At this site the fallopian tube empties into the uterine cavity before being implanted into the wall of the uterine cavity (fifth to sixth day following fertilization).

442. The answer is d. *(Moore, Anatomy, 4/e, pp 377–378.)* The mesosalpinx, mesovarium, and suspensory ligament are all continuous with the broad ligament, which is a reflection of peritoneum over the female reproductive organs. The mesovarium attaches the ovary to the broad ligament. The suspensory ligament of the ovary runs from the pelvic brim to the lateral pole of the ovary. It contains the ovarian artery, ovarian vein, ovarian lymphatics, and ovarian nerves (ovarian neurovascular bundle). Volvulus of the ovary (usually associated with an ovarian tumor) may constrict the neurovascular bundle with ovarian infarct and pain referred to the inguinal and hypogastric regions.

443. The answer is b. *(April, 3/e, pp 457–458.)* The bulbourethral glands, lying in the deep pouch, drain into the penile urethra. Spermatozoa mature in the epididymis. Emission moves the spermatozoa to the ampulla of the vas, where they are stored prior to ejaculation. On receiving the duct from the seminal vesicle, the passage becomes the narrow ejaculatory duct, which passes through the prostatic parenchyma to empty into the prostatic urethra.

444. The answer is d. *(April, 3/e, pp 449, 473–475.)*

Pelvic Visceral Afferent Innervation			
Organ	**Afferent Pathway**	**Level**	**Referral areas**
Kidneys Renal pelvis Upper ureters	Aorticorenal plexus, least splanchnic nerve, white ramus of T12, subcostal nerve	T12	Subcostal and pubic regions
Descending colon Sigmoid colon Midureters Urinary bladder Oviducts Uterine body	Aortic plexus, lumbar splanchnic nerves, white rami of L1–L2, spinal nerves L1–L2	L1–L2	Lumbar and inguinal regions, anterior mons and labia, anterior scrotum, anterior thigh
None	No white rami between L3–S1	L3–S1	No visceral pain refers to dermatomes L3–S1
Cervix Pelvic ureters Epididymis Vas deferens Seminal vesicles Prostate gland Rectum Proximal anal canal	Pelvic plexus, pelvic splanchnic nerves, spinal nerves S2–S4	S2–S4	Perineum, thigh, lateral leg and foot

445. The answer is a. *(Moore, Anatomy, 4/e, pp 396–398.)* The anterior portion of the deep transverse perineal muscle (A) is closely associated with the urethra and forms the external urethral sphincter. Voluntary control of this muscle is mediated by the pudendal nerve. The muscles of the superficial pouch generally are associated with the penis or clitoris. The deep perineal pouch is formed by the deep transverse perineal muscle (A). This muscle, along with its inferior and superior fascial layers, forms the urogenital diaphragm. Extending from the ischiopubic ramus to meet its counterpart of the opposite side in a midline raphe, the deep transverse perineal muscle reinforces the urogenital hiatus of the pelvic diaphragm formed by the central defect in the levator ani muscle (C). Although the obturator internus muscle (B), a lateral rotator of the thigh, does not contribute to the support of the pelvic viscera, the tendinous arch of the obturator fascia provides an origin for the levator ani muscle. The bulbospongiosus muscle (E), which overlies the erectile tissue of the corpus spongiosus urethrae, functions to compress the penile urethra to expel residual urine. The ischiocavernosus muscles (D), which overlie the corpora cavernosa, along with the bulbospongiosus muscle, may assist in maintenance of erection by retarding venous return from the erectile tissue.

446 to 447. The answers are 446-b, 447-b. *(April, 3/e, pp 419–421, 453–55.)* The vestibular bulbs, underlying the urethral folds, are homologous to the male corpus spongiosum. Fusion of the urethral folds in the male results in the fusion of the underlying erectile tissue into the single bulb of the penis, through which the penile urethra passes. The glans clitoris is formed by the conjoined anterior terminal portions of the left and right vestibular bulbs. It is thus homologous to the glans penis, which is the terminal portion of the male corpus spongiosum. The labia majora and the scrotum both develop from the labial-scrotal folds of the undifferentiated external genitalia. In the male the scrotal folds fuse along the scrotal raphe to form the scrotum.

The vestibule of the vulva, lying within the labia minora, represents the persistent urogenital sinus of the undifferentiated external genitalia. In the developing male, the urethral folds (homologous to the labia minora) fuse over the urogenital sinus to form the penile urethra. Therefore, the vestibule and the penile urethra are homologous.

448 to 449. The answers are 448-d, 449-d. *(April, 3/e, pp 434–435, 457, 469, 472.)* The superficial lymphatics of the penis drain toward the superficial inguinal nodes, whereas the deep penile lymphatics drain into the internal iliac nodes. The gonads develop high in the abdominal cavity and descend with their neurovascular supply. Thus, the testes and ovaries drain directly to the para-aortic lymph nodes in the vicinity of the renal vessels. The pelvic portions of the urethra, uterus, cervix, and deep vagina drain to the internal iliac nodes. Lymph from the lower abdominal wall, the inferior part of the anal canal, as well as most of the superficial perineum (including the scrotum and vulva), drains to the superficial inguinal nodes. The lymphatics of the lower extremity drain to the deep inguinal nodes.

Extremities

Questions

DIRECTIONS: Each item below contains a question or incomplete statement followed by suggested responses. Select the **one best** response to each question.

450. The scapula is formed by

a. Splanchnic lateral plate mesoderm
b. Neural crest cells
c. Axial mesoderm
d. Somatic lateral plate mesoderm
e. Somitic mesoderm

451. Innervation to the rotator cuff muscle that medially rotates the arm is provided by the

a. Axillary nerve
b. Suprascapular nerve
c. Thoracodorsal nerve
d. Upper and lower subscapular nerves

452. The structure that is most often associated with bursitis at the shoulder is the

a. Acromioclavicular joint capsule
b. Glenohumeral joint capsule
c. Subacromial bursa
d. Subdeltoid bursa

453. The accompanying x-ray shows the shoulder of an 11-year-old female who fell off the monkey bars, extending her arm in an attempt to break her fall. The small arrows indicate a fracture in the area of the surgical neck of the humerus. The large arrows indicate

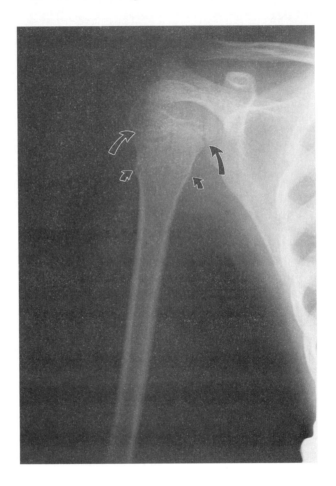

a. A fracture at the anatomic neck of the humerus
b. The glenohumeral joint
c. The joint space between the proximal humerus and the acromion of the scapula
d. The proximal humeral epiphyseal plate
e. What is commonly called a shoulder separation

454. A patient presents in her fifth pregnancy with a history of numbness and tingling in her right thumb and index finger during each of her previous four pregnancies. Currently, the same symptoms are constant, although generally worse in the early morning. Symptoms could be somewhat relieved by vigorous shaking of the wrist. Neurologic examination revealed atrophy and weakness of the abductor pollicis brevis, the opponens pollicis, and the first two lumbrical muscles. Sensation was decreased over the lateral palm and the volar aspect of the first three digits. Numbness and tingling were markedly increased over the first three digits and the lateral palm when the wrist was held in flexion for 30 s. The symptoms suggest damage to

a. The radial artery
b. The median nerve
c. The ulnar nerve
d. Proper digital nerves
e. The radial nerve

Questions 455 to 457

A 52-year-old man is brought to the emergency room after being found in the park, where apparently he had lain overnight after a fall. He complains of severe pain in the left arm. Physical examination suggests a broken humerus that is confirmed radiologically. The patient can extend the forearm at the elbow, but supination appears to be somewhat weak; the hand grasp is very weak compared with the uninjured arm. Neurologic examination reveals an inability to extend the wrist (wristdrop). Because these findings point to apparent nerve damage, the patient is scheduled for a surgical reduction of the fracture.

455. The observation that extension at the elbow appears normal but supination of the forearm appears weak warrants localization of the nerve lesion to the

a. Posterior cord of the brachial plexus in the axilla
b. Posterior divisions of the brachial plexus
c. Radial nerve at the distal third of the humerus
d. Radial nerve in the midforearm
e. Radial nerve in the vicinity of the head of the radius

456. Wristdrop results in a very weak hand grasp. The strength of the grasp is greatest with the wrist in the extended position because the

a. Flexor digitorum superficialis and profundus muscles are stretched when the wrist and metacarpophalangeal joints are extended
b. Lever arms of the interossei are longer when the metacarpophalangeal joints are extended
c. Lever arms of the lumbrical muscles are longer when the metacarpophalangeal joints are extended
d. Line of action of the extensor digitorum muscle is most direct in full extension
e. Radial half of the flexor digitorum profundus muscle is paralyzed because it is innervated by the radial nerve

457. On examination of muscle function at the metacarpophalangeal (MP), proximal interphalangeal (PIP), and distal interphalangeal (DIP) joints, the findings expected in the presence of radial nerve palsy would include which of the following?

a. Inability to abduct the digits at the MP joint
b. Inability to adduct the digits at the MP joint
c. Inability to extend the MP joint only
d. Inability to extend the MP, PIP, and DIP joints
e. Inability to extend the PIP and DIP joints

458. In the upper extremity, each major nerve passes between two heads of a muscle. The median nerve passes between the

a. Long and medial heads of the triceps brachii muscle
b. Medial and posterior division of the coracobrachialis muscle
c. Ulnar and humeral heads of the flexor carpi ulnaris muscle
d. Ulnar and humeral heads of the pronator teres muscle

Questions 459 to 460

Refer to the x-ray below.

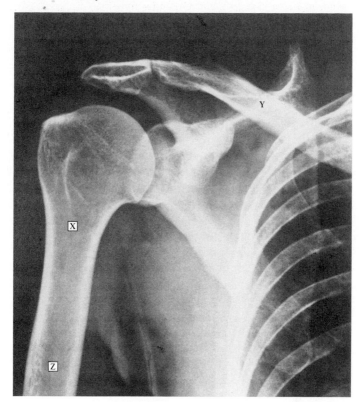

(Reproduced, with permission, from Wicke L: Atlas of Radiological Anatomy, 6/e. Baltimore, MD: Williams & Wilkins, 1998.)

459. A spiral fracture of the humerus in the region marked "Z" on the accompanying radiograph had severely injured a major nerve that passes over the dorsal aspect of the bone. Which of the following is most likely to occur as a result of this injury?

a. Wristdrop palsy
b. Total clawing of the hand
c. Waiter's tip palsy
d. Clawing of digits 4 and 5
e. Dupuytren's contracture

460. Fracture of the humerus in the region marked "X" could result in paralysis of which of the following muscles?

a. Subscapularis
b. Pectoralis major
c. Teres major
d. Deltoid
e. Supraspinatus

Questions 461 to 462

A 45-year-old plumber presented in the clinic complaining of long-standing pain in the elbow. Subsequent examination revealed normal flexion/extension at both the elbow and the wrist but weakened abduction of the thumb and extension at the metacarpophalangeal joints of the fingers. These symptoms were found to be caused by entrapment of the posterior interosseus nerve.

461. Which of the following muscles could be expected to demonstrate normal contraction?

a. Extensor indices
b. Extensor digitorum
c. Extensor carpi radialis longus
d. Abductor pollicis longus
e. Extensor digit minimi

462. Which of the following muscles could itself cause entrapment of the posterior interosseus nerve?

a. Extensor carpi ulnaris
b. Extensor indices
c. Anconeus
d. Extensor digitorum
e. Supinator

Questions 463 to 467

A 67-year-old woman slipped on a scatter rug and fell with her right arm extended in an attempt to ease the impact of the fall. She experienced immediate severe pain in the region of the right collar bone and in the right wrist. Painful movement of the right arm was minimized by holding the arm close to the body and by supporting the elbow with the left hand.

463. There is marked tenderness and some swelling in the region of the clavicle about one-third of the distance from the sternum. The examiner can feel the projecting edges of the clavicular fragments. The radiograph confirms the fracture and shows elevation of the proximal fragment with depression and subluxation (underriding) of the distal fragment. Traction by which of the following muscles causes subluxation (the distal fragment underrides the proximal fragment)?

a. Deltoid muscle
b. Pectoralis major muscle
c. Pectoralis minor muscle
d. Sternomastoid muscle
e. Trapezius muscle

464. Internal bleeding can be a complication if the subluxed bone fragment tears a vessel and punctures the pleura. Which of the following vascular structures is particularly vulnerable in a clavicular fracture?

a. Axillary artery
b. Brachiocephalic artery
c. Lateral thoracic artery
d. Subclavian artery
e. Thoracoacromial trunk

465. Marked swelling is noted about the palmar aspect of the wrist. Persistent flexion of the fingers and apparent shortening of the middle finger is seen. There is paresthesia (sensory dullness) over the palmar aspect of the thumb, index finger, middle finger, and a questionable portion of the ring finger, yet when the wrist is gently flexed, intense pain spreads over this area. Sensation over the palm seems normal. The partial flexion of the fingers in this case is best explained by

a. Compression of the radial artery
b. Compression of the recurrent branch of the median nerve
c. Impingement of the flexor tendons by a dislocated carpal bone
d. Paralysis of the dorsal interossei muscles
e. Paralysis of the flexor digitorum superficialis muscle

466. The carpal bone that is most likely to dislocate anteriorly and cause a form of carpal tunnel syndrome is the

a. Capitate
b. Hamate
c. Lunate
d. Navicular
e. Scaphoid

467. The fractured clavicle was reduced and the shoulder bandaged. The lunate bone was surgically reduced. After eight weeks the bone had healed, but the patient was found to have persistent loss of hand function. In addition to the region of original paresthesia (palmar aspects of the thumb, index, and middle fingers as well as a portion of the ring finger), which of the areas listed below should also exhibit paresthesia?

a. Dorsal aspect of the distal phalanges of the index and middle fingers
b. Dorsal web space between the thumb and index finger
c. Medial aspect of the fifth digit
d. Skin over the central palm

Questions 468 to 469

Refer to the x-ray below.

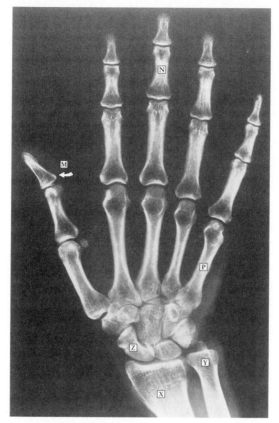

(Reproduced, with permission, from Wicke L: Atlas of Radiological Anatomy, 6/e. Baltimore, MD: Williams & Wilkins, 1998.)

468. Which of the following muscles inserts on the bony protuberance marked "M"?

a. First dorsal interosseus
b. First lumbricale
c. Flexor pollicis longus
d. First palmar interosseus
e. Opponens pollicis

469. "Z" marks the location of which frequently fractured carpal bone?

a. Lunate
b. Triquetral
c. Trapezium
d. Scaphoid
e. Pisiform

Questions 470 to 471

After a night of fraternity parties, a 20-year-old college sophomore came to the ER the following morning complaining that she could not raise her wrist. There was no history of trauma. On examination, the patient could not extend her fingers or wrist but could flex them. She could also both flex and extend her elbow normally. There were no other motor deficits.

470. The symptoms suggest damage to the

a. Median nerve
b. Ulnar nerve
c. Radial nerve
d. Axillary nerve
e. Musculocutaneous nerve

471. Which of the following muscles is spared by the type of injury described above?

a. Extensor digitorum communis
b. Extensor carpi radialis
c. Extensor pollicis longus
d. Triceps
e. Anconeus

472. A female patient falls on an icy sidewalk and complains of her thumb hurting. You take her x-ray and show her there are no fractures. However, she asks what the small light circles (arrow) on the x-ray are. You explain they are sesamoid bones in the tendon of the

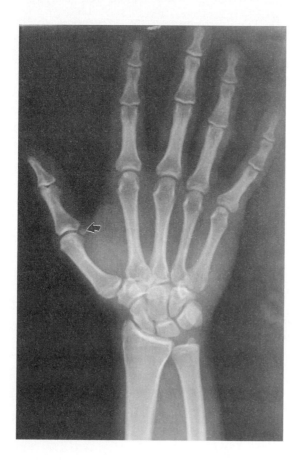

a. Flexor pollicis longus
b. Flexor pollicis brevis
c. Adductor pollicis
d. Abductor pollicis longus
e. Abductor pollicis brevis

Questions 473 to 474

A workman accidentally lacerated his wrist as shown in the accompanying diagram. On exploration of the wound, a vessel and nerve are found to have been severed, but no muscle tendons were damaged.

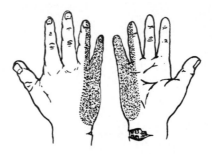

473. From the indicated location of the laceration, the involved nerve is the

a. Median nerve
b. Recurrent branch of the median nerve
c. Superficial branch of the radial nerve
d. Ulnar nerve

474. Which of the following thumb movements would be abolished?

a. Abduction
b. Adduction
c. Extension
d. Opposition

Questions 475 to 476

On the advice of a lawyer, a 27-year-old casino employee visited her personal physician because she found she could no longer flex her thumb and was unable to deal cards. Examination revealed weakness at the interphalangeal joint of the thumb as well as difficulty in bending the tips of the index and middle fingers. She could make a fist but had some difficulty in pinching with the thumb and index finger. There was some forearm pain but no tingling or numbness.

475. These symptoms indicate damage to the
a. Posterior interosseus branch of the radial nerve
b. Palmar branch of the ulnar nerve
c. Recurrent branch of the median nerve
d. Anterior interosseus branch of the median nerve
e. Digital branches of the ulnar nerve

476. What type of joint is the interphalangeal joint?
a. Ball and socket
b. Ginglymus
c. Gomphosis
d. Saddle
e. Ellipsoidal

477. The type of femoral fracture most likely to result in avascular necrosis of the femoral head in adults is
a. Acetabular
b. Cervical
c. Intertrochanteric (between the trochanters)
d. Subtrochanteric
e. Midfemoral shaft

478. Paresthesia, hyperesthesia, or even painful sensation in the anterolateral region of the thigh may occur in obese persons. It results from an abdominal panniculus adiposus that bulges over the inguinal ligament and compresses the underlying
a. Femoral branch of the genitofemoral nerve
b. Femoral nerve
c. Iliohypogastric nerve
d. Ilioinguinal nerve
e. Lateral femoral cutaneous nerve

479. Your patient just took up jogging in the evening for exercise and complains that after a mile or so his left "leg" begins to hurt. You question him on regions of the body or movements that do or do not evoke pain and find that it is widespread throughout his left lower limb. Based on the location of the constriction of the artery (indicated by the arrow), what compartment or movement would you think would be least affected by the reduced arterial blood flow?

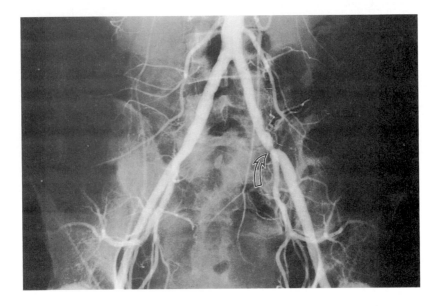

a. Gluteal region
b. Flexion of the thigh
c. Extension of the leg
d. Posterior thigh
e. Plantar flexion of the foot

Questions 480 to 481

Refer to the x-ray below.

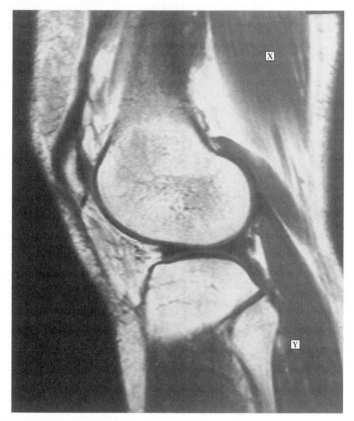

(Reproduced, with permission, from Wicke L: Atlas of Radiologic Anatomy, 6/e.
Baltimore, MD: Williams & Wilkins, 1998.)

480. Which of the following muscles, indicated by "X", inserts on the lateral aspect of the fibular head?

a. Gracilis
b. Adductor magnus
c. Biceps femoris
d. Semimembranosus
e. Adductor longus

481. What type of movement is caused by contraction of the muscle labeled "Y"?

a. Dorsiflexion
b. Plantar flexion
c. Inversion
d. Eversion
e. Flexion of the first metatarsophalangeal joint

482. The process of unlocking the fully extended knee in preparation for flexion requires initial contraction of the

a. Gastrocnemius, soleus, and plantaris muscles
b. Hamstring muscles
c. Popliteus muscle
d. Quadriceps femoris muscle
e. Sartorius muscle and short head of the biceps femoris muscle

483. A 22-year-old male who belongs to a weekend football league presents in the ER. He was running with the ball when a defender tackled him in the midthigh. The patient reports that when he got up, his thigh hurt, so he sat out the rest of the game. When walking to the car, his posterior thigh was extremely painful and swollen. After his shower, he noticed it was becoming discolored with increased swelling. You are concerned about the presence of a hematoma and a disruption of the arterial blood flow to the hamstring muscles. An arteriogram is performed and the vessels in question (arrows) show good filling by contrast. These blood vessels are

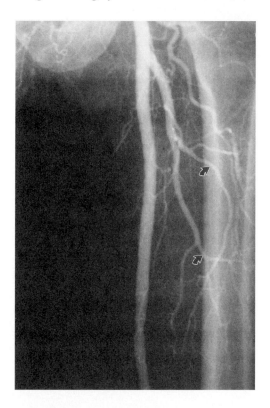

a. Descending branches of the inferior gluteal artery
b. Perforating branches of the deep femoral artery
c. Perforating branches from the obturator artery
d. Perforating branches of the femoral artery
e. Posterior femoral artery

Questions 484 to 485

484. A patient experienced a prolonged stay in one position during a recent surgery and postoperative recovery that resulted in compression of the common peroneal nerve against the fibular head. Which of the following motor deficits would be most likely to occur?

a. Loss of extension at the knee
b. Loss of plantar flexion
c. Loss of flexion at the knee
d. Loss of eversion
e. Loss of medial rotation of the tibia

485. In the above scenario, inversion of the foot is still intact although weakened. Which of the following muscles supplies this action?

a. Tibialis posterior
b. Plantaris
c. Peroneus longus
d. Extensor digitorum longus
e. Quadratus plantae

486. The muscles of the anterior compartment of the leg are innervated primarily by which of the following nerves?

a. Deep fibular
b. Lateral sural cutaneous
c. Saphenous
d. Superficial fibular
e. Sural

487. The tendon of which of the following muscles is involved when the tuberosity of the fifth metatarsal bone is avulsed in an inversion fracture?

a. Abductor digiti minimi
b. Peroneus brevis
c. Peroneus longus
d. Tibialis anterior
e. Tibialis posterior

Questions 488 to 489

Refer to the x-ray below.

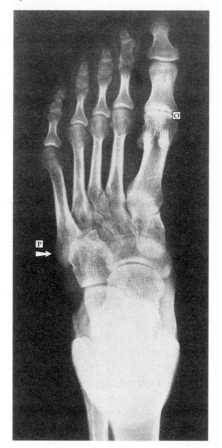

(Reproduced, with permission, from Wicke L: Atlas of Radiological Anatomy, 6/e. Baltimore, MD: Williams & Wilkins, 1998.)

488. Which of the following maladies occurs preferentially at the site marked "O"?

a. Pes planus
b. Claw toe
c. Gout
d. Talipes

489. A fracture of the bone marked "P" in the radiograph will result in avulsion of the tendon of which muscle?

a. Tibialis anterior
b. Peroneus (fibularis) brevis
c. Abductor digiti minimi
d. Plantaris
e. Tibialis posterior

490. A 27-year-old man was admitted for neurologic evaluation of a gunshot wound received five days previously. A 9-mm bullet had passed through both the medial and lateral heads of the gastrocnemius muscle. The exit wound on the lateral head of the muscle was somewhat deeper than the entrance wound in the medial head. The bullet had not struck bone or significant arteries although significant tissue damage, suppuration, and swelling were found around the exit wound. Neurologic examination revealed losses of dorsiflexion and eversion of the left foot. The patient could not feel pinprick or touch on the dorsum of the left foot or anterolateral surface of the left leg. Which nerve was most likely involved in the injury?

a. Sciatic nerve
b. Femoral nerve
c. Sural nerve
d. Common peroneal nerve
e. Tibial nerve

491. In a presurgical patient, the great saphenous vein was cannulated in the vicinity of the ankle. During the procedure, the patient experienced severe pain that radiated along the medial border of the foot. Which of the following nerves was accidentally included in a ligature during this procedure?

a. Medial femoral cutaneous nerve
b. Saphenous nerve
c. Superficial fibular nerve
d. Sural cutaneous nerve
e. Tibial nerve

492. A pulse in the dorsalis pedis artery may be palpated

a. Between the tendons of the extensor digitorum longus and peroneus tertius muscles
b. Between the tendons of the extensor hallucis and extensor digitorum muscles
c. Between the tendons of the tibialis anterior and extensor hallucis longus muscles
d. Immediately anterior to the lateral malleolus
e. Immediately posterior to the medial malleolus

493. The odontoid process (dens) is correctly described by which of the following statements?

a. It articulates with the occipital portion of the skull
b. It is separated from the atlas by an intervertebral disk
c. It projects from the inferior surface of the atlas
d. It represents the vertebral body of the first cervical vertebra

Questions 494 to 495

Refer to the x-ray below.

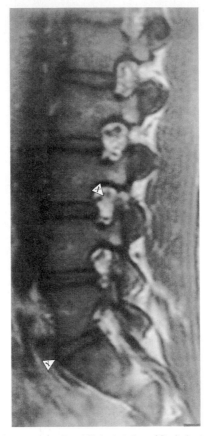

(Reproduced, with permission, from Wicke L: Atlas of Radiological Anatomy, 6/e.
Baltimore, MD: Williams & Wilkins, 1998.)

494. Herniation of the nucleus pulposus in the area marked "X" would compress which of the following?

a. Sensory root of the lumbar spinal nerve
b. Motor root of the lumbar spinal nerve
c. The lumbar spinal nerve
d. Dorsal primary ramus of the lumbar spinal nerve
e. Ventral primary ramus of the lumbar spinal nerve

495. The anterior displacement of the fifth lumbar vertebra over the sacrum (S1 vertebra) at the spot marked "Y" constitutes which of the following?

a. Spondylolysis
b. Spondylolisthesis
c. Ankylosis
d. Kyphosis
e. Scoliosis

496. A 22-year-old male who belongs to a weekend football league was running with the ball when a defender tackled him mid-lower limb from the side. After the tackle, he felt that the knee was hurt and went to the emergency room. From an MRI of the knee, the lateral meniscus is uniformly black; however, the medial meniscus has a tear (lucent area within the meniscus). Which of the following is the reason why the medial meniscus is more susceptible to damage than the lateral meniscus?

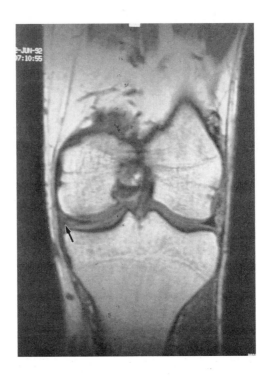

a. The medial meniscus is attached to the popliteus muscle tendon, which can move into a position making it more susceptible.
b. The medial meniscus is attached to the medial (tibial) collateral ligament, which holds it relatively immobile, making it more susceptible.
c. The medial meniscus is attached to the anterior cruciate ligament, which holds it relatively immobile, making it more susceptible.
d. The only reason the medial meniscus is more susceptible to damage is that the knee usually gets hit laterally, causing more torsion on the medial meniscus.

497. The muscles of the back receive motor innervation from

a. Dorsal roots
b. Dorsal primary rami
c. Gray rami communicantes
d. Splanchnic nerves

498. A physician examines a patient who complains of pain and paresthesia in the left leg. The distribution of the pain—running down the medial aspect of the leg and the medial side of the foot and including the great toe—is suggestive of a herniated intervertebral disk. The physician links the distribution of symptoms with nerve L4 and concludes that herniation has occurred at which location?

a. L3–L4 intervertebral disk
b. L4–L5 intervertebral disk
c. L5–S1 intervertebral disk
d. S1–S2 intervertebral disk
e. Insufficient data to determine

499. Landmarks useful in determining the proper location for a spinal tap include the

a. Hiatus of the sacral canal
b. Iliac crests
c. Posterior superior iliac spines
d. Vertebra prominens

500. Intervertebral disks have a tendency to herniate into the intervertebral foramen because the

a. Annulus fibrosus is attenuated in the posterolateral regions
b. Interspinous ligament reinforces the disks anteriorly and anterolaterally
c. Ligamentum flavum reinforces the intervertebral disks posteriorly
d. Lumbar intervertebral disks are thicker posteriorly than anteriorly
e. Posterior longitudinal ligament is stronger and more complete posteriorly than posterolaterally

Extremities

Answers

450. The answer is d. (*Moore, Developing Human, 6/e, pp 434–435.*) Somatic lateral plate mesoderm gives rise to the connective tissue, cartilage, and bones of the appendages, including the shoulder and pelvis. The muscles of the appendages, however, originate from somitic mesoderm (myotome). Neural crest cells contribute to the connective tissue of the head but not the appendages. Axial mesoderm forms the notochord, whereas splanchnic lateral plate mesoderm forms the smooth muscle and connective tissue associated with the viscera.

451. The answer is d. (*Moore, Anatomy, 4/e, pp 698–699.*) The upper and lower subscapular nerves innervate the subscapularis muscle, which is the only muscle of the rotator cuff group that medially rotates the arm. The lower subscapular nerve also innervates the teres major muscle, which is not part of the rotator cuff group. The suprascapular nerve innervates the supraspinatus and infraspinatus muscles that abduct and laterally rotate the arm, respectively. The teres minor muscle, innervated by the axillary nerve, also laterally rotates the arm. The thoracodorsal nerve, originating from the posterior cord between the upper and lower subscapular nerves, innervates the latissimus dorsi muscle.

452. The answer is c. (*Moore, Anatomy, 4/e, pp 698–699.*) Shoulder bursitis is often the result of calcium deposits associated with the subacromial bursa, which separates the acromion process from the underlying supraspinatus muscle, or within the suprajacent supraspinatus tendon. The subdeltoid bursa separates the deltoid muscle from the head of the humerus and the insertions of the rotator cuff muscles.

453. The answer is d. (*Moore, Anatomy, 4/e, pp 669–670, 810.*) The large arrows indicate the proximal humeral epiphyseal plate. The young girl was only 11 and still growing. The epiphyseal plates show up on x-rays as radiolucent cartilage and should not be confused with a fracture. The epiphysis is located at the anatomic neck of the humerus but is not discoid-shaped like many epiphyseal plates in long bones. This plate is tent-shaped, which is why it is not clearly visible all the way across the proximal humerus.

454. The answer is b. (*Moore, Anatomy, 4/e, pp 775, 821–822.*) The patient has a classic case of carpal tunnel syndrome, in which the median nerve is compressed as it passes through the carpal tunnel formed by the flexor retinaculum in the wrist. Evidence for involvement of the median nerve is weakness and atrophy of the thenar muscles (abductor pollicis brevis, opponens pollicis) and lumbricals 1 to 3. Sensory deficits also follow the distribution of the median nerve. The median nerve enters the hand, along with the tendons of the superficial and deep digital flexors, through a tunnel framed by the carpal bones and the overlying flexor retinaculum. Symptoms are worse in the early morning and in pregnancy because of fluid retention, resulting in swelling that entraps the median nerve. Flexing the wrist for an extended period exaggerates the paresthesia ("Phelan's" sign) by increasing pressure on the median nerve.

Neither the ulnar nerve, radial nerve, nor radial artery passes through the carpal tunnel. The ulnar nerve supplies the third and fourth lumbricals and only the short adductor of the thumb. The radial nerve innervates mostly long and short extensors of the digits and the dorsal aspect of the hand. Proper digital nerves lie distal to the carpal tunnel but are only sensory.

455. The answer is c. (*Moore, Anatomy, 4/e, p 731.*) The clinical signs and findings in the patient presented in the question indicate radial nerve damage. The evidence that extension at the elbow appeared normal while supination appeared weak can be used to localize the lesion. The innervation to the medial and long heads of the triceps brachii, principal extensor of the arm, arises from the radial nerve (in the axilla) as the medial muscular branches. The innervation to the lateral head, and to a smaller portion of the medial head, arises from the radial nerve as it passes along the musculospiral groove at mid-humerus. The supinator muscle is innervated by muscular twigs from the deep branch of the radial nerve in the forearm, just before the radial nerve reaches the supinator muscle. Thus, paralysis of the supinator muscle, but not of the triceps brachii, localizes the fracture to the distal third of the humeral shaft between the elbow and musculospiral groove.

456. The answer is a. *(April, 3/e, p 96.)* Muscles are most powerful (disregarding leverage factors) when stretched by extension of the joint(s) over which they pass, because this places the sarcomeres at the optimum tension-producing length in the length-tension relationship. Thus, hand grasp is strongest when the wrist joint and metacarpophalangeal joints are extended, which stretches the digitorum superficialis and profundus flexors to their optimum position. Paralysis of the radial nerve with subsequent wristdrop will weaken hand grasp because the extrinsic flexor muscles are compelled to operate in a nonoptimum region. The lever arms of the lumbricals and interossei are greatest when the metacarpophalangeal joints are flexed, a consideration that does not apply to the patient presented in the question. The median nerve innervates the radial side of the flexor digitorum profundus.

457. The answer is c. *(April, 3/e, pp 90–92.)* Radial nerve palsy produces an inability to extend the metacarpophalangeal joints, owing to paralysis of the extensor digitorum communis muscle. However, the lumbrical and interossei muscles, which are served by the median and ulnar nerves and insert into the dorsal expansions (extensor hoods) of the proximal phalanges, are able simultaneously to flex the metacarpophalangeal joints and to extend the interphalangeal joints. Also, abduction of the digits, a function of the dorsal interossei, and adduction, a function of the palmar interossei, are both mediated by the ulnar nerve and, therefore, unaffected.

458. The answer is d. *(Moore, Anatomy, 4/e, p 757.)* In the arm, the musculocutaneous nerve passes through the coracobrachialis muscle. The radial nerve, which lies in the musculospiral groove, passes between the long and medial heads of the triceps brachii muscle in company with the profunda brachii artery. It is here that the nerve and artery are in jeopardy in the event of a midhumeral fracture. In the forearm, the median nerve courses between the humeral and ulnar heads of the pronator teres. As the ulnar nerve courses behind the medial epicondyle, it passes between the humeral and ulnar heads of the flexor carpi ulnaris as it enters the forearm. In each instance, the nerve innervates the muscle that it pierces.

459. The answer is a. *(Moore, Anatomy, 4/e, p 731.)* The area marked "Z" points to the approximate location of the spiral (radial) groove. This shallow depression, on the posterior (dorsal) aspect of the humeral shaft, accommodates the radial nerve and the deep (profunda) brachial vessels. A midline fracture of the humerus may rupture the blood vessels, causing a hematoma that would compress and impair the ability of the radial nerve to conduct information to the extensor muscles of the wrist and digits. A more severe fracture may transect the radial nerve, causing paralysis of the same muscles, resulting in wristdrop. These muscles include the following: brachioradialis, extensor carpi radialis longus, extensor carpi radialis brevis, extensor digitorum communis, extensor digiti minimi, extensor carpi ulnaris, supinator, abductor pollicis longus, extensor pollicis longus, extensor pollicis brevis, and the extensor indicis. The causes of other palsies listed in this question are injuries due to the nerves within parentheses: total claw hand palsy (median and ulnar nerves); clawing of digits 4 and 5 (ulnar nerve); waiter's tip palsy (C5, C6 roots of the brachial plexus; upper trunk of the brachial plexus; and Erb-Duchenne palsy). Dupuytren's contracture is caused by a thickening of the palmar aponeurosis.

460. The answer is d. *(Moore, Anatomy, 4/e, p. 696.)* The area marked "X" gives the location of the surgical neck of the humerus, which is the narrow area located distal to the head and anatomical neck of the humerus. On the posterior (dorsal aspect), the surgical neck is transversed by the axillary nerve (C5, C6; posterior/dorsal cord of the brachial plexus) and the accompanying posterior circumflex humeral vessels. A fracture of the surgical neck may rupture the posterior circumflex humeral vessels, causing either the compression of the axillary nerve or transection of the same nerve. Injury to this nerve causes weakness (paresis) or paralysis of the deltoid and teres minor muscles. The nerve supply to the other muscles mentioned is shown in parentheses: subscapularis (upper and lower subscapular nerves); pectoralis major (medial and lateral pectoral nerves); teres major (lower subscapular nerve); and supraspinatus (suprascapular nerve).

461. The answer is c. *(Moore, Anatomy, 4/e, pp 731, 742, 761.)* All of the muscles listed above are innervated by the posterior interosseus branch of the radial nerve (the terminal part of the deep radial nerve). Extensor carpi radialis longus, however, is innervated by a muscular branch of the radial nerve proximal to the origin of the deep branch. Its function would, therefore, be preserved in entrapment of the posterior interosseus nerve.

462. The answer is e. *(Moore, Anatomy, 4/e, pp 731, 742, 761.)* Each of the muscles listed above is innervated by the deep branch of the radial nerve or its terminal portion, the posterior interosseus nerve. The deep radial nerve passes between the deep and superficial layers of the supinator muscle and lies on a bare area of the radius where it may be compressed by action of the supinator or damaged by a fracture of the radius.

463. The answer is b. *(April, 3/e, p 57.)* The horizontal direction of the fibers of the clavicular head of the pectoralis major muscle draws the humerus medially and causes the distal fragment of the bone to sublux. The sternal head of this muscle also has the effect of pulling the arm medially, an effect that is normally offset by the strutlike action of the clavicle.

464. The answer is d. *(April, 3/e, p 65.)* Because large and important neurovascular structures pass between the clavicle and first rib, including the subclavian artery, clavicular fracture may produce life-threatening bleeding into the pleural cavity. The axillary artery is the continuation of the subclavian after it has cleared the first rib, so neither this vessel nor its thoracoacromial branch is likely to be threatened by clavicular fracture. There is no brachiocephalic artery on the left side, and on the right its terminal point is marked by its bifurcation into common carotid and subclavian arteries proximal to the fracture site.

465. The answer is c. *(Moore, Anatomy, 4/e, p 807.)* A fall on the extended hand will frequently dislocate the lunate bone anteriorly. This dislocated bone may then impinge on the tendons of the extrinsic digital flexor muscles and thereby prevent flexion of the fingers. Compression of the median nerve in the carpal tunnel cannot explain this observation because the prime flexors of the digits are the extrinsic flexors (flexors digitorum superficialis and profundus), which receive their innervation in the forearm, well proximal to the injury. The dorsal interossei, innervated by the ulnar nerve, are digital extensors. The recurrent branch of the median nerve innervates the thenar muscles.

466. The answer is c. *(April, 3/e, pp 86, 102. Moore, Anatomy, 4/e, pp 748–749.)* The lunate bone tends to dislocate anteriorly into the transverse carpal arch, thereby entrapping the tendons of the extrinsic digital flexors and compressing the median nerve. The capitate is frequently fractured but does not tend to dislocate into the carpal arch. The hamate provides an anchor for the transverse carpal ligament and is, therefore, located lateral to the carpal tunnel. The navicular (scaphoid) bone has a tendency to fracture but does not dislocate into the carpal tunnel.

467. The answer is a. *(Moore, Anatomy, 4/e, pp 774–777.)* In addition to supplying sensation to the palmar aspects of the thumb, index, and middle fingers as well as the radial portion of the ring finger, the median nerve also supplies the dorsal aspect of the terminal phalanx of those fingers. The dorsal web space between the thumb and index finger is supplied exclusively by the radial nerve. The fifth finger is supplied completely by the ulnar nerve. The central region of the palm is supplied by the superficial branch of the median nerve that arises proximal to the carpal tunnel and is not compromised by carpal tunnel syndrome because it passes superficial to the flexor retinaculum.

468. The answer is c. *(Moore, Anatomy, 4/e, p 737.)* M points to the base of the distal phalanx on the palmar (volar) aspect. This is the area indicating the insertion of the flexor pollicis longus, which flexes the interphalangeal joint; it also flexes the metacarpophalangeal joint of the thumb. The median nerve controls the contraction of the flexor pollicis longus. This muscle is important in facilitating power and precision grips. Thus, it plays a significant role in manipulatory movements, the ultimate objective of the upper limb. The insertions of the other muscles in this question are in parentheses: first dorsal interosseus (proximal phalanx of the index digit); first lumbrical (extensor expansion tendon of the index finger); first palmar interosseus (proximal phalanx of the thumb); and opponens pollicis (metacarpal of the thumb).

469. The answer is d. *(Moore, Anatomy, 4/e, pp 748–749.)* The carpal bone marked Z is the scaphoid (it is clinically still called the "navicular"; thus, the fracture of the scaphoid is often called the "navicular fracture"). The scaphoid is important because it is the most commonly fractured short bone of the carpus (wrist). It is the largest of the proximal row of the carpal bones (the others being the lunate, triquetral, and the pisiform). Because it supports the trapezium—contributory to the saddle-shaped carpometacarpal joint of the thumb—its fracture can curtail thumb function, which, in turn, compromises the manipulatory capacity of the hand. The other bone that frequently fractures in this region is the distal, flared end of the radius; this is clinically called Colles' fracture.

470. The answer is c. (*Moore, Anatomy, 4/e, pp 696, 731, 758–759.*) The radial nerve innervates extensors of the upper extremity. Damage to the radial nerve in the radial groove is frequently caused by supporting the arm in an outstretched position as may be encountered when an inebriated college student passes out on her friend's sofa. This is sometimes referred to as "Saturday night palsy." The median nerve supplies the pronators (teres and quadratus) and the flexors of the fingers, thumb, and wrist. The ulnar nerve supplies the flexor carpi ulnaris and a portion of flexor digitorum profundus. The axillary nerve innervates the deltoid and teres minor and is thus involved in abduction of the arm. The musculocutaneous nerve innervates flexors of the elbow joint (e.g., biceps brachii).

471. The answer is d. (*Moore, Anatomy, 4/e, p 731.*) When the radial nerve is compressed in the radial groove (e.g., by supporting the outstretched arm on a hard object), only the triceps is spared because the branch of radial nerve supplying this muscle originates proximal to the nerve's position in the groove. Branches to all the other muscles innervated by the radial nerve occur distal to that point and thus would be affected by compression of the nerve in the groove.

472. The answer is b. (*Moore, Anatomy, 4/e, p 15.*) The flexor pollicis brevis has two heads and there is a sesamoid bone associated with each of the tendons of these heads. Sesamoid bones are isolated islands of bone that may occur in tendons passing over joints. The patella is the classic example. The adductor pollicis also has two heads (transverse and oblique), but they are not associated with sesamoid bones.

473. The answer is d. (*Moore, Anatomy, 4/e, p 774–777.*) The ulnar nerve descends along the postaxial (ulnar) side of the forearm. It passes lateral to the pisiform bone and under the carpal volar ligament, but superficial to the transverse carpal ligament. In the hand it divides into superficial and deep branches. The median nerve lies deep to the transverse carpal ligament where it is protected from superficial lacerations. Emerging from the carpal tunnel, it gives off the vulnerable recurrent branch to the thenar eminence. The superficial branch of the radial nerve supplies the dorsolateral aspects of the wrist and hand.

474. The answer is b. *(Moore, Anatomy, 4/e, p 776.)* The ulnar nerve innervates two of the intrinsic thenar muscles: the adductor pollicis and frequently the deep head of the flexor pollicis brevis. Because of the actions of the flexor pollicis longus and the superficial head of the flexor pollicis brevis, there would probably be no noticeable deficit in flexion. However, the ability to adduct the thumb would be lost with ulnar nerve injury.

475. The answer is d. *(Moore, Anatomy, 4/e, pp 757–758.)* The anterior interosseus branch arises from the posterior portion of the median nerve in the cubital fossa and innervates the flexor pollicis longus, pronator quadratus, and portion of the flexor digitorum profundus inserting in the index and middle fingers. Thus, it mediates flexion of both the thumb and distal interphalangeal joints of the index and middle fingers. In addition, the anterior interosseus branch has no sensory distribution. The posterior interosseus branch of the radial nerve supplies abductors of the thumb and extensors of the thumb and fingers. The palmar branch of the ulnar nerve is purely sensory. The recurrent branch of the median nerve innervates muscles of the thenar compartment (e.g., flexor pollicis brevis), and damage may result in some difficulty in flexion of the thumb, but not of the index and middle fingers. The digital branches of the ulnar nerve supply the ring and little fingers and are sensory.

476. The answer is b. *(Moore, Anatomy, 4/e, pp 21–26.)* A joint between phalanges is termed a ginglymus or "hinge" joint. It allows movement in only one plane (flexion and extension are opposite movements in the same plane). The hip joint is typical of a ball and socket joint. This type of joint permits movement in all three axes and in a combination termed circumduction. A gomphosis is the type of joint made by a tooth with bone. The carpometacarpal joint of the thumb typifies a saddle joint. It permits movement in two axes. The radiocarpal joint at the wrist is an example of an ellipsoidal joint. It is biaxial, but the excursion of movement is longer in one axis.

477. The answer is b. *(Moore, Anatomy, 4/e, p 511, 614–615.)* Fractures of the femoral neck will completely interrupt the blood supply to the femoral head in adults. If the capsular retinaculum also is torn, avascular necrosis of the head will certainly occur because the only remaining blood supply to the head (through the ligamentum teres) is inadequate to sustain it. The nearer the fracture to the femoral head, the more likely will be disruption of the retinacular blood supply.

478. The answer is e. *(April, 3/e, p 199.)* The lateral femoral cutaneous nerve passes beneath the inguinal ligament just medial to the anterior superior iliac spine. It innervates the lateral aspect of the thigh. The iliohypogastric nerve innervates a portion of the gluteal, inguinal, and pubic regions. The ilioinguinal nerve and the femoral branch of the genitofemoral nerve supply the upper portions of the anterior thigh. The sensory distribution of the femoral nerve is the anterior thigh and medial leg.

479. The answer is b. *(Moore, Anatomy, 4/e, pp 189, 350–351.)* Flexion of the thigh would be least affected. The lesion involves the common iliac artery just proximal to its division into the internal and external iliac branches. Blood flow would be compromised to the external iliac artery and its downstream branches including the femoral, deep femoral, popliteal, tibial, fibular, and plantar arteries. Blood flow would also be diminished to branches of the internal iliac artery, including gluteal and visceral arteries. One of the most powerful flexors of the thigh is the psoas muscle, which originates from the lumbar vertebrae and receives most of its blood from the aorta and common iliac artery and thus would be unaffected by the lesion.

480. The answer is c. *(Moore, Anatomy, 4/e, p 263.)* The muscle marked "X" is the biceps femoris as it approaches its insertion on the lateral aspect of the fibular head. The bone that is located anterior to this muscle is the distal femur, which is seen articulating with the proximal extremity of the tibia. It articulates with the fibular head at the proximal tibiofibular joint. The (long heads of) biceps femoris muscle belongs to the hamstring group, which also includes the semitendinosus and semimembranosus. The hamstring muscles extend the hip joint and flex the knee joint. They are supplied by the tibial division of the sciatic nerve (the short head of the biceps femoris is *not* a hamstring muscle; it receives a branch from the common fibular nerve). When the hamstrings are paralyzed, the person tends to fall forward because the remaining extensor of the hip joint, the gluteus maximus, is not strong enough to maintain erect posture. The insertions of the other muscles in this question are in parentheses: gracilis (medial surface of the tibia); adductor magnus (femur); semimembranosus (medial condyle of tibia); and adductor longus (linea aspera-medial third).

481. The answer is b. (*Moore, Anatomy, 4/e, pp 586–588.*) The muscle marked "Y" is the lateral head of the gastrocnemius. This is evident from its location close to the head of the fibula (tibiofibular joint). The two heads of the gastrocnemius, the soleus and plantaris, form the calcaneal (Achilles) tendon, which inserts on the posterior surface of the calcaneus. Contraction of these muscles causes plantar flexion at the ankle. The muscles of the calcaneal tendon receive branches of the tibial nerve. The muscle(s) that cause the other movement in this question are in parentheses: dorsiflexion (tibialis anterior, extensor digitorum longus, extensor hallucis longus, and fibularis tertius); eversion (fibularis longus and fibularis brevis); inversion (tibialis anterior); and flexion of the first metatarsophalangeal joint (flexor hallucis longus and flexor hallucis brevis).

482. The answer is c. (*Moore, Anatomy, 4/e, pp 621–622.*) To unscrew a knee from its locked and slightly hyperextended position, the popliteus muscle contracts and causes medial rotation of the tibia or, if the foot is planted, lateral rotation of the femur. This movement frees the medial femoral condyle from its posterior position on the tibial condylar surface. The quadriceps femoris then relaxes, and knee flexion occurs by contraction of the hamstring muscles, assisted by the short head of the biceps femoris, sartorius, gracilis, and gastrocnemius muscles.

483. The answer is b. (*Moore, Anatomy, 4/e, pp 546, 561.*) Perforating branches of the deep femoral artery are the principal blood supply to the posterior thigh. The other arteries supply anterior, medial, and gluteal regions of the thigh.

484. The answer is d. (*Moore, Anatomy, 4/e, pp 540–543.*) Compression of the common peroneal nerve would affect all muscles innervated by this nerve, including tibialis anterior, peroneus longus, and extensor digitorum longus. Loss of dorsiflexion and eversion is usually complete. The extensors of the knee joint (quadriceps femoris) are supplied by the femoral nerve, whereas the flexors of the knee joint (the hamstrings and gracilis) are supplied by the tibial nerve and obturator nerve, respectively. The gastrocnemius and soleus muscles are the principal plantar flexors of the foot and are innervated by the tibial nerve. The popliteus is the prime medial rotator of the tibia and is also innervated by the tibial nerve.

485. The answer is a. (*Moore, Anatomy, 4/e, pp 582–585.*) Following compression injury of the common peroneal nerve, eversion is usually completely impaired, whereas loss of inversion is only partial. Tibialis posterior is a powerful inverter of the foot and is innervated by the tibial nerve; therefore, its action would remain. The peroneus longus is an everter of the foot, and its action is lost by compression of the common peroneal nerve. The extensor digitorum longus is innervated by the common peroneal nerve but is an everter of the foot. The quadratus plantae is a flexor of the toes and is innervated by the lateral plantar branch of the tibial nerve.

486. The answer is a. (*April, 3/e, p 208.*) The common fibular (peroneal) nerve bifurcates into superficial and deep branches. The deep fibular nerve innervates all muscles of the anterior compartment of the leg. The superficial fibular nerve emerges from the deep fascia and descends in the lateral compartment, where it innervates the peroneus longus and brevis muscles before dividing into median dorsal cutaneous and intermediate dorsal cutaneous nerves, which supply the distal third of the leg, dorsum of the foot, and all the toes. The saphenous nerve (the terminal branch of the common femoral nerve) distributes cutaneous branches to the anterior and medial aspects of the leg as well as to the dorsomedial aspect of the foot. The sural nerve follows the course of the lesser saphenous vein and becomes the lateral sural cutaneous nerve to supply the anterolateral aspect of the foot.

487. The answer is b. (*April, 3/e, p 207.*) The peroneus (fibularis) brevis, a pronator and everter of the foot, inserts into the tubercle at the base of the fifth metatarsal. The peroneus longus passes under the tarsal arch to insert onto the plantar aspect of the first metatarsal. The tibialis posterior inserts onto the navicular bone, whereas the tibialis anterior inserts into the first cuneiform and first metatarsal. The abductor digiti minimi inserts onto the proximal phalanx of the fifth toe.

488. The answer is c. (*Moore, Anatomy, 4/e, p. 645.*) Severe pain, swelling, and redness of the first metatarsophalangeal joint (podagra) are among the diagnostic symptoms of gout (crystal arthropathy). The serum uric acid level is high, and when the joint is aspirated, the fluid contains needle-shaped crystals of monosodium urate monohydrate (uric acid). Although pain may also occur in other joints, it is the first tarsometatarsal joint that is most frequently affected; the reason for this is open to conjecture. The other conditions listed are as follows: pes planus (flat foot); talipes (club foot); and claw toe (due to hyperextension of metatarsophalangeal joint and the flexion of the interphalangeal joint).

489. The answer is b. (*Moore, Anatomy, 4/e, p. 645.*) The prominence P is located on the lateral aspect of the base of fifth metatarsal (basal tuberosity). It is the site of insertion of the peroneus brevis muscle. A sudden, forceful inversion of the foot can cause the avulsion fracture of the prominence marked P. A very painful swelling results, and support and walking are impaired. The patient has great difficulty in everting the foot.

490. The answer is d. (*Moore, Anatomy, 4/e, pp 579, 582.*) The common peroneal (fibular) nerve is the lateral terminal branch of the sciatic nerve. After arising near the apex of the popliteal fossa, it descends on the popliteus muscle and winds superficially around the fibular neck. It is extremely vulnerable in this position and is the most often injured nerve in the lower extremity. The common peroneal nerve innervates all muscles in the anterior and lateral compartments of the leg. In addition, it provides sensory innervation to the dorsum of the foot and the anterolateral surface of the legs via the superficial and sural/lateral sural cutaneous nerves, respectively. The tibial nerve innervates plantar flexors of the posterior compartment. The sciatic nerve generally divides into the tibial and common peroneal nerves superior to the popliteal fossa. Damage to it might result in deficits in both plantar flexion and dorsiflexion. The femoral nerve innervates the quadriceps muscles of the anterior thigh. Damage to it would impair flexion of the thigh at the hip.

491. The answer is b. (*Moore, Anatomy, 4/e, pp 541–542.*) The saphenous nerve accompanies the great saphenous vein along the medial aspect of the leg and foot as far as the great toe. The superficial fibular nerve innervates the central portion of the dorsum of the foot. The sural cutaneous nerve innervates the lateral aspect of the foot. The medial and lateral plantar branches of the tibial nerve supply the sole of the foot.

492. The answer is b. *(April, 3/e, p 211.)* The dorsal pedal artery, a continuation of the anterior tibial artery, passes onto the dorsum of the foot between the tendons of the extensor hallucis longus and extensor digitorum longus muscles. The dorsal pedal pulse may be palpated here before the artery passes beneath the extensor hallucis brevis muscle. The posterior tibial artery passes behind the medial malleolus, where the posterior tibial pulse is normally palpable.

493. The answer is d. *(Moore, Anatomy, 4/e, pp 439, 460.)* The odontoid process (dens) of the axis, the second cervical vertebra, is the remnant of the body of the first cervical vertebra (atlas). Developing from a separate ossification center, it fused to the body of the axis. The fact that there is no intervertebral disk between the atlas and axis probably facilitates the fusion. The dens, projecting from the superior surface of the axis, provides a pivot about which rotation occurs at the atlantoaxial joint. Fracture and posterior dislocation of the dens may crush the spinal cord with fatal results.

494. The answer is c. *(Moore, Anatomy, 4/e, pp 452–453.)* The opening marked "X" is the intervertebral foramen. It allows passage of the spinal nerve and vessels. Herniation of the nucleus pulposus into the intervertebral foramen may compress the spinal nerve, causing lumbago or sciatica. This is due to the fact the lower true back muscles, the gluteal muscles, and the muscles of the back of the thigh are supplied by the lumbar spinal nerves shown by this MRI.

495. The answer is b. *(Moore, Anatomy, 4/e, pp 462–463.)* Sudden vehicular accidents or a fall can cause the laminae of the lumbar vertebrae to fracture. This leads to the unmooring of the bodies of the lumbar vertebrae. The lumbosacral joint is a vulnerable site owing to the sudden dorsal angulation of the sacrum. This is clinically known as spondylolisthesis. The meanings of the other terms are as follows: spondylolysis (fracture of the vertebral laminae); ankylosis (ossification of the synovial articular joints); kyphosis (excessive curvature of the thoracic spine); and scoliosis (lateral curvature of the spine).

496. The answer is b. (*Moore, Anatomy, 4/e, pp 621, 626.*) The medial meniscus is attached to the medial collateral ligament. It is relatively immovable and, therefore, unable to evade damage such as occurred in this case. The medial meniscus is clearly not attached to the popliteus muscle or to the anterior cruciate ligament.

497. The answer is b. (*Moore, Anatomy, 4/e, pp 467–473.*) The axial musculature of the back receives innervation from the dorsal primary rami of the spinal nerves. The ventral primary rami contribute to the cervical plexus, brachial plexus, intercostal nerves, and the lumbosacral plexus. The dorsal roots convey sensation to the spinal cord. The splanchnic nerves and gray rami communicantes are components fo the sympathetic division of the autonomic nervous sytem.

498. The answer is a. (*April, 3/e, pp 133, 140.*) The deep incisure in the inferior border of the pedicle ensures that the spinal nerve associated with that vertebra will exit through the intervertebral foramen well above the intervertebral disk so that it will not be affected by a herniation at that level. However, a posterolateral herniation (the usual direction) will impinge on the next lower nerve as it courses toward its associated intervertebral foramen. In this case, pain was distributed along the medial side of the leg and foot as far as the great toe—the distribution of the saphenous branch of the femoral nerve (L4). Herniation of the third lumbar intervertebral disk between vertebral bodies L3–L4 would affect nerve L4.

499. The answer is b. (*April, 3/e, p 155.*) The most superior extent of the iliac crests defines the level of the fourth lumbar vertebra. Thus, the spinous process felt beneath a line connecting the left and right iliac crests must be L4. The preferred location for a spinal tap or introduction of spinal or epidural anesthesia is at the level of the L4–L5 interspace for two reasons: the spinal cord usually ends by the L2 level (except in newborn infants and extremely short-statured adults), which eliminates the possibility of spinal cord injury; and the horizontal orientation of the L4 spinous process provides ample access to the dural sac. The posterior inferior iliac spines and the coccyx provide landmarks for the location of the hiatus of the sacral canal.

500. The answer is e. (*Moore, Anatomy, 4/e, pp 451–453.*) Intervertebral disks are strongly reinforced ventrally and laterally by the anterior longitudinal ligaments. The posterior longitudinal ligament, although it is denticulate and attenuated laterally, reinforces the posterior aspect of the intervertebral disk. Because the posterolateral region of the disk is supported least by ligamentous structures, a nucleus pulposus that is herniated through the annulus fibrosus of the intervertebral disk will take the line of least resistance and move posterolaterally into the intervertebral foramen. In so doing, the herniation is apt to impinge on a spinal nerve of the next lower vertebral level.

Abbreviations and Acronyms

ACTH	adrenocorticotropic hormone
ADH	antidiuretic hormone
ANP	atrial natriuretic peptide
ANS	autonomic nervous system
ATP	adenosine triphosphate
Cdk proteins	cyclin-dependent kinases
cGMP	guanosine 3'5'-cyclic monophosphate
CNS	central nervous system
DNA	deoxyribonucleic acid
ER	endoplasmic reticulum
FSH	follicle-stimulating hormone
GH	growth hormone
GI	gastrointestinal
hCG	human chorionic gonadotropin
IVC	inferior vena cava
LH	luteinizing hormone
MSH	melanocyte-stimulating hormone
PNS	peripheral nervous system
PTH	parathyroid hormone
RER	rough endoplasmic reticulum
RNA	ribonucleic acid
SER	smooth endoplasmic reticulum
TSH	thyroid-stimulating hormone
UV	ultraviolet

Bibliography

Alberts B, Bray D, Lewis J, et al: *Molecular Biology of the Cell,* 3/e. New York, Garland, 1994.

April EW: *Clinical Anatomy.* 3/e. New York, John Wiley & Sons, 1997.

Avery JK (ed): *Oral Development and Histology,* 2/e. New York, Thieme, 1994.

Braunwald E, Fauci AS, Kasper DL, Hauser SL, Longo DL, Jameson JL (eds): *Harrison's Principles of Internal Medicine,* 15/e. New York, McGraw-Hill, 2001.

Brust JCM: *The Practice of Neuroscience.* New York, McGraw-Hill, 2000.

Carpenter MB: *Core Text of Neuroanatomy,* 4/e. Baltimore, Williams & Wilkins, 1991.

Coe FL, Favus MJ (eds): *Disorders of Bone and Mineral Metabolism.* New York, Raven, 1992.

Fawcett DW: *The Cell,* 2/e. Philadelphia, Saunders, 1981.

Gilbert SF: *Developmental Biology,* 6/e. Sunderland, MA, Sinauer, 2000.

Greenspan FS, Gardner DG: *Basic & Clinical Endocrinology,* 6/e. New York, McGraw-Hill, 2001.

Guyton AC, Hall JE: *Textbook of Medical Physiology,* 10/e. Philadelphia, Saunders, 2000.

Hollinshead WH, Rosse C: *Textbook of Anatomy,* 5/e. New York, Harper & Row, 1997.

Johnson LR (ed): *Physiology of the Gastrointestinal Tract,* 3/e. New York, Raven, 1994.

Junqueira LC, Carneiro J, Kelley RO: *Basic Histology,* 9/e. Stamford, CT, Appleton & Lange, 1998.

Kandel ER, Schwartz JH, Jessell TM: *Principles of Neural Science,* 4/e. New York, McGraw-Hill, 2000.

Kumar, V, Cotran RS, Robbins SL. *Basic Pathology,* 6/e. Philadelphia, Saunders, 1997.

Larsen WJ: *Human Embryology,* 2/e. New York, Churchill Livingstone, 1997.

Lebenthal E: *Human Gastrointestinal Development.* New York, Raven, 1989.

Male D: *Immunology: An Illustrated Outline,* 3/e. St. Louis, Mosby, 1998.

Mayne R, Burgeson RE (eds): *Structure and Function of Collagen Types.* New York, Academic, 1987.

McKenzie, JC, Klein RM: *Basic Concepts in Cell Biology and Histology.* New York, McGraw-Hill, 2000.

Moore KL, Persaud TVN: *Before We Are Born,* 5/e. Philadelphia, Saunders, 1998.

Moore KL, Persaud TVN: *The Developing Human,* 6/e. Philadelphia, Saunders, 1998.

Moore KL, Dalley AF: *Clinically Oriented Anatomy,* 4/e. Baltimore, Lippincott, Williams & Wilkins, 1999.

Newell FW: *Ophthalmology: Principles and Concepts,* 8/e. St. Louis, Mosby-Year Book, 1996.

Noback CR, Strominger NL, and Demarest RJ: *The Human Nervous System,* 4/e. Philadelphia, Lea & Febiger, 1991.

Paul WE (ed): *Fundamental Immunology,* 4/e. New York, Raven, 1999.

Roitt I, Brostoff J, Male D: *Immunology,* 5/e. St. Louis, Mosby, 1998.

Sadler TW: *Langman's Medical Embryology,* 8/e. Baltimore, Williams & Wilkins, 2000.

Sweeney L: *Basic Concepts in Embryology: A Student's Survival Guide.* New York, McGraw-Hill, 1998.

Vaughn D, Asbury T, Riordan-Eva P: *General Ophthalmology,* 15/e. East Norwalk, CT, Appleton & Lange, 1999.

Waxman SG: *Correlative Neuroanatomy,* 24/e. New York, McGraw-Hill, 2000.

Wicke L: *Atlas of Radiologic Anatomy,* 6th Eng. ed. Baltimore, Williams & Wilkins, 1998.

Yen SSC, Jaffe RB, Barbieri RL: *Reproductive Endocrinology,* 4/e. Philadelphia, Saunders, 1991.

Young B, Heath JW: *Wheater's Functional Histology,* 4/e. New York, Churchill Livingstone, 2000.

Index